Social Indicators Research Series

Volume 77

This series aims to provide a public forum for single treatises and collections of papers on social indicators research that are too long to be published in our journal *Social Indicators Research*. Like the journal, the book series deals with statistical assessments of the quality of life from a broad perspective. It welcomes the research on a wide variety of substantive areas, including health, crime, housing, education, family life, leisure activities, transportation, mobility, economics, work, religion and environmental issues. These areas of research will focus on the impact of key issues such as health on the overall quality of life and vice versa. An international review board, consisting of Ruut Veenhoven, Joachim Vogel, Ed Diener, Torbjorn Moum, Mirjam A.G. Sprangers and Wolfgang Glatzer, will ensure the high quality of the series as a whole.

More information about this series at http://www.springer.com/series/6548

Adele Bianco • Paola Conigliaro • Michela Gnaldi
Editors

Italian Studies on Quality of Life

Springer

Editors
Adele Bianco
Department of Psychological,
Health and Territorial Sciences
University G. D'Annunzio Chieti-Pescara
Chieti, Italy

Paola Conigliaro
ISTAT
National Institute of Statistics
Rome, Italy

Michela Gnaldi
Department of Political Sciences
University of Perugia
Perugia, Italy

ISSN 1387-6570 ISSN 2215-0099 (electronic)
Social Indicators Research Series
ISBN 978-3-030-06021-3 ISBN 978-3-030-06022-0 (eBook)
https://doi.org/10.1007/978-3-030-06022-0

This Springer imprint is published by the registered company Springer Nature Switzerland AG.
The registered company address is: Gewerbestrasse 11, 6330 Cham, Switzerland

Acknowledgments

Antonio Alaminos, University of Alicante
Silvia Bacci, University of Perugia
Alberto Baldissera, University Torino
Adele Bianco, University of Chieti-Pescara
Rainer Bruggemann, Leibniz-Institute of Freshwater Ecology and Inland Fisheries
Aviana Bulgarelli, INAAP
Lars Carlsen, Roskilde University - Forskning
Andrew Clark, Paris School of Economics
Benedetta Castiglioni, University of Padova
Paola Conigliaro, ISTAT, Sapienza University of Rome
Federica Cornali, University of Torino
Carlo Cristini, University of Brescia
Maria Amparo Cruz-Saco Oyague, Connecticut College, Economics
Enrico Di Bella, University of Genova
Cinzia Di Novi, University of Pavia
Simone Di Zio, University of Chieti-Pescara
Viviana Egidi, Sapienza University of Rome
Massimo Finocchiario Castro, Mediterranea University of Reggio Calabria
Nadia Fiorino, University of L'Aquila
Lara Fontanella, University of Chieti-Pescara
Carlo Francescutti, Azienda per l'Assistenza Sanitaria, Regione Friuli Venezia Giulia
Francesca Gagliardi, University of Siena
Emma Galli, Sapienza University of Rome
Margherita Giannoni, University of Perugia
Michela Gnaldi, University of Perugia
Giorgio Gosetti, University of Verona
Heinz-Herbert Noll, Formerly Social Indicators Research Center of GESIS, Mannheim
Roberta Maeran, University of Padova
Nicola Mammarella, University of Chieti-Pescara

Matteo Mazziotta, ISTAT - Rome
Michele Mosca, University of Napoli
Annarita Paiano, University of Bari
Paola Passafaro, Sapienza University of Rome
Alessandro Porrovecchio, Université de Lille 2
Laura Ravazzini, Université de Neuchâtel
Dino Rizzi, University Ca' Foscari Venezia
Aldo Rosano, Istituto Superiore di Sanità - Rome
Paola Ungaro, ISTAT - Rome
Francesco Vidoli, Sose S.p.A., University of Roma Tre
Moreno Zago, University of Trieste

Contents

Italian Studies on Quality of Life: An Interdisciplinary Overview

Adele Bianco, Paola Conigliaro, and Michela Gnaldi

The volume collects a selection of the papers presented at the conferences of the Italian Association for Quality of Life Studies (AIQUAV), held in Florence in 2015 and 2016. The aim is to offer an overview of the ways the Italian school of quality of life studies addresses various topics both in terms of content and quality.

Italy is known around the world for its artistic, natural and landscape beauties, for its good culinary art, and more generally for its aesthetic sense and good taste. "Made in Italy" is synonymous with high-quality manufacturing products, characterized by care and elegance. In the opinion of most people, Italy is the country of the "dolce vita" and because of these characteristics it can therefore be considered a natural and social laboratory of well-being and quality of life.

Despite this, Italy is affected by difficulties and suffers from a restriction of its potential development. After the global financial crisis of 2008–2013, Italy is recovering more slowly in comparison to other advanced countries (OECD 2011).

According to the OECD (2017), Italy seems to be a very contradictory country. Italy faces difficulties in the labor market—e.g. the employment rate of women and young people is one of the lowest among the OECD countries (https://data.oecd.org/emp/employment-rate.htm)—but in spite of it the level

A. Bianco (✉)
Department of Psychological, Health and Territorial Sciences, University G. D'Annunzio Chieti-Pescara, Chieti, Italy
e-mail: adele.bianco@unich.it

P. Conigliaro
Sapienza University of Rome, Rome, Italy

Italian National Institute of Statistics, Rome, Italy
e-mail: paola.conigliaro@istat.it

M. Gnaldi
Department of Political Sciences, University of Perugia, Perugia, Italy
e-mail: michela.gnaldi@unipg.it

A. Bianco et al. (eds.), *Italian Studies on Quality of Life*, Social Indicators Research Series 77, https://doi.org/10.1007/978-3-030-06022-0_1

of wealth among Italian families is relatively high. The Italian population is one of the most long-lived. Recently the National Institute of Statistics (ISTAT, https://www.istat.it/it/archivio/204917) published evidence that healthy life expectancy is rising among people over sixty. More generally, Italians experience a good state of health. Nevertheless, they are dissatisfied with regards to work and school, environmental and living conditions, and safety. On the other hand, familial relationships and friendship networks are very satisfying and seem to be a "social capital" (Granovetter 1973; Bourdieu 1980; Godechot and Mariot 2004, pp. 243–282), a resource that can be used in case of need. The social sciences suggest possible welfare measures to improve these situations, as already suggested by Maggino and Nuvolati (2012).

Although they are very different from each other, the papers presented here offer an overview of the richness, breadth of the topics and of the multidisciplinary approach of Italian scholars engaged in these issues. These researchers and experts in different research fields come from Italian universities, public research centers such as ISTAT or CNR (National Research Council) and other associations.

The volume is structured as follows. The first part is devoted to *methods and indicators for research on the quality of life*, the second one to *social sustainability, lifestyles, cultural aspects and local applications* and the third section concerns *economy, welfare and quality of life.*

The topics covered in the first section range from the social inclusion of disadvantaged people, to economic aspects, to the quality of Italian provincial life, to issues related to transparency, corruption and its prevention. Despite the thematic heterogeneity the papers of the section share the same methodological rigor. This makes it possible to place the Italian contribution on the quality of life in the broader international scene.

In the first article of the first section, the contribution by Fattore and Zenga deals with new methods for the evaluation of complex traits, with data on financial literacy. The paper develops an innovative procedure for reducing the dimensionality of multidimensional ordinal data, by using the concept of "embedded scale": that is, deriving an evaluation scale against which to assess the individual level of literacy in the financial field. The procedure tries to pick-up the scale that minimizes the information loss in the dimensionality reduction process, in the logic of Principal Component Analysis, while carefully preserving the ordinal nature of the data. In this respect, the paper advances the development of a statistical toolbox for the treatment of multidimensional systems of ordinal attributes.

Mazziotta, Pallara and Solipaca focus on the theme of social inclusion of people with a disability, a key objective of the EU and the ONU Development Sustainable Goals. In this paper, the multidimensional and complex nature of social inclusion of people with a disability is handled through a synthetic measure of disparity, obtained through the Adjusted Mazziotta Pareto Index, between disabled and non-disabled people in EU15 countries. The aims are yielding a measurement of active inclusion of persons with disabilities and describing the interactions between health conditions and contextual factors affecting inclusion. The results show that there is a disparity between the two subpopulations throughout Europe, even though the situation across member states varies significantly.

The next paper by Costa, Declich, Marchesich and Osti proposes the use of the Mazziotta-Pareto Index to compare the well-being of Italian provinces. The Authors report results with province-based rankings and maps that allow identification of distinctive characteristics of well-being in various territories for comparative purposes, both within single domains and globally. The snapshot of Italy they show is not fully consistent with the stereotype of the rich North vs. poor South.

The subsequent three contributions of the first section deal with the measurement of corruption and transparency. In his paper, Carloni frames the issue of measuring corruption by discussing corruption indicators in the context of Italian prevention policies. The discussion starts by stressing the inadequacy of commonly adopted corruption indicators—such as "perception-based", objective and judicial measures—and concentrates on new indicators of administrative corruption, indicators of abnormality and risk of corruption, which signal a shift from a repressive enforcement approach, typical of traditional measures of corruption, to a broader and preventative approach. The development of these last measures arises from the acknowledgement that it is not as important to measure corruption, as to understand where it emerges from, and to issue an alert when such conditions arise. In the Italian context, the annual report filled in by the prevention-of-corruption supervisor within the "Piano Triennale per la Prevenzione della Corruzione" (PTPC) has to be considered one of such latest measures of corruption prevention, and is the object of analysis of the subsequent article by Gnaldi and Del Sarto. The Authors provide a synthetic measure of corruption prevention—the Composite Indicator of Corruption Prevention (CICP)—for a sample of 232 Italian municipalities. Afterwards, they classify and qualify them into homogeneous groups as regards to the adopted anti-corruption measures, relying on a Latent Class approach. They show that despite a general tendency to comply with the corruption prevention law, it is possible to identify a group of least virtuous municipalities showing very low values for the CICP, deserving special attention by the Italian Anticorruption Authority (ANAC).

Closely related to the issue of corruption prevention is that of transparency, which is the focus of the paper by Galli, Rizzo and Scaglioni who propose a first integrated study of transparency and Equitable and Sustainable Well-being (BES, https://www.istat.it/en/well-being-and-sustainability/the-measurement-of-well-being) indicators at the Italian regional level. Based on four different dimensions—transparency, digital, social and political—the Authors specifically assess whether transparency of public administrations is correlated with the quality of the socio-political environment. They provide initial evidence that there is a relationship between transparency and some BES indicators: that is, the intensity of Internet use, trust in institutions, social participation and, to a lower extent, civic and informal political participation and women's participation in municipal councils.

BES indicators are also at the core of the contribution proposed by Cataldo et al., who investigate the relative weight of some BES dimensions in shaping the perceived quality of life of citizens of the historic centre of Naples, an Italian southern city whose town centre has been recognized by UNESCO as a world heritage site. Within a Structural Equation Model approach, the Authors show that while quality of services, safety and social relations have a low impact on quality of life perception, tourism—a dimension investigating citizens' views as regard to the effects of tourist flows in the area at issue—has the strongest impact among all dimensions.

In the article entitled "The incidence of sin taxes: evidence from Italy", di Bella, Gandullia, Leporatti and Montefiori discuss the fairness of the Italian taxation system as regards to sin goods (products such as tobacco, alcohol, and gambling), whose consumption is considered self-destructive for individuals and source of negative outcomes for the entire society. After investigating the Italian taxation on such goods, the Authors analyse and compare their degree of regressiveness using data from the Italian Household Budget Survey (HBS). Results show that, among such goods, those on gambling taxes can be considered the most regressive form of taxation, followed by cigarettes and beer, and that lower income households spend a larger proportion of their income on risky behaviours than higher income ones.

The article by Ravazzini and Piekałkiewicz closes the section and addresses the general question of whether gender should be included as a characteristic for the definition of reference groups, by focusing on an application on the impact of income comparisons on subjective well-being and using as data three pretests of the German Socio-Economic Panel. The Authors show that in any specifications, the effect of income comparisons on subjective well-being is better explained with the regression constructed without gender in the reference group than including gender and conclude that reference groups for income comparisons should not include gender as a relevant characteristic.

The second section is focused on the topic of social sustainability, lifestyles, and culture in Italy. A first group of contributions is devoted to the BES and a second one to food, an important element of Italian culture. This section is closed by contributions on the quality of life of the elderly population and on the Italian natural and landscape beauties.

The paper of Bachelet, Riccardini, Maggino focuses on how the concepts of vulnerability and resilience may be employed in the analysis of the sustainability of human well-being. The Authors propose an approach focusing on an individual dimension of well-being, considering single persons' exposure to risk and their ability to recover. Using data provided by the National Institute of Statistics (ISTAT), they offer an example of how to analyze the subjective aspects of wellbeing in terms of sustainability.

The contribution of Salustri and Viganò gives a multi-stakeholders' analysis of BES data. It concerns some subjective indicators on health regarding citizens based in Bozen (South Tyrol). The aim is to show convergences and divergences among four selected classes of agents (citizens, local stakeholders, central administrations and for-profit institutions), interdependencies among data on well-being and economic development, and the gap between the institutional indicators and a subjective approach, based on satisfaction surveys. It could help policy makers in promoting quality of life.

At the time of EXPO 2015, food has been the core of many studies. The subsequent three contributions of the second section deal with this basic aspect of our life. Corazziari, Facioni, Maggino show the close relationship between the quality of life and the food habits of Italians, using data provided by the National Institute of Statistics.

Di Francesco focuses on the dietary habits of European university students in a comparative way. He points out that inappropriate dietary habits are associated with a set of behaviors (almost a syndrome) such as substance and / or medicines abuse, excessive use of social networks, frequent breaking of the sleep / waking cycle, psycho-physical disorders, irregular and excessively fatiguing forms of sports activities.

Corvo focuses on the link between food waste and quality of life. He points out that food waste is a feature of advanced countries and that this is a function of the productive system. After providing some official data on food waste, the Author shows that the dramatic consequences of the economic crisis are leading to a waste reduction.

A third group of contributions in the second section of the volume focuses on the ageing Italian population. In fact, Italy, as along with Germany and Japan, has the highest proportion of old people in the world. The papers by Cristini, Cesa-Bianchi and Dryjanska, Giua are respectively devoted to the standard of living of the elderly population and to the relationship between generations. The first two Authors show the close connection between culture, creativity and age. The history of art confirms this link. Michelangelo, for example, made his last masterpiece, the *Rondanini Pietà* at 89. Neuroscientific researches confirm that culture plays a role in mitigating neuropsychiatric diseases. The Authors point out that culture and creativity might perform various functions such as: (a) facilitate aging; (b) constitute a model for cross-generational relationships; (c) represent a therapeutic tool for the elderly patient, including those with dementia.

Dryjanska and Giua focus on intergenerational solidarity as the way to prevent cognitive decline and improve the quality of life. Considering the positive effects on the physical and cognitive level, the Authors report a case study based in Rome. The intergenerational relationship makes it possible to improve the quality of life of all the participants.

Intergenerational relationships are also addressed by Albanese and Bocci in their contribution dedicated to sustainable tourism. This paper is part of a series of research and experimental projects in intergenerational tourism started in 2000. The quality of tourism is related to natural and socio-cultural resources and could solve specific local problems and promote social-cultural learning experiences between participants of different generations. In particular, intergenerational holiday activities are focused on the local area, its history and environment with the aim of promoting it.

Ferrari, Bocci, Lepisto, Cavallero and Rombai draw attention to the perception and evaluation of the features of Italian natural and landscape beauties. In so doing they contribute to the study of environmental psychology and show that the topic is closely linked to the quality of life also in developing personal identity and the sense of belonging to a social group.

The third section of the volume deals with the quality of life related to economic and welfare aspects. Ciani Scarnicci, Laino, Belcaro and Vita examine in an original way the correlation between economic growth and indicators of quality, lifestyles and sustainability. Their starting point is that GDP is not an indicator of well-being and they propose to consider alternative indicators such as the Equitable and Sustainable Well-being. The environmental factors improving equity and sustainability should be considered in evaluating the evolution of a community.

The paper by Coli and Pacini deals with the new organization of Welfare systems experienced in the last 20 years. They discuss whether the administrative decentralization process has increased poverty in Europe.

Concerning the link between the quality of work and psycho-physical well-being, Conigliaro underlines the increasing relevance of working conditions in term of social sustainability, both for workers' and for clients' quality of life. She considers three clusters of features: universal rights, job quality, including general working conditions, and well-being in relation to work, also in terms of organizational well-being.

Giammanco and Gitto and Mussino and Cosmai address in two different papers the topic of health and lifestyles. Giammanco and Gitto focus on the quality of life of cancer patients. This is a relevant and sensitive topic due to the spread of the disease and its impact on quality of life. There are many different styles of application of therapeutic protocols in healthcare. The Authors present a study carried out at four operating units of the Oncology center of Catania Hospital. The 300 cancer patients were involved in a customer satisfaction survey. The results suggest that the uncertainty in illness impacts on patient satisfaction as well as patient participation and other service-related aspects.

Mussino and Cosmai make a comparison of active lifestyles within Europe. The importance of practicing sports for well-being and health is recognized. Regular physical activity can also be considered an investment in health and therefore a saving of welfare costs. The Authors compare the quantity and quality of sports practice with the different welfare models in Europe.

Borrelli's paper deals with the issue of sustainable energy sources. The Author focuses attention on the social acceptance of key technologies and its governance. Attention is devoted by him to the link between policies at macro (international and national) and micro (local) level. The sustainability of energy policies depends at the local level on the dialogue between citizens and decision-makers and between businesses and decision-makers.

Bianco's paper closes the volume. The question is whether per capita income and level of consumption could be considered the key indicators to describe the rise of the middle class and the improvement of the quality of life in developing countries. Evidences show that the condition for the rise of the middle class are a modern economic system and a social context where gender gaps are reduced and where women are respected and empowered.

The contributions collected here show that Italian studies on quality of life are interdisciplinary, fruitful and open to the complexity of the globalized world.

The curators—who shared the commitment and responsibility in implementing this volume and therefore are strictly alphabetically ordered—would like to thank the Authors and the reviewers who have collaborated on this volume.

Last but not least, a special thanks to our AIQUAV President Prof. Filomena Maggino for having supported us in the making of this volume.

References

Bourdieu P. (1980). Le capital social – Notes provisoire. *Actes de la recherche en sciences sociales*, 31.

Godechot, O. & Mariot, N. (2004). Les deux formes du capital social: Structure relationnelle des jurys de thèses et recrutement en science politique. *Revue française de sociologie*, vol. 45,(2), 243–282. doi:https://doi.org/10.3917/rfs.452.0243.

Granovetter M. (1973). The strength of weak ties. *American Journal of Sociology*, 78, 1360–1380.

Maggino F. & Nuvolati G. (2012). *Quality of Life in Italy*. New York: Springer.

OECD (2011) *OECD Economic Surveys: Italy 2011*. Paris: OECD Publishing. https://doi.org/10.1787/eco_surveys-ita-2011-en.

OECD (2017). *How's Life in Italy?*, https://www.oecd.org/italy/Better-Life-Initiative-country-note-Italy.pdf. Accessed 25 April 2018

Part I
Methods and Indicators for Quality of Life Research

Quantification of Partially Ordered Data and the Evaluation of Financial Literacy

Marco Fattore and Mariangela Zenga

Abstract In this paper, we address the problem of the quantification of partially ordered data arising from multi-indicator systems of binary attributes and develop a procedure for the evaluation of Financial Literacy, on a real dataset pertaining to Italy. The procedure is based on the concept of "quantification" of chains (i.e. on the assignment of non-negative scores to sequences of comparable elements), in the poset arising from the attribute system, and aims at providing a two-dimensional representation of the data, in the spirit of a dimensionality reduction procedure. Due to the existence of incomparabilities in the poset, statistical units can be assessed only to some degree of indeterminacy and the goal of the procedure is to find out the "coordinate axes" that maximally reduce such indeterminacy.

Introduction

The use of Partially Ordered Set (poset) theory (Neggers and Kim 1998; Schröder 2002), in evaluation studies, has been recently investigated by several authors (Bachtrögler et al. 2014; Badinger and Reuter 2015; Bruggemann et al. 2014; Bruggemann and Patil 2011; Carlsen and Bruggemann 2016; Di Bella et al. 2016; Fattore et al. 2011, 2016; Fattore 2016; Fattore and Arcagni 2016; Iglesias et al. 2016; Patil and Taillie 2004), as a way to overcome the inconsistencies of composite indicators, particularly when ordinal attributes are involved. Following this stream, here we propose a procedure to quantify partially ordered data derived from multidimensional systems of attributes, in view of providing numerical evaluations of complex socio-economic traits. The idea is to map the elements of the poset associated to the attribute system into a bidimensional real space, by identifying a pair of "coordinate axes", as in classical data reduction algorithms. Here, however, axes coincide with suitable sequences of ordered profiles (chains), which get

---

M. Fattore (✉) · M. Zenga
University of Milano-Bicocca, Milan, Italy
e-mail: marco.fattore@unimib.it; mariangela.zenga@unimib.it

A. Bianco et al. (eds.), *Italian Studies on Quality of Life*, Social Indicators Research Series 77, https://doi.org/10.1007/978-3-030-06022-0_2

exogenously quantified (see (Knuth and Bahreyni 2014)), to serve as embedded measurement scales for the quantification of all poset elements (notice that our aim is not to reduce the complexity of the poset itself, like in the POSAC algorithm (Di Bella et al. 2016), but to quantify, in a parsimonious way, poset elements). As a first step in this direction, we focus on a particular class of posets, namely on product orders of binary attributes, since binary data are often encountered in socio-economics and since their mathematical features lead to powerful results that deserve a specific mention. To make the treatment as plain as possible, we develop the procedure on a real dataset pertaining to Financial Literacy, in Italy. Data are presented in section "Financial literacy data and the knowledge poset"; section "Chain quantification in product orders of binary attributes" introduces the concept of chain quantification; section "Data reduction through chain quantifications" develops the data reduction procedure; section "Bidimensional representation of knowledge data" introduces the bidimensional representation of financial data; section "Some technical comments on chain quantification" provides a brief discussion on some technical aspects related to quantification and section "Conclusion: open questions and further research" concludes. A final Appendix provides a pictorial example of the kind of posets employed in the paper.

Financial Literacy Data and the Knowledge Poset

The data used in this paper are extracted out of a survey on Financial Literacy, held in Italy in 2013 (see (VV.AA 2014)). The survey involved a sample of 1247 individuals and collected data on three main domains, namely *Financial Attitude*, *Financial Knowledge* and *Financial Behavior*. Financial Attitude refers to attention to medium/long term financial planning; Financial Knowledge pertains to basic technical competencies and to the comprehension of essential financial concepts; Financial Behaviour regards the way subjects choose financial instruments, make expenditure choices, manage their savings and the like. Socio-demographic data are also collected, for subpopulation analysis. Here, as a leading example to develop the posetic procedure, we focus on the Knowledge domain, which comprises six binary attributes related to the comprehension of the following items: (i) inflation, (ii) simple interest, (iii) compound interest, (iv) relation between risk and return, (v) investment diversification and (vi) investments comparison, based on risk-return profiles. Based on their knowledge (yes/no) of these concepts, statistical units are assigned binary sequences of six digits (0 = "no"; 1 = "yes"), in the following called *Knowledge profiles* (or, simply, profiles). These $2^6 = 64$ profiles are then structured into a partially ordered set, the *Knowledge poset*, according to the following criterion: *profile "a" has equal or less financial knowledge than profile "b", written* $a \trianglelefteq b$*, if and only if all of the scores of "a" are not higher than the*

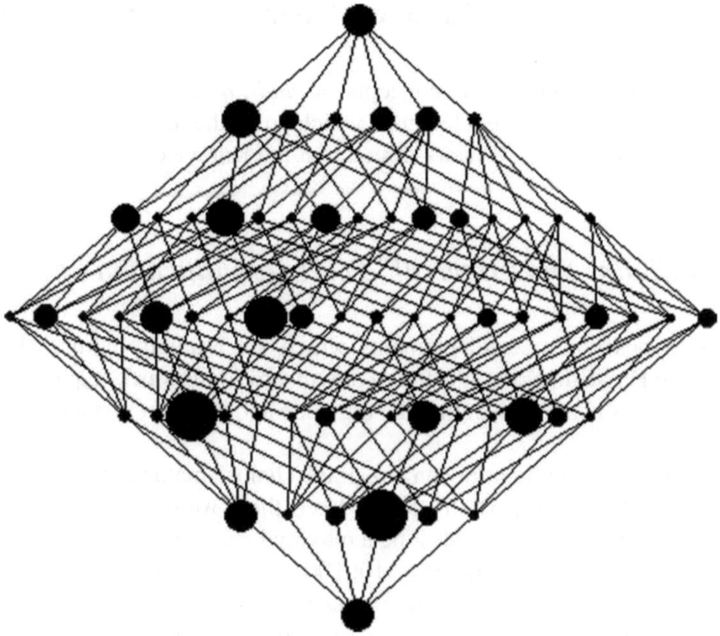

Fig. 1 Hasse diagram of the Knowledge poset (the greater the diameter of the node, the higher the frequency of the corresponding profile in the dataset)

corresponding scores of "b". This partial ordering criterion is very natural and is called the *product order* of (linear orders associated to) the input binary attributes (notice that this product order is also a lattice). Figure 1 depicts the Hasse diagram (see (Bruggemann et al. 1995)) of the Knowledge poset, where "better" profiles (represented as nodes) are linked to "worse" profiles by edges, to be read as downward oriented. Profiles not linked by downward sequences of edges are, instead, incomparable. The bottom element is profile 000000 (the respondent answered incorrectly to all of the questions), the top is profile 111111 (the respondent was able to correctly answer to all of the questions). Profiles on the same level of the Hasse diagram share the same number of 0s and 1s (the latter increases from bottom to top). For sake of readability, profiles have not been explicitly shown in the diagram (see Appendix for an example with profile labels); anyway, the picture is intended just to give an overall impression of the data structure. Each profile is realized by a different number of respondents; to visually account for that, the diameter of a node increases with the relative frequency associated to it. Only profile 011001 is not observed in the dataset (we notice, that this profile would correspond to a somehow incoherent set of answers, where one declares knowledge of investment comparison based on risk-return analysis, but not on what the relation between risk and investment is).

Chain Quantification in Product Orders of Binary Attributes

In this section, we introduce the concepts of *chain quantification* and of *induced interval quantification* of poset elements, which are at the heart of the data reduction procedure. To be concrete, we work directly on the Knowledge poset.

Maximal Chains and "Interval" Poset Quantification

A *chain* in a poset is a set of elements which are mutually comparable; in the corresponding Hasse diagram, it is thus a downward (or upward) sequence of nodes, linked by edges. A chain connecting the top node and the bottom node is here called a *maximal chain*.

We first define quantification on maximal chains, making them *measurement scales* embedded into the partially ordered set; then, we extend the quantification to the whole poset. To this goal, let γ be a maximal chain in the Knowledge poset Π (e.g., in Fig. 2, 000000 – 000100 – 100100 – 100110 – 110110 – 111110 – 111111, which is the maximal chain passing through the nodes with greatest diameters in Fig. 1). Let us *quantify* γ, defining a *monotone positive valuation* (from now on, a *valuation*), i.e. an order preserving map $v(\bullet)$ from Π to $[0, 1]$, so that $a \trianglelefteq b$ implies $v(a) \leq v(b)$. To make things simple, for $p \in \gamma$, we define $v(p)$ as the fraction of 1s in the profile (e.g. $v(010010) = 1/3$) and call it the *canonical quantification*; once defined $v(\bullet)$, any element a in the poset gets quantified, by the interval $\Delta_a(\gamma) = \left[v\left(\gamma_a^-\right), v\left(\gamma_a^+\right)\right]$, where γ_a^- is the greatest element of γ less than a and γ_a^+ is the lowest element of γ greater than a (see Fig. 2). Elements γ_a^+ and γ_a^- are also called *forward* and *backward projections* (see (Knuth and Bahreyni 2014)) of a on γ. Notice that if $a \in \gamma$, then $\gamma_a^- = \gamma_a^+ = a$ and the quantification interval is $[v(a), v(a)]$. In summary, given the quantification of γ, different profiles are assessed to different indeterminacy degrees, i.e. with different interval widths. This is a consequence of data multidimensionality that, in posets, reflects into the existence of incomparabilities among profiles. In particular, there are elements of the Knowledge poset which are quantified as $[0, 1]$. Consider, for example, profile $a = 010000$, whose forward and backward projections on γ are $\gamma_a^+ = 111111$ and $\gamma_a^- = 000000$, respectively. It should be clear that any profile p having 0 where the second element (from bottom) of γ has 1 and having 1 where the sixth element of γ has 0 is assigned the interval [0, 1] by γ[1]. So, for example, the entire chain $\lambda = 000000 - 000001 - 000011 - 001011 - 011011 - 111011 - 111111$ is composed of elements all of which are quantified as $[0, 1]$ (with the exception of 000000 and 111111, which are valuated as 0 and 1, respectively). In this case, we say that chain γ is uninformative on chain λ. On the whole, in the Knowledge

[1]More formally, this is true since the join between such p and any element of γ is 111111 and the meet is 000000.

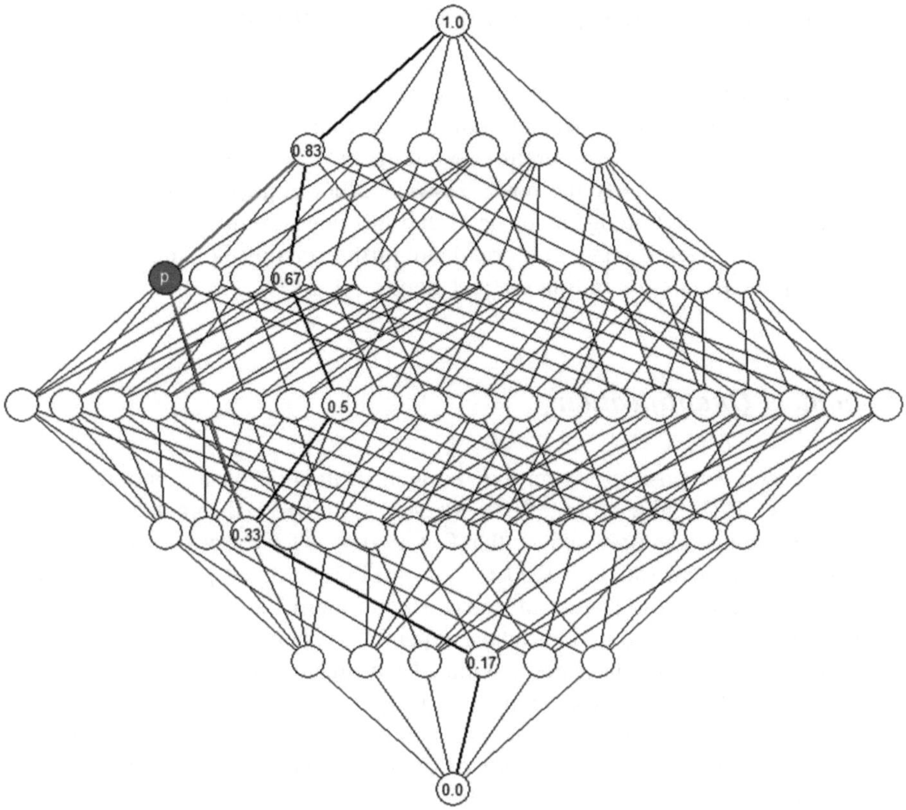

Fig. 2 Example of chain and profile quantification in the Knowledge poset. Given the chain γ_{max}, highlighted in black with valuations in white, profile p is assigned the valuation interval [0.33, 0.83]

poset there are 24 chains on which γ is uninformative (in a general product order of k binary attributes, for each maximal chain there are $(k-2)!$ chains on which the former is uninformative). Finally, it is easy to see that uninformativeness is a symmetric relation, i.e. if γ is uninformative on λ, then λ is uninformative on γ (to see this, let be γ uninformative on λ: if λ would be informative on γ, there would exist $q \in \lambda$ and $p \in \gamma$, both different from 000000 and 111111, such that $\gamma_p^+ = q$, or $\gamma_p^- = q$; but then certainly either $p \trianglelefteq \gamma_q^-$, or $\gamma_q^+ \trianglelefteq p$, i.e. γ would be informative on λ).

To summarize, in product orders of binary attributes, quantifying a maximal chain allows to assign quantification intervals to each poset element and, also, to identify a subset of maximal chains which are mutually uninformative with it.

Data Reduction Through Chain Quantifications

The Knowledge poset Π is highly symmetric, in that its structure and the shape of its Hasse diagram do not depend upon the way attributes are listed. As a result, no maximal chain has any preferred role and there is no *a priori* criterion to pick one up, in order to quantify the poset. However, the frequency distribution of the statistical units is not homogeneous on Π and this does provide a way to break the symmetry and to identify one, or more, distinguished chains. For simplicity's sake, we develop the discussion in four distinct steps.

Canonical Quantification

As a first step, suppose to assign the following valuation on the bottom and the top profiles of Π only: $v(000000) = 0$; $v(111111) = 1$. From this "baseline" quantification, one can only deduce that $0 \leq v(a) \leq 1$, for every knowledge profile a (since any of them satisfies $000000 \leq a \leq 111111$). Each profile is (possibly) realized by one or more statistical units, which inherit the quantification interval $[0, 1]$ as well. Suppose now to introduce a quantified chain. A generic profile a and the statistical units sharing it get associated the quantification interval $\Delta_a(\gamma) = \left[v\left(\gamma_a^-\right), v\left(\gamma_a^+\right)\right]$, where in general $0 \leq v\left(\gamma_a^-\right) \leq v\left(\gamma_a^+\right) \leq 1$ (we can think of $\Delta(\gamma)$ as a map from Π to intervals comprised in $[0, 1]$). Thus, introducing a quantified chain reduces the width of quantification intervals (indeterminacy) associated to profiles and statistical units.

In view of data reduction, it is then natural to search for the quantified chain that maximally reduces the population indeterminacy, given the frequency distribution on Π. Such a chain will be called a *maximum information chain*. Here, however, an issue arises. The indeterminacy reduction induced by a chain depends upon (i) the chain itself and (ii) how it is quantified. In principle, one could quantify the chain so as to reflect exogenous evaluation criteria or, in Bayesian terms, some prior knowledge. When developing an evaluation procedure to be used by "domain experts", the possibility to fix the embedded scale should be highly appreciable. Here, however, we simply look for a "neutral" rule; we thus quantify profiles canonically, from 0 to 1, assigning to each profile the frequency of 1s in it, as we did in the previous example.

Indeterminacy Reduction Power of a Quantified Chain

With the quantification choice discussed in the previous paragraph, we search for the maximum information chain on the Knowledge poset, by listing all of the maximal chains (their number being $6! = 720$) and comparing their Indeterminacy Reduction Power *IRP*, defined as:

$$IRP(\gamma) = 1 - \frac{\sum_{a \in \Pi} \left[v\left(\gamma_a^+\right) - v\left(\gamma_a^-\right) \right] \cdot n_a}{\sum_{a \neq \bot, a \neq \top} n_a} \tag{1}$$

In the above expression, the numerator is the sum of profiles' interval widths along γ, weighted by the number of statistical units in the profiles, and the denominator is the same for the baseline quantification (since, in this case, the score range associated to profiles is 1, but for the bottom ($\bot$) and top ($\top$) profiles, which are scored with no indeterminacy). Figure 3 shows the *IRP*s of all of the maximal chains, sorted in a decreasing way. The chain γ_{max} with maximum *IRP* (0.656) turns out to be 000000 – 000100 – 100100 – 100110 – 101110 – 111110 – 111111. By projecting poset profiles on γ_{max}, we get different valuation intervals for different profiles. In particular, 7 profiles (those on the identified chain) are quantified with no indeterminacy, 5 profiles have quantification ranges equal to $0.\overline{3}$, 8 profiles have ranges equal to 0.5, 12 equal to $0.\overline{6}$, 16 equal to $0.8\overline{3}$ and 16 equal to 1 (Fig. 4). The latter ones are profiles over which chain γ_{max} is uninformative and whose existence was anticipated in the previous paragraph.

Indeterminacy Reduction Power of a Pair of Quantified Chains

After extracting chain γ_{max}, it would be natural to search for a second chain, which quantifies with a small indeterminacy degree profiles and statistical units "badly" (i.e. with wide intervals) quantified by the maximum information chain.

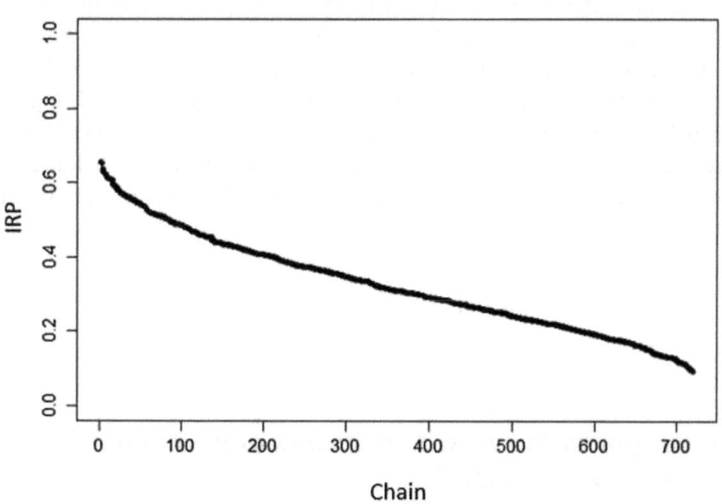

Fig. 3 Indeterminacy reduction power of maximal chains of the Knowledge poset, sorted in a decreasing way

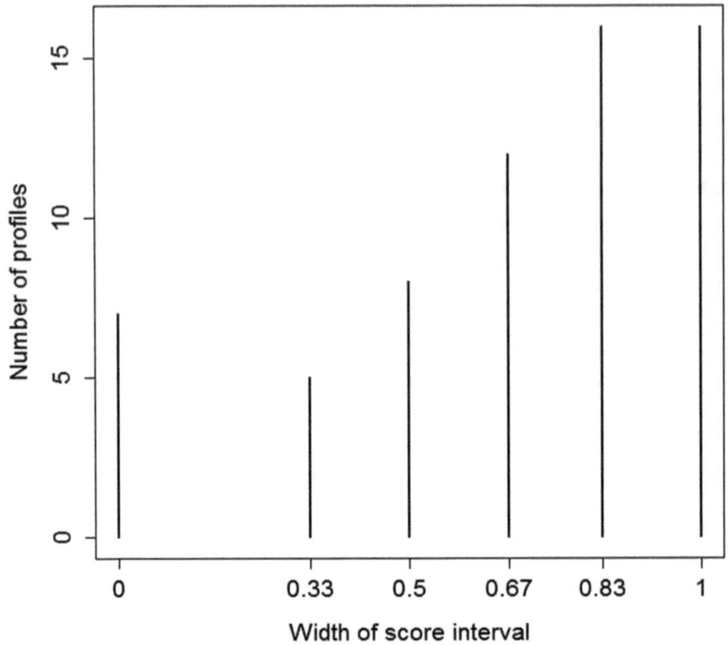

Fig. 4 Frequency distribution of the width of score intervals against γ_{max}

Profiles with wide intervals on the first chain (i.e. on which the first chain is uninformative or almost uninformative), could get narrower intervals on the second chain, so reducing the overall indeterminacy of the poset quantification. To make this idea formal, however, we first have to define a way to measure quantification indeterminacy, when two chains are involved. Suppose $\Delta_a(\gamma_1)$ and $\Delta_a(\gamma_2)$ are the interval quantifications of element a on two chains γ_1 and γ_2. The most natural way to define the global quantification indeterminacy of a is through the geometric mean $\Delta_a(\gamma_1\gamma_2) = \sqrt{\Delta_a(\gamma_1)\,\Delta_a(\gamma_2)}$ (see (Knuth and Bahreyni 2014)). Analogously to what done before, we define the *IRP* of the pair of chains γ_1 and γ_2 as:

$$IRP(\gamma_1\gamma_2) = 1 - \frac{\sum_{a\in\Pi}\Delta_a(\gamma_1\gamma_2)\cdot n_a}{\sum_{a\neq\perp,a\neq\top} n_a}.$$

Mutual Uninformativeness: Differences and Analogies with Classical Data Analysis

Among all pairs of maximal chains, it is natural to search for that maximizing the *IRP* and such that the two chains are mutually uninformative; otherwise, the second chain could be "redundant", quantifying with narrow intervals profiles and statistical units already "well" quantified by the first chain. In a sense, this is analogous to what is typically done in euclidean data analysis, where orthogonal (or uncorrelated) components are often looked for. In euclidean data analysis the measure of total variation (e.g. total variance) can be reconstructed optimally, by choosing suitable orthogonal components, extracted in sequence. In the poset case, however, there is no concept of "variance decomposition" and we cannot minimize the global indeterminacy of the resulting quantification $\Delta_a(\gamma_1\gamma_2)$, by searching γ_2 among the maximal chains uninformative with respect to the maximum information chain γ_{max}. In order to minimize $\Delta_a(\gamma_1\gamma_2)$, we have to search directly among all of the pairs of maximal, and mutually uninformative, chains. To this goal, for each maximal chain of the Knowledge poset, we first computed the set of 24 corresponding uninformative chains; then, we searched for the best pair. The pair of chains γ_1 and γ_2 which minimizes the global indeterminacy is composed of $\gamma_1 = 000000 - 100000 - 100100 - 100110 - 110110 - 110111 - 111111$ and $\gamma_2 = 000000 - 001000 - 001100 - 001110 - 011110 - 011111 - 111111$ (see Fig. 5). The indeterminacy reduction power $IRP(\gamma_1\gamma_2)$ of this pair is equal[2] to 0.678. We see that, in this case, the improvement over $IRP(\gamma_{max})$ is negligible. However, the choice of two chains has the positive effect to make profile uncertainties much more homogeneous, than in the single chain case. In fact, no profile has indeterminacy equal to 1 and, in general, the indeterminacy distribution is much less spread, as shown in Fig. 6. Moreover, as discussed later, the "financial" interpretation of the result becomes much easier.

Bidimensional Representation of Knowledge Data

Chains γ_1 and γ_2 can be used as two axes, on which to represent financial literacy data. To each statistical unit, an interval on γ_1 and an interval on γ_2 correspond, providing an insight on the levels and the indeterminacy of its quantification. Since the Knowledge poset comprises 64 profiles, statistical units are grouped and there are 64 different possible pairs of intervals on the two axes. Figure 7 shows the width of the intervals along γ_1 and γ_2 for each profile (some jittering has been added

[2]The minimum IRP equals 0.311, thus showing that the range of possible IRP values across mutually uninformative chain pairs is quite wide.

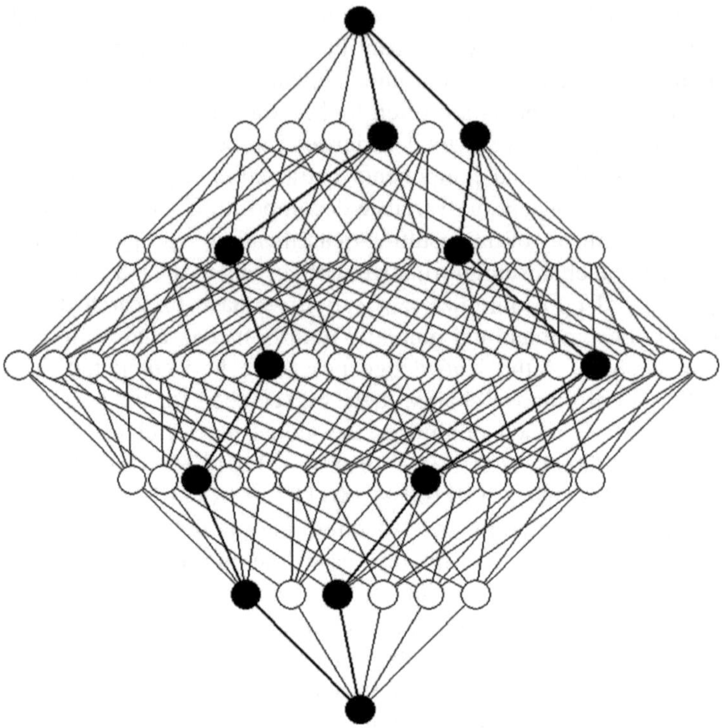

Fig. 5 Maximum information chain pair; the chain on the left, in the poset, is γ_1; that on the right is γ_2

to show them in a distinct way), weighted by the corresponding frequencies[3]. The only profiles with no indeterminacy on both chains are 000000 and 111111; the other elements of γ_1 and γ_2 have indeterminacy 0 on one axis and indeterminacy 1 on the other. All of the other knowledge profiles have different indeterminacy levels and one can identify "badly", i.e. with great indeterminacy, quantified elements (right upper corner) and better, i.e. with low indeterminacy, quantified ones (towards the center of the plot).

A different representation of the Knowledge profiles is provided in Figure 8. There, profiles are represented as rectangles, whose sides are the score intervals on chains γ_1 and γ_2, respectively. Thus, the plot conveys information on both the level and the indeterminacy of profiles' quantification (clearly, when indeterminacy is high, profile level is not informative). In view of communication to decision-makers,

[3]To ease visualization, weights are actually proportional to frequencies at power 0.6; the plot is meant just to provide a general idea of the frequency distribution.

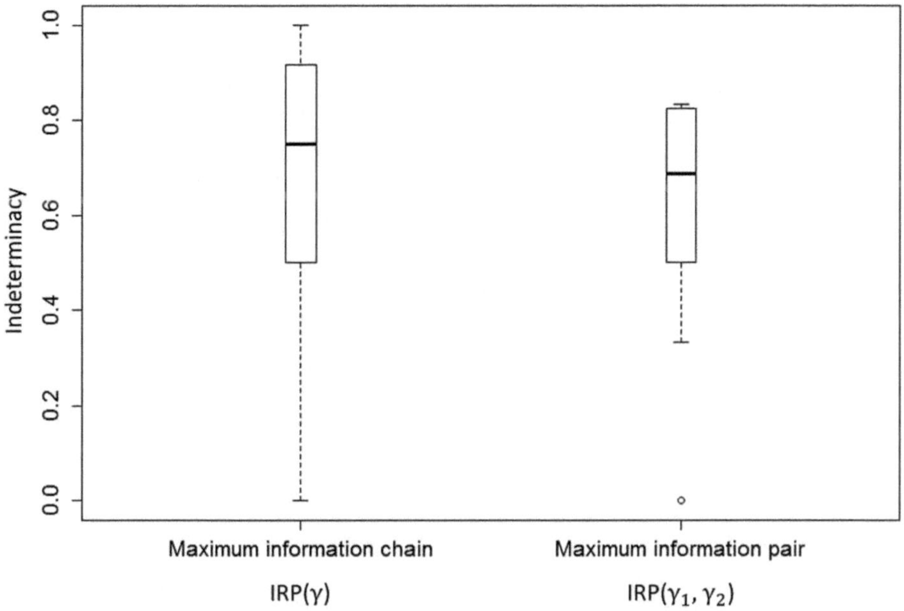

Fig. 6 Boxplot of indeterminacy distributions for the maximum information chain ($\gamma = \gamma_{max}$) and the maximum information chain pair γ_1 and γ_2

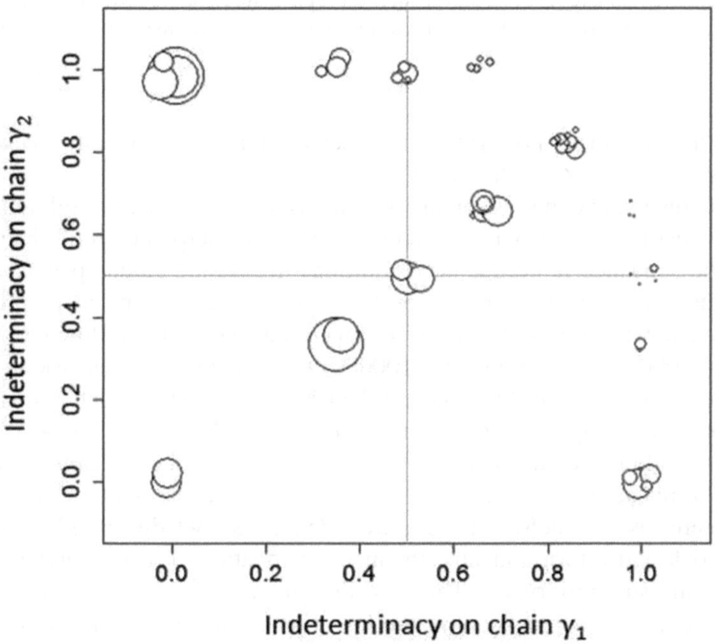

Fig. 7 Width of intervals associated to Knowledge profiles, by quantification on the best pair of chains γ_1 and γ_2 (the bigger the circle, the higher the observed frequency of that profile)

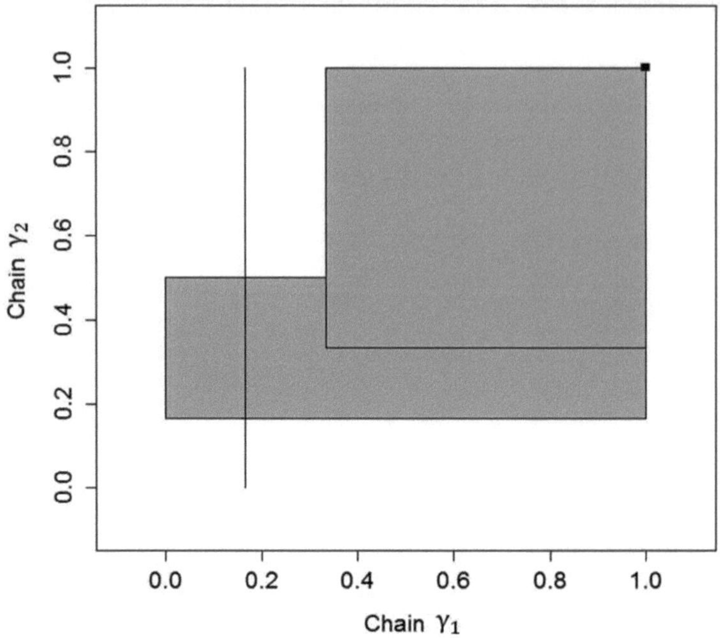

Fig. 8 Plot of profiles against chains γ_1 and γ_2. Each profile is represented as a rectangle (possibly degenerate) whose sides are the score intervals on the axes. To ease readability, just a few profiles have been plotted, namely: 111111 (the small black square top right); 001010 (the large horizontal rectangle, partly hidden), 100000 (the vertical line, i.e. a degenerate rectangle); 111100 (the large square)

such an "indeterminacy-preserving" representation is likely to be more useful than providing classical composite scores.

It is interesting to comment on the two chains γ_1 and γ_2, seen as reference scales for the evaluation of Financial Literacy. To give an interpretation of chain γ_1, we look at the sequence of competence additions, from the "no competencies at all" profile (the bottom of the Knowledge poset) to the "full competence" profile (the top of the Knowledge poset). The competence sequence is the following: "no competencies" (000000) $\rightarrow$ "inflation" (100000) $\rightarrow$ "relation between risk and return" (100100) $\rightarrow$ "investment diversification" (100110) $\rightarrow$ "simple interest" (110110) $\rightarrow$ "investments comparison, based on risk-return profiles" (110111) $\rightarrow$ "compound interest" (111111). Read the other way around, the sequence can be seen as a chain of implications; for example, if a respondent declares knowledge of what simple interest is, then he/she also declares adequate knowledge of inflation, relation between risk and return and investment diversification. The interpretation of the chain is quite straightforward. The first three items refer to qualitative aspects of finance, ordered by sophistication; the last three items are of a more quantitative nature and, again, ordered by "difficulty". So chain γ_1 can be read as a scale ranging from knowledge of easier qualitative concepts to knowledge of more difficult quantitative terms, i.e. as a "general Financial Knowledge scale". Such a clear interpretation lacks for chain γ_2, whose upward sequence of declared competencies seems to identify outliers or somehow strange respondents (for example, knowledge of compound interest comes before knowledge of simple interest). Maybe this kind of answers could be classified as erroneous, but it is not of concern, here, to go into the issue of survey quality. We limit ourselves to notice that the proposed chain extraction procedure identifies a main axis, whose interpretation is clear, and a residual one. This is quite similar to what often happens with principal component analysis, particularly when data matrices with non-negative entries are dealt with: the first principal component can usually be easily interpreted, while the other components are less clear in their meaning.

Some Technical Comments on Chain Quantification

In this section we briefly discuss some technical aspects, related to the extraction and quantification of chains; for readability's sake, we enumerate them.

1. *Larger sets of mutually uninformative maximal chains*. After extracting the best chain pair, it would be natural to go on, searching for larger sets of mutually uninformative chains, as in principal component analysis one extracts more components. Unfortunately, such larger sets do not exist, as can be easily seen from the discussion provided in previous sections. In fact, it turns out that in the Knowledge poset no more than two chains can be mutually uninformative. In a sense, "there is not enough space", for three chains not to quantify each other, at the same time. In summary, if the aim is to reduce data complexity by uninformative maximal chains, we can only look for bidimensional representations (things would change, if non-maximal chains would be allowed).
2. *Uniqueness of the best chain pair*. Uniqueness depends upon the shape of the frequency distribution of statistical units over the poset. Trivially, in the case of uniform distribution, any pair of mutually uninformative chains would have the same *IRP*; anyway, in real cases uniqueness is guaranteed.
3. *Indeterminacy associated to chain pairs*. In this paper, we have measured the indeterminacy associated to profiles by a pair of chains, employing the geometric mean of the widths of the intervals on each chain separately. This choice can be maintained in different ways (see (Knuth and Bahreyni 2014) for a deep discussion on why geometric means are natural in this context); here, it may suffice to notice that if a profile is quantified with no indeterminacy on one of the two chains, so that one of the two intervals has width 0, then the overall

indeterminacy should be 0 as well (this property would be assured also by the min(•,•) operator, which, however, is too rigid, not being sensitive to changes in the greater of the two arguments).

Conclusion: Open Questions and Further Research

The ideas of chain quantification, induced intervals and embedded scales seem promising, in order to develop effective procedures for measurement and data reduction on multidimensional systems of ordinal attributes. What we have illustrated in the paper is nothing but a first exploration of these ideas, which leaves many questions open for further developments, investigations and research. We list some of them in the following. First, the uninformativeness relation is perhaps the most interesting concept presented in the paper, but its interpretation as the analogous of "orthogonality" or "incorrelation" is not that clear yet; moreover, it cannot be trivially carried over to posets built from non-binary attributes. The concept might then be extended in terms of "degree" of uninformativeness of two chains over each other, so as to make it more useful for data reduction, and possibly considering not only maximal chains. Second, the way indeterminacy is quantified and measured deserves more investigation. Although deep arguments are given in (Knuth and Bahreyni 2014), in favour of the use of geometric means in poset quantification, in statistical applications other formulas could be explored. A third important issue pertains to the interpretation of the chains. As in other dimensionality reduction tools, statistical optimality may well be at odds with clearness of interpretation. A way to improve the latter could be to restrict the set of candidate chains to those respecting some suitable constraints (e.g. not to pass through some profiles, considered by the analyst as "incoherent" or likely to express errors of the respondents). Finally, in this paper we have dealt with a small poset, where it is possible to list all of the maximal chain pairs and to look for the best. But in larger posets, this is not possible and some more sophisticated algorithm is needed, to perform the search.

Appendix

In this section, we simply report the Hasse diagram of a product order built upon four binary attributes, inserting profile labels into the nodes so as to better exemplify the structure of this kind of posets. The Knowledge poset is more complex than the one here described, but its structure is analogous (Fig. 9).

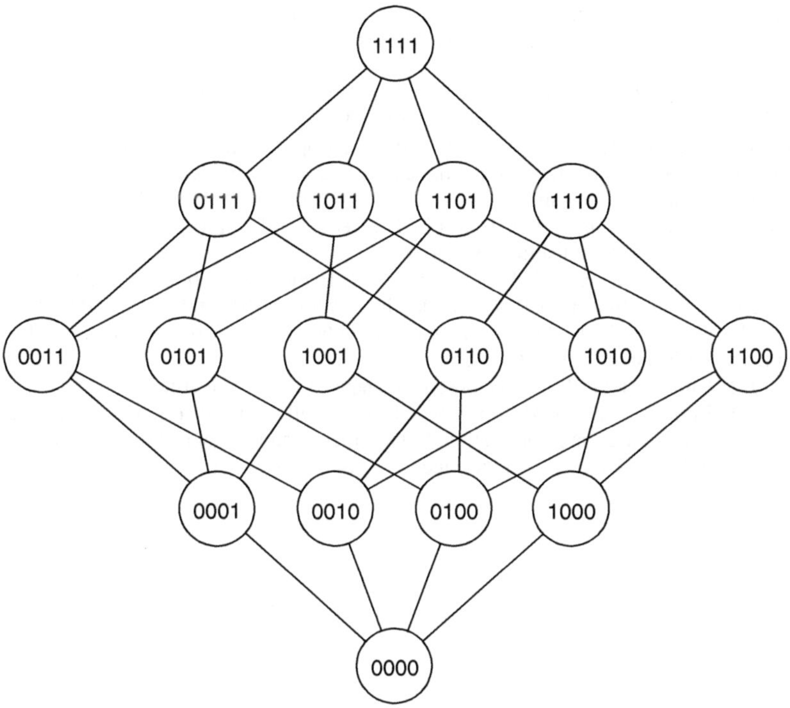

Fig. 9 Hasse diagram of a product order built on four binary variables

References

Bachtrögler, J., Badinger, H., Fichet de Clairfontaine, A., Reuter, W. H. (2014). Summarizing Data using Partially Ordered Set Theory: An Application to Fiscal Frameworks in 97 Countries, Department of Economics Working Paper Series, 181, WU Vienna University of Economics and Business.

Badinger, H. & Reuter, W. H. (2015). Measurement of Fiscal Rules: Introducing the Application of Partially Ordered Set (POSET) Theory. Journal of Macroeconomics, 43, 108–123.

VV.AA. (2014). Le Competenze economico-finanziarie degli Italiani, Rome: Bancaria.

Bruggemann, R., Schwaiger, J., Negele, R. D. (1995). Applying Hasse diagram technique for the evaluation of toxicological fish tests. Chemosphere, 30(9), 1767–1780.

Bruggemann, R., Carlsen, L., Wittmann, J. (Eds.). (2014). Multi-Indicator Systems and Modelling in Partial Order. New York: Springer-Verlag.

Bruggemann, R. & Patil, G. P. (2011). Ranking and Prioritization for Multi-indicator Systems. New York: Springer-Verlag.

Carlsen, L. & Bruggemann, R. (2016). Fragile State Index: Trends and Developments. A Partial Order Data Analysis. Social Indicators Research. doi:https://doi.org/10.1007/s11205-016-1353-y.

Di Bella, E., Gandullia, L., Leporatti, L., Montefiori, M., Orcamo, P. (2016). Ranking and Prioritization of Emergency Departments Based on Multi-indicator Systems. Social Indicators Research. doi:https://doi.org/10.1007/s11205-016-1537-5.

Fattore, M., Maggino, F., Greselin, F. (2011). Socio-economic evaluation with ordinal variables: integrating counting and poset approaches, Statistica & Applicazioni, Special Issue 2011, 31–42.

Fattore, M. (2016). Partially ordered sets and the measurement of multidimensional ordinal deprivation. Social Indicators Research, 128(2), 835–858.

Fattore, M. & Arcagni, A. (2016). A Reduced Posetic Approach to the Measurement of Multidimensional Ordinal Deprivation. Social Indicators Research, 136(3), 1053–1070.

Fattore, M., Maggino, F., Arcagni, A. (2016). Non-aggregative assessment of subjective wellbeing, In G. Alleva, A. Giommi (Eds.). Topics in Theoretical and Applied Statistics (pp. 227–237). Springer International Publishing Switzerland.

Iglesias, K., Suter, C., Beycan, T., Vani, B. P. (2016). Exploring multidimensional well-being in Switzerland. Social Indicators Research. doi: https://doi.org/10.1007/s11205-016-1452-9.

Knuth, H. K. & Bahreyni, N. (2014). A potential foundation for emergent space-time. Journal of Mathematical Physics 55, 112501 1–35.

Neggers, J. & Kim, S. H. (1998). Basic posets. Singapore: World Scientific.

Patil, G. P. & Taillie, C. (2004). Multiple indicators, partially ordered sets, and linear extensions: Multicriterion ranking and prioritization. Environmental and ecological statistics, 11, 199–228.

Schröder, B. (2002). Ordered set. An introduction. Basel: Birkhäuser.

Using a Composite Index to Measure Social Inclusion of People with Disabilities

Matteo Mazziotta, Alessandro Pallara, and Alessandro Solipaca

Abstract Measuring disability is a very challenging task, because of its complexity and multidimensionality. Indeed, data from different statistical sources may vary both for the aspects of disability surveyed and for the way they identify a person as belonging to the population with disability. We present an empirical study with a comparison among EU countries between conditions of disabled and non-disabled people, using individual indicators on people's major life domains (education, training, labor market participation, living conditions, social participation, health conditions) obtained from different surveys. We handle the inherently multidimensional nature of disability through a synthetic measure of disparity between disabled and non-disabled people obtained using the methodology on composite indices, which allows to find suitable combination of the individual indicators, aiming at measuring active inclusion of persons with disabilities in EU countries. We consider a non-compensatory composite index, that is based on the assumption of non-substitutability of the individual indicators.

Introduction

Disability is a complex, evolving and multi-dimensional concept. Disabilities affect people's life in many areas, such as mobility and the use of transport equipment; access to goods and services; participation in education and training, the labor market and leisure activities; social contacts and economic independence.

According to the United Nation's Convention on the Rights of People with Disabilities (CRPD) (United Nations 2007), people with disabilities include those who have long-term physical, mental, intellectual or sensory impairments which, in interaction with various barriers, may hinder their full and effective participation in society on an equal basis with others. Indeed, this definition of disability is coherent

M. Mazziotta · A. Pallara (✉) · A. Solipaca
Istituto Nazionale di Statistica, Rome, Italy
e-mail: pallara@istat.it

A. Bianco et al. (eds.), *Italian Studies on Quality of Life*, Social Indicators Research Series 77, https://doi.org/10.1007/978-3-030-06022-0_3

with the conceptual framework introduced by the International Classification of Functioning, Disability and Health (ICF) (WHO 2001), which conceives disability (and *functioning*[1]) just as a dynamic interaction between health conditions and contextual factors, both personal and environmental. Under this perspective, health is then "a state of complete physical, mental and social well-being and not merely the absence of disease or infirmity".[2] Indeed, while CRPD points out the idea of disability as a inequality in participation, ICF vision emphasizes the role of the environment in enabling or disabling people with health conditions.

The capability approach developed by Sen (1993, 1999) is, as well, a useful framework for defining disability and understanding its social and economic causes and consequences. With reference to the capability approach, disability can be deemed as a deprivation of practical opportunities (a *lack of capability*) for persons with disabilities. Such deprivation may result from the interaction between the resources available to the person, personal characteristics like impairment, age or gender, and the environmental barriers (physical, social, cultural, political, and economic). According to this view, (social) inclusion is thus a process which ensures that each person with a disability gains opportunities and resources necessary to participate fully in economic, social, political and cultural life and enjoy his own desired state of well-being. The European Commission (2004) points out this concept as the right for people at risk of poverty and social exclusion (including people with disabilities) to a certain basic standard of living and a right to participate to most social and occupational experiences common to an ordinary life: education, employment, housing, health care, ... Whereas CRPD emphasizes this idea as the need for persons with disabilities to be guaranteed full and equal enjoyment of all human rights and fundamental freedoms.

Measuring disability is, therefore, a very challenging task, because of its complex nature and multidimensionality. Indeed, when considering the main sources of statistical data on disability, the different surveys vary for the particular aspect of disability investigated, either health conditions (*European health interview survey*, EHIS) or income, living conditions and social inclusion (EU-SILC) or employment of disabled people (*ad hoc* module of the Labor Force Survey handled in 2011). Measurement of disability in EHIS is based on the presence of limitations concerning the main *Instrumental Activities of Daily Living* (IADL), according to the ICF (European Commission 2013). In Italy, an *ad-hoc* module was administered in 2013 to a sub-sample of respondents to the Multipurpose Health Status and Health Service Utilization Survey, aimed at measuring disability as defined by CPRD.

In this paper we present an empirical study with a comparison among EU countries between conditions of disabled and non-disabled people, using individual

---

[1] "Functioning is an umbrella term encompassing all body functions, activities and participation; similarly, disability serves as an umbrella term for impairments, activity limitations or participation restrictions" (WHO 2001, p. 3).

[2] *Constitution of the World Health Organization*. New York, July 22, 1946, p. 1 (http://apps.who.int/gb/bd/PDF/bd47/EN/constitution-en.pdf).

indicators on people's major life domains (education and training, labor market participation, poverty and/or living conditions, social participation, health conditions) obtained from different surveys.

We handle the inherently multidimensional nature of disability through a synthetic measure of disparity between disabled and non-disabled people based on the methodology on composite indices (OECD 2008), which allows us to find suitable combination of the individual indicators, aimed at yielding a measurement of active inclusion of persons with disabilities in EU countries. We consider a non-compensatory composite index, that is based on the assumption of non-substitutability of the individual indicators, i.e. they have all the same weight and no compensation is allowed among them.

The paper is organized as follows. In section "A common perspective on social inclusion: CRPD, European Disability Strategy and the SDG's" the development of international frameworks for defining disability is briefly reviewed, trying to account for the multiplicity of the views on social inclusion of disabled people, as well as, in section "Data and methodologies for measuring disability", the ways disability is currently measured in statistical surveys. The application is then presented, in section "A composite indicator for rating inequality conditions of people with disabilities": the composite index employed is briefly described in section "Methodology on composite indicators: AMPI", while in section "An application to social inclusion of disabled people: indicators selected" we present the data and the individual indicators utilized and, in section "Empirical results", the results obtained for the synthetic measure of active inclusion of disabled people in EU countries. Finally, section "Discussion and concluding remarks" contains a short discussion and some concluding remarks.

A Common Perspective on Social Inclusion: CRPD, European Disability Strategy and the SDG's

The UN Convention on the Rights of People with Disabilities (CRPD), adopted in December 2006 (United Nations 2007), is the first international legal agreement setting minimum standards for rights of people with disabilities in UN Member States. CRPD came into effect in the EU on January 2011. Indeed, formal approval of CRPD was the ultimate accomplishment of a course of action ruled by UN and other international organizations over a long period of time, which dated back to early thru mid-1980s. Definitely, one of the most important step along the pathway to CRPD was the approval in 1993 of the *United Nations Standard Rules on the Equalization of Opportunities for Persons with Disabilities*,[3] which, although not

[3]The *Standard Rules* (http://www.un.org/esa/socdev/enable/dissre00.htm) were adopted on 20 December 1993 by the United Nations General Assembly, during its 48th session (Resolution *A/RES/48/96*).

compulsory, represented a first strong moral and political commitment of Member States to promote equal rights and opportunities for people with disabilities.

The purpose of the CRPD is "to promote, protect and ensure the full and equal enjoyment of all human rights and fundamental freedoms by all persons with disabilities, and to promote respect for their inherent dignity" (art. 1). CRPD identifies the main dimensions of social inclusion, recognizing the rights attached to it and setting out some general principles that States must follow and continuously monitor. Indeed, art. 24 and art. 27 recognize the right to school education and work for persons with disabilities; art. 25 identifies healthy condition as a main right and establishes that the States have to ensure the full access to health care, while art. 28 recognizes the right to an adequate standard of living, ensuring access by persons with disabilities to social protection and poverty reduction programs. Furthermore, CRPD urges the States Parties (art. 31) "to collect appropriate information, including statistical and research data, to enable them to formulate and implement policies to give effect to the (present) Convention".

The core elements of the CRPD are also reflected in the European Disability Strategy 2010–20 (EDS, European Commission 2010) which cover eight priority areas for promoting active inclusion and the full participation of people with disabilities: Accessibility, Participation, Equality, Employment, Education and training, Social protection, Health and External action. The goal of the EDS is to empower people with disabilities so that their rights and social participation can be safeguarded. EDS promotes the equality through contrasting of discrimination based on disability and promoting equal opportunities. The EU strategy aims at raising significantly the share of persons with disabilities working in the open labor market and promotes inclusive education and lifelong learning for students and pupils with disabilities in order to ensure them to participate fully in society and to improve their quality of life. Other challenges are to foster decent living conditions for disabled persons, contrasting poverty and social exclusion and favoring equal access to health services and related facilities. The EDS encourages national measures to monitor the policies on disability and it also identifies the support needed for funding, research, awareness-raising, statistics and data collection. CRPD and EDS have then a common vision, emphasizing the social inclusion as the main target and monitoring to ensure compliance with the commitments.

The UN 2030 Agenda on Sustainable Development, adopted by the UN General Assembly in September 2015 (United Nations 2015), is another internationally agreed upon framework which addresses active inclusion of persons with disabilities. The 2030 Agenda proposes principles and actions for providing a global response to the challenges raised by poverty eradication and favoring sustainable development in its three dimensions: economic, social and environmental, with the ultimate goal of ensuring, by 2030, an adequate quality of life for all people in vulnerable situations, including disabled people. The 2030 Agenda is detailed in a set of 17 Sustainable Development Goals (SDGs) and 169 related targets.

Indeed, goals and targets in the SDGs include seven targets which explicitly refer to persons with disabilities and have strong relation with the priority areas identified by the EDS. The goals and targets will be followed up and reviewed using a set of global indicators agreed upon at the 47th session of the UN Statistical Commission, in 2016.[4]

All member States are then urged to providing indicators at regional and national levels, disaggregated by all relevant targets and giving equal weight to all targets, in accordance with the Fundamental Principles of Official Statistics. Therefore, the targets which explicitly refer to disability must include disability related indicators. See Table 1 for the full list of such targets and indicators.

Table 1 Goals, targets and indicators in SDG's explicitly referring to disability

Goal	Target	Indicator
1. End poverty in all its forms everywhere	*1.3 Implement nationally appropriate social protection systems and measures for all, including floors, and by 2030 achieve substantial coverage of the poor and the vulnerable*	1.3.1 Proportion of population covered by social protection floors/systems, by sex, distinguishing children, unemployed persons, older persons, persons with disabilities, ...
4. Ensure inclusive and equitable quality education and promote lifelong learning opportunities for all	4.5 By 2030, eliminate gender disparities in education and ensure equal access to all levels of education and vocational training for the vulnerable, including persons with disabilities [. . .]	4.5.1 Parity indices (disability/no disability) for education indicators
	4.a Build and upgrade education facilities that are child, disability and gender sensitive [. . .]	4.a.1 Schools with access to:[. . .] (d) adapted infrastructure and material for students with disabilities
8. Promote sustained, inclusive and sustainable economic growth, full and productive employment and decent work for all	8.5 By 2030, achieve full and productive employment and decent work for all women and men, including for young people and persons with disabilities, and equal pay for work of equal value	8.5.1 Average hourly earnings of female and male employees, by occupation, age and persons with disabilities 8.5.2 Unemployment rate, by sex, age and persons with disabilities
10. Reduce inequality within and among countries	10.2. By 2030, empower and promote the social, economic and political inclusion of all, irrespective of age, sex, disability, race, ethnicity, origin, religion or economic or other status	10.2.1 Proportion of people living below 50 per cent of median income, by age, sex and persons with disabilities

(continued)

[4]UNECE Statistical Commission, *Report of the Inter-Agency and Expert Group on Sustainable Development Goal Indicators*. https://unstats.un.org/unsd/statcom/47th-session/documents/2016-2-IAEG-SDGs-E.pdf

Table 1 (continued)

Goal	Target	Indicator
11. Make cities and human settlements inclusive, safe, resilient and sustainable	11.2 By 2030, provide access to safe, affordable, accessible and sustainable transport systems for all, [. . .], with special attention to the needs of those in vulnerable situations, [. . .] persons with disabilities and older persons	11.2.1 Proportion of population that has convenient access to public transport, by sex, age and persons with disabilities
	11.7 By 2030, provide universal access to safe, inclusive and accessible, green and public spaces, in particular for women and children, older persons and persons with disabilities	11.7.1 Average share of the built-up area of cities that is open space for public use for all, by sex, age and persons with disabilities 11.7.2 Proportion of persons victim of physical or sexual harassment, by sex, age, disability status
16. Promote peaceful and inclusive societies for sustainable development, [. . .] build effective, accountable and inclusive institutions at all levels	*16.7 Ensure responsive, inclusive, participatory and representative decision-making at all levels*	16.7.1 Positions (by sex, age, persons with disabilities and population groups) in public institutions [. . .] compared to national distributions 16.7.2 Proportion of population who believe decision-making is inclusive and responsive, by sex, age, disability and population group
17. Strengthen the means of implementation and revitalize the global partnership for sustainable development	17.18 By 2020, [. . .] increase significantly the availability of high-quality, timely and reliable data disaggregated by [. . .] disability, [. . .] and other characteristics relevant in national contexts	17.18.1 SDG indicators at national level with full relevant disaggregation, when relevant to the target, in accordance with the Fundamental Principles of Official Statistics

Note that indicators 1.3.1, 16.7.1 and 16.7.2 has to be disaggregated for people with disabilities, although their corresponding target (appearing in italics in Table 1) does not explicitly refer to persons with disabilities

Data and Methodologies for Measuring Disability

As it is clear from the 'ICF model' as well as the other frameworks previously introduced, when looking at social inclusion of people with disabilities it is important to be aware of the contextual factors. Unfortunately, the 'ICF model' is not implemented by statistical tools and the debate to translate the ICF definition in the statistical survey language is yet open at international level and a suitable solution is far to be reached (Sebastiani and Solipaca 2014).

The challenge is, therefore, building-up proper statistical measurements of the domains of social inclusion indicated by CRPD and the other internationally agreed agenda. From a statistical point of view, concepts like accessibility, active inclusion or participation are theoretical concepts not directly measurable, consequently to monitor the social inclusion we have to implement statistical indicators suitable to approximate the different dimensions of these concepts.

The approach herein adopted is trying to measure social inclusion of disabled people comparing, between disabled and non-disabled people, the value of statistical indicators on aspects of social inclusion, such as those put across in the EDS. More inclusion will exist to the extent that the indicators observed in the two sub-populations have similar values.

There are two main sources for comparable data between disabled and non-disabled people in (most) EU countries using coherent methodology and definitions harmonized within the European Statistical System (ESS): the European Statistics of Income and Living Conditions (EU-SILC) survey and the *ad hoc* module on employment of disabled people in the 2011 labour force survey (LFS).

The EU-SILC survey is the reference source for comparative statistics on income distribution and social exclusion at European level. The survey covers all individuals aged 16 years old and over living in private households. Persons living in collective households and in institutions are generally excluded from the target population.

Definition of disability used in EU-SILC. The EU-SILC survey contains a small module on health, including three questions on general health status. The questions on the general health status represent the so-called Minimum European Health Module (MEHM, Cox et al. 2009) and are proposed to be used in any EU health survey or survey module, in order to link results among surveys. The three questions are about (*i*) self-perceived health, (*ii*) chronic (longstanding) illnesses or conditions and (*iii*) limitation in activities due to health problems.

The data on limitation in activities due to health problems refer to the auto-evaluation by the respondents of the extent to which, because of health problems, they are limited, for at least in the last 6 months, in activities people usually do. The measurement is based on the Global Activity Limitation Instrument (GALI, Jagger et al. 2010). The exact question is "*Limitation in activities people usually do because of health problems for at least the last 6 months*" and possible answers are: 1. *Severely limited*, 2. *Limited but not severely* and 3. *Not limited at all.*

Therefore, the EU-SILC term (activity limitation) does not expressly take into account any 'interactions with barriers' which is typical of the social (ICF) model approach. On the other end, in 2011, the European Union Labor Force Survey (EU-LFS) included an *ad hoc* module (AHM) on employment of disabled people. The AHM consisted of a number of questions dealing with:

- Health problems and difficulties in basic activities;
- Limitations in work caused by health problems/difficulties in basic activities;
- Special assistance needed or used by people with health problems/difficulties in basic activities;
- Limitations in work because of other reasons.

Definition of disability in AHM. The results of AHM were presented using two definitions of disability, as either (*i*) people having a basic activity difficulty (such as seeing, hearing, walking, communicating), which have lasted or be expected to last for 6 months or more or (*ii*) people having a work limitation caused by a longstanding health condition (i.e. a permanent health condition or disease which is expected to require a long period of care or personal assistance) and/or a basic activity difficulty. Limitations are deemed as: (*a*) in the amount of work (i.e. the number of hours); (*b*) in the type of work (for instance, having problems in carrying heavy loads, working outdoors, sitting for a long time); (*c*) getting to and from work.

In order to run surveys and ensure the international comparability of statistics on disability, within the domain of European disability statistics, the GALI question has been currently included in EU social surveys, such as EU-SILC (as well as in EHIS).

A Composite Indicator for Rating Inequality Conditions of People with Disabilities

The 'ICF model' defines components of health as well as some health-related components of well-being, such as education and employment, then disability (and active inclusion of people with disabilities) has to be examined through these various dimensions. Pursuing the goal of social inclusion for people with disabilities may refer to the kinds of activities, relationships, and environments that the various frameworks presented in section "A common perspective on social inclusion: CRPD, European Disability Strategy and the SDG's" encompass.

As mentioned previously, the purpose of this paper is to analyze the lack of activities and social participation through the differences observed between the sub-populations of people with and without limitations with respect to several dimensions of social inclusion, such as those indicated as priority areas in the EDS.

Indeed, given the multiple dimensions to be considered at once in the measurement of the latent construct, the idea is bringing in a synthetic representation of the distinct features of social inclusion, using the methodology of composite indicators (OECD 2008). Composite indices have become recently very popular in order to synthesizing multidimensional phenomena in economic, social and policy domains. The literature offers a wide range of aggregation methods, which, however, need to meet in some cases assumptions either not desirable or difficult to satisfy.

Methodology on Composite Indicators: AMPI

Given the matrix $\mathbf{X} = \{x_{ij}\}$, whose generic element x_{ij} represents the value of the indicator j for the i-th statistical unit, let Inf_{x_j} and Sup_{x_j} be, respectively, the overall minimum and maximum values of the indicator *j* across all units and all time periods considered. Denoting with Ref_{x_j} a reference values for the indicator *j*, the minimum and the maximum value of the possible range for each indicator (*goalposts*) are defined (Mazziotta and Pareto 2016) as:

$$\begin{cases} \mathrm{Min}_{x_j} = Ref_{x_j} - \Delta \\ \mathrm{Max}_{x_j} = Ref_{x_j} + \Delta \end{cases}$$

where $\Delta = \left(Sup_{x_j} - Inf_{x_j}\right)/2$.

In typical socio-economic applications, the elementary indicators considered are correlated either positively (i.e. they have positive *polarity*) or negatively (negative polarity) with the phenomenon to be measured. Therefore, it can be useful to normalize the indicators so that an increase in the normalized indicators corresponds to an increase in the composite index, regardless of their polarity.

Given the matrix $\mathbf{X} = \{x_{ij}\}$, a normalized matrix $\mathbf{R} = \{r_{ij}\}$ is then computed, where the generic element r_{ij} is obtained as follows (in the case of positive polarity of the indicator *j*):

$$r_{ij} = \frac{\left(x_{ij} - \mathrm{Min}_{x_j}\right)}{\left(\mathrm{Max}_{x_j} - \mathrm{Min}_{x_j}\right)} 60 + 70 \tag{1}$$

where Min_{x_j} and Max_{x_j} are the *goalposts* for the indicator *j* (Mazziotta and Pareto 2016). Indeed, if the indicator *j* has negative polarity, the complement of (1) with respect to 200 is used for computing the normalized value. In both cases, the range of the normalized values is [70; 130], where 100 corresponds to the reference value.

Denoting with M_{r_i} and S_{r_i}, respectively, mean and standard deviation of the normalized values of the unit *i*, the generalized form of AMPI (*Adjusted* Mazziotta Pareto Index) is given by:

$$AMPI_i^{+/-} = M_{r_i} \pm S_{r_i} cv_i$$

where $cv_i = S_{r_i}/M_{r_i}$ is the coefficient of variation for the unit *i*. In order to make interpretation of the results straightforward, it is recommended to choose the goalposts so that 100 represents a reference value (e.g., the average in a given year). If the composite index is 'increasing' or 'positive', i.e., it is expected that increasing values of the index correspond to positive variations of the phenomenon, then AMPI^- will be used; AMPI^+ is used, instead, if the composite index is 'decreasing' or 'negative', i.e., increasing values of the index correspond to negative variations of the underlying construct. For further details, cfr. Mazziotta and Pareto (2016).

An Application to Social Inclusion of Disabled People: Indicators Selected

In accordance with the EDS, we focus our attention on: education and training, health status, employment, risk of poverty, housing condition and social participation. These dimensions of social inclusion are coherent with those identified in the CRPD as the most relevant in order to guarantee to people with disabilities full enjoyment of their fundamental rights. Hence, one indicator, calculated using data from either LFS or EU-SILC, has been picked out for representing each of the above dimensions.

As for the selection of the individual indicators, the basic criteria which were followed are that each indicator should be robust and statistically validated and should permit a sufficient level of cross countries comparability, namely using internationally harmonized definitions and data collection standards. See Table 2 for the full list of variables and indicators selected for the application.

The selected individual indicators have the property of non-substitutability, i.e. they are assumed having the same conceptual importance and that there are no compensative effects among indicators that are relevant to the description of the latent construct (i.e. *social inclusion* of disabled people). Moreover, since the measurement model is based on a formative approach (i.e. causality relation is deemed from the indicators to the underlying construct), the correlations among the individual indicators have no relevance (Mazziotta and Pareto 2017).

In order to analyze the social inclusion in a harmonized way among EU countries the indicators related to poverty, housing conditions, social participation and health consider as belonging to the subpopulation of disabled people a person with some or severe limitation due to health problems, while the indicators on education and training and employment calculated for disabled people refer to persons having a basic activity difficulty.

For time consistency with the data obtained from the *ad hoc* module of LFS on disabled people, all indicators from EU-SILC survey have been considered for 2011 as the reference year, except for the frequency of getting together with friends, which is taken from the 2006 *ad-hoc* module of EU-SILC on social participation.[5]

[5]The analysis and comparisons among countries and between the two subpopulations of disabled and nondisabled persons can be affected by countries' different demographical structure – particularly for elderly people – notably for three elementary indicators used in the calculation of the composite index: *AROPE*, *Bad_dwelling* and *S_P_health*. Likewise, the small number of observations available for each age class does not allow age-standardization of indicators. In order to reduce the influence on the analysis of different age-structure in the population, these indicators have then been considered for the subpopulation within 16–64 age group, which shows comparable demographic structures between countries.

Table 2 Data and variables selected for the application

Domain (EDS targets)	Ref. CRPD	Variable/indicator	Variable_ID	Source	Details on data/definitions used
Education and training	artt.3, 24	Percentage of young people neither in employment nor in further education or training	NEET	LFS	Subpopulation of disabled people: persons having a basic activity difficulty. Age group: 15–24
Employment	artt.3, 27	Employment rate	Emp_rate	LFS	Subpopulation of disabled people considered: persons having work limitation caused by a longstanding health condition and/or a basic activity difficulty. Age group: 20–64
Poverty/social protection	artt.3, 5, 19, 26, 28	Share of the total population which is at risk of poverty or social exclusion	AROPE	EU-SILC	The indicator refer to persons who are either (i) at risk of financial poverty, or (ii) severely materially deprived, or (iii) living in households with very low work intensity. Subpopulation of disabled people: persons having some or severe activity limitation due to health problems. Age group: 16–64.
Housing conditions	art.19	Percentage of population living in a dwelling with a leaking roof, damp walls, floors or foundation, or rot in window frames of floor	Bad_dwelling	EU-SILC	Subpopulation of disabled people: persons having some or severe activity limitation due to health problems. Age group: 16–64.

(continued)

Table 2 (continued)

Domain (EDS targets)	Ref. CRPD	Variable/indicator	Variable_ID	Source	Details on data/definitions used
Social participation	art.30	Frequency of getting together (spending time) with friends, at home or elsewhere.	Friends	EU-SILC	Data from the 2006 ad-hoc module on social participation of EU-SILC. The module was surveyed on the same sample as the main questionnaire. Several different possible answer for frequency of getting together, frequency selected: every day. Subpopulation of disabled people: persons having some or severe activity limitation due to health problems. Age group: 16–29
Health	art.25	Self-perceived health condition	S_P_health	EU-SILC	The indicator is calculated for respondents stating that their health status is “good” or “very good”. Subpopulation of disabled people: persons having some or severe activity limitation due to health problems. Age group: 16–64.

Empirical Results

In this section the methodology and the indicators introduced in sections "Methodology on composite indicators: AMPI" and "An application to social inclusion of disabled people: indicators selected" have been employed to yield a cross-country comparison of social inclusion of person with disabilities in EU countries. The observed values of the indicators are listed in Table 3, distinguishing between disabled and non-disabled people. Because of constraints with the availability of the underlying data, we focused on EU15 Member States (the Member States before the 2004 enlargement of the EU to Central and Eastern European countries). The overall (disabled and non-disabled) average for EU27 has been used, instead, as a reference value (final row in Table 3) for calculating the composite index.

The observed values of the indicators show a marked disadvantage of people with disability with respect to people without disabilities, for each dimension of social inclusion considered. However, the situation across Member states differs significantly. Indeed, we find wide disparities across Europe for each of the individual indicators, with observed values across Southern Europe typically showing even less favorable conditions for disabled people than across most of Northern and North-Western Europe. With peculiarities observed in some countries for specific indicators.

In 2011, the share of young people with disability aged 15–24 who were not in employment, education or training (denoted as *NEET* in Tables 2 and 3) varied across the EU between slightly more than 10,5% and 45,9%, a figure which is more or less four times higher than the average over all countries (EU27). The lowest NEET rates were in Sweden, Austria, Germany, Luxembourg and Denmark. At the other end of the spectrum, NEET rates were the highest in some southern EU Member States, such as Italy and Greece, where almost half of the persons with disabilities in the age group between 15 and 24 years fell into the NEET category. The NEET rate for people without disabilities range from 2,6% in Netherlands to the highest figures in Italy and Spain, where something less then every fifth person aged 15 through 24 years fell into the NEET category.

The employment rate (*Emp_rate*) of people with disability ranged in 2011 from as low as 22% in Ireland to more than 60% in France (61%) and Sweden (64%), with the corresponding figure for people without disabilities ranging from less than two-thirds in Southern Europe countries (Greece, Italy, Spain) to more than 80% in Nordic countries (Denmark, Sweden, Finland) and some of North Western countries (Netherlands and Austria). For comparison, notice that the headline target of Europe 2020 for overall (disabled and non-disabled) employment rate is 75%.[6] Furthermore, comparing, for each country, the figures for disabled and non-disabled, it is also noteworthy the large disparity (>40%) in some North Western countries (Ireland, Netherlands, United Kingdom, Germany) between the two subpopulations.

[6]http://ec.europa.eu/eurostat/web/europe-2020-indicators/europe-2020-strategy/headline-indicators-scoreboard

Table 3 Indicators for disabled and non-disabled people – EU15

Country	NEET		Emp_rate		AROPE		Bad_dwelling		Friends		S_P_health	
	Disabled	Not disabled	Disabled	Not disabled	Disabled	Not disabled	Disabled	not disabled	Disabled	Not disabled	Disabled	Not disabled
Belgium	20,6	9,2	34,0	74,0	38,5	16,2	28,2	19,7	29,5	38,2	25,2	91,8
Denmark	15,4	5,2	41,8	83,5	28,1	17,7	21,8	15,0	24,6	31,3	37,0	86,6
Germany	14,8	7,9	36,2	77,8	34,1	15,7	18,8	13,1	30,8	46,3	22,7	89,5
Ireland	40,3	17,5	22,0	67,8	50,8	27,9	17,2	9,9	34,4	43,8	36,3	94,3
Greece	44,6	15,8	30,1	63,8	46,6	30,3	24,2	13,2	47,4	69,9	17,4	95,2
Spain	26,7	19,1	34,3	65,9	41,3	26,3	21,7	15,0	32,4	49,7	23,9	93,9
France	19,8	10,7	61,0	74,7	31,7	17,4	14,4	10,7	29,2	29,4	27,2	86,1
Italy	45,9	18,0	37,6	64,0	37,7	26,8	31,5	21,1	30,1	47,4	28,1	89,0
Luxembourg	15,1	4,5	49,8	73,6	28,1	16,3	16,7	15,8	45,6	57,6	31,9	86,1
Netherlands	17,3	2,6	39,7	83,2	28,6	14,2	17,5	14,8	24,1	30,7	39,3	93,0
Austria	12,7	6,7	48,4	80,7	29,1	12,6	17,8	13,0	22,1	27,2	29,1	89,8
Portugal	23,5	10,7	44,8	76,0	35,9	20,5	27,8	18,2	35,7	64,9	13,4	72,1
Finland	18,1	6,4	51,4	81,0	26,6	14,9	8,6	4,8	43,4	50,8	43,1	90,2
Sweden	10,6	6,5	64,0	83,4	25,5	14,3	13,2	8,3	26,7	35,6	37,6	91,6
United Kingdom	28,6	15,2	36,4	79,7	39,4	18,0	22,6	15,6	36,3	41,3	31,9	92,2
EU–27	***12,9***		***68,6***		***25,0***		***15,7***		***41,7***		***77,0***	

The at-risk-of-poverty or social exclusion (*AROPE*) rate[7] is one of the three indicators used for monitoring progress towards the Europe 2020 social inclusion target. In 2011 one-fourth of all persons aged 16 through 64 years in the EU27 countries lived in households which were at risk of poverty or social exclusion. Concerning people with disabilities aged 16 through 64 years, the lowest AROPE rates were found in Sweden, Finland and Denmark (and Luxembourg). On the other hand, high percentages (from 35% up to just about 40%) were found in Southern Europe countries (Italy, Spain, Portugal) but also in some North Western countries (United Kingdom, Belgium), up to a highest rate of more and less than one-half in Ireland (50,8%) and Greece (46,5%). High gaps between persons with and without disabilities can be found in Ireland (22,9%), Belgium (22,3%) and United Kingdom (21,4%).

As for the housing conditions, the share of total population living in a dwelling with a leaking roof, damp walls, floors or foundation, or rot in window frames of floor (*Bad_dwelling*) has high rates (between 27,8% and 31,5%) for households with disabled people in Italy, Belgium and Portugal, with respect to an average rate of 15,7% for EU27 countries, thus worsening deprivation conditions for persons with disabilities.

The frequency of getting together with friends (i.e. spending time, at home or elsewhere, with nonfamily members, *Friends*) has been selected as an indicator of the quality of social interaction and the degree of involvement in communities. Note that for the total of population aged 16 or over the most common answer for this variable is "*Every week*", with exceptions for some countries (Greece, Portugal) where the most frequent answer is *'Daily'* (maybe because of cultural differences on the degree of community participation in Southern Europe countries). Indeed, for this indicator, Greece and Portugal (and, to some minor extent, Italy and Spain) show, as well, the highest gaps between persons with and without disabilities in the age group 16 through 29. It should also be highlighted the relatively high level of '*not applicable*' for this variable, which corresponds to the answer *'no friends*', among persons with disability in Italy (11,1%) and Greece (11,6%).

Finally, the indicator on health status (*S_P_health*) refers to the individuals who answered "*good*" or "*very good*" to the question on self-perceived general health. This indicator is a subjective perception but it is taken as a good proxy for true health conditions concerning the different dimensions of health, i.e. physical, social and

[7]Eurostat defines a person *at risk-of-poverty or social exclusion* (AROPE) as: *1.* Persons with an equalized disposable income below the risk-of-poverty threshold, which is set at 60% of the national median equalized disposable income (after social transfers) and/or *2.* Severely materially deprived persons, which have living conditions severely constrained by a lack of resources, i.e. they experience at least 4 out of 9 following deprivations items: cannot afford (i) to pay rent or utility bills, (ii) keep home adequately warm, (iii) face unexpected expenses, (iv) eat meat, fish or a protein equivalent every second day, (v) a week holiday away from home, (vi) a car, (vii) a washing machine, (viii) a colour TV, or (ix) a telephone and/or *3.* People living in households with very low work intensity, namely people aged 0–59 living in households where the adults (aged 18–59) worked less than 20% of their total work potential during the past year.

Table 4 Composite index of social inclusion: disabled and non-disabled people

Country	Disabled		Non-disabled	
	Index	Ranking	Index	Ranking
Belgium	74,2	*27*	104,4	*9*
Denmark	82,3	*22*	106,4	*6*
Germany	79,7	*23*	104,7	*8*
Ireland	68,8	*28*	102,7	*12*
Greece	67,0	*30*	100,2	*13*
Spain	75,0	*26*	104,0	*10*
France	85,6	*19*	108,1	*4*
Italy	68,1	*29*	93,8	*15*
Luxembourg	88,8	*18*	107,1	*5*
Netherlands	83,1	*21*	112,9	*3*
Austria	83,1	*20*	106,0	*7*
Portugal	75,3	*25*	97,5	*14*
Finland	92,6	*16*	116,2	*1*
Sweden	91,0	*17*	113,1	*2*
United Kingdom	77,1	*24*	103,2	*11*
EU-27	100.0			

emotional functioning. Regarding people with disabilities aged 16 through 64 years, the lowest rates can be found in Portugal, Greece and Germany. As it is expected, this indicator shows high gaps between disabled and non-disabled people, with the largest disparity observed in Southern Europe countries (Spain and Greece) and, as well, in some North-Western countries (Belgium and Germany).

The results for the calculation of the composite index described in section "Methodology on composite indicators: AMPI" are displayed in Table 4. As mentioned in section "Methodology on composite indicators: AMPI", the methodology is based on a reference value (i.e., overall average for EU27 countries). In this way, it is straightforward to compare the countries in relative terms and, at the same time, compare their performances for disabled and non-disabled people. The values taken from the composite index appear in the second and fourth columns of Table 4 for disabled and non-disabled people, respectively, with the resulting countries' rank in the adjacent column.

As it might be expected, the value of the composite index confirms that there is a gap between the two subpopulations throughout Europe, as, indeed, the computed values for the non-disabled take up the positions from 1 to 15, while the values for disabled rank 16 through 30. Moreover, some of the Southern countries (Italy, Greece, and, particularly for non-disabled people, Portugal) and some of North-Western countries (Ireland, Belgium, especially for disabled, and, to some extent, United Kingdom) tend to occupy lower positions in the list, for both the subpopulations. On the other end, two Northern countries (Finland, Sweden) have the highest value of the index for both disabled and non-disabled people.

Note that for two countries (Italy and Portugal) the value taken from the composite index for non-disabled people is lower than the reference value. Instead, comparing, for each country, the index for the two subpopulations, the lowest difference can be found in Luxembourg, Sweden, Portugal, France and Austria, while the highest discrepancies are observed in Ireland, Greece, and Belgium. Note also that the largest difference of the index between two consecutive values in the ordered list of countries is between position 3 (Netherlands, non-disabled people) and 4 (France, non-disabled); however, large gaps between consecutive values of the composite indicator can also be found between positions 1 (Finland, non-disabled) and 2 (Sweden, non-disabled), as well as between countries ranking 14th (Portugal, non-disabled) and 15th (Italy, non-disabled).

Finally, a sensitivity analysis has been made to assess the robustness of the synthetic indicator, primarily to understand the implicit weight of each individual indicator on the composite index. The sensitivity measure employed is the average shift in country rankings, obtained as the average of the absolute differences in countries' rankings calculating the composite indicator with the full matrix of m elementary indicators and its reduced form, with $m-1$ indicators, attained by removing iteratively each elementary indicator.

The average shift of country rankings for this application is comprised within the interval [0,47–0,93]. This confirms that the implicit weight of the selected indicators is rather similar. The highest weight is held by two elementary indicators: *Emp_rate* and *Friends*; indeed, if one of these indicators is removed from the calculation of the composite index, each country changes, in average, less than one position in the ranking. If any other indicator is removed from the matrix $\mathbf{X}$ of elementary indicators, each country ranking changes even less on average, down to a lowest value of 0,47 for *S_P_health*.

Discussion and Concluding Remarks

Social inclusion and/or participation of people with disabilities is a complex construct which, actually, does not have a clear-cut definition. Meanwhile, conceptual difficulty has encouraged a large flow of literature which considers different approaches to the definition of social inclusion, e.g. identifying the scope of inclusion/participation through the kind of activities relationships and environments that it embraces and/or trying to capture the structural and functional components behind it (cfr. Whiteneck and Dijkers 2009; United Nations 2010; Simplican et al. 2015). The multiple definitions may, in turn, influence the main dimensions to be considered when trying to measure social inclusion and the selection of indicators calculated from surveys and/or secondary data for carrying on concrete analysis of social inclusion. Indeed, the variations between definitions leads to insufficient data about its effective implementation.

In this paper the inherently multidimensional nature of social inclusion of people with disability has been handled through a synthetic measure of disparity between disabled and non-disabled people in EU15 countries (the 'old' EU Member States) based on the methodology of composite indices; using these techniques we realize a suitable combination of individual indicators on different aspects of disability conditions, aimed at yielding a measurement of active inclusion of persons with disabilities in EU countries.

This study is not meant as an attempt to implementing the ICF model or the capability approach, but rather proposes a simple instrument to describe the interactions between health conditions and a multiplicity of contextual factors, which may cause the lack of social inclusion of people with disability.

The composite index considered, AMPI [*Adjusted* Mazziotta Pareto Index, Mazziotta and Pareto (2016)], such as all techniques used for synthesizing multi-dimensional phenomena, has its *pros* and *cons*. Among main advantages: (*i*) the index may be divided into two components: the average (*compensatory*) effect and the *penalty* (unbalanced) effect; (*ii*) the composite index is applicable to any single indicator, varying the penalty sign, so that the variance term in the calculation of the composite index can be summed up or subtracted from the average; (*iii*) in order to calculate the composite index of each statistical unit it is not necessary to know the values of the other units (namely, the method is *absolute*); (*iv*) the index can be applied to aggregate values of the indicators, i.e. it is straightforward to calculate the composite index of composite indices; (*v*) absolute comparisons of unit values over time can be done. The main disadvantage is that the method does not completely remove extra-variability of the elementary indicators since the denominator of the normalizing function (1) is the range of the elementary indicator.

The results of the empirical study confirm that there is a disparity between the two subpopulations throughout Europe, even though the situation across Member states may vary significantly, with most of the Southern Europe countries and some of North-Western countries (Belgium, Ireland) having lower value of the composite indicator for both disabled and non-disabled people and, at the same time, the largest difference in each country's index for the two subpopulations. Finland and Sweden, instead, show the highest value of the composite index for both sub-populations. Sensitivity analysis allowed to explore also the influence of each individual indicators on the composite index. The results of sensitivity analysis essentially confirm that the implicit weights of the elementary indicators selected are rather similar.

Future developments of the present work will consider extending the empirical study to other countries in the ESS and different variables representing the dimensions of social inclusion, possibly to be analyzed over a time-span. Hence, more extensive measurements of the underlying phenomenon would be worthwhile, e.g. using the indicators on the SDG's targets presented in Table 1 once suitable disaggregation for disabled people will be delivered.

References

Cox, B., Van Oyen, H., Cambois, E., Jagger, C., Le Roy, S., Robine, J.M., & Romieu, I. (2009). The reliability of the Minimum European Health Module. *International Journal of Public Health,* 54, 55–60. doi: https://doi.org/10.1007/s00038-009-7104-y.

European Commission (2010). European Disability Strategy 2010–2020: A Renewed Commitment to a Barrier-Free Europe. COM(2010) 636 final. Brussels, 15.11.2010. European Commission. https://eur-lex.europa.eu/legal-content/EN/TXT/PDF/?uri=CELEX:52010DC0636&from=EN. Accessed 8 June 2018.

European Commission (2004). *Joint Report on Social Inclusion. Report* 7101/04; Brussels: European Commission. http://ec.europa.eu/employment_social/soc-prot/soc-incl/final_joint_inclusion_report_2003_en.pdf. Accessed 8 June 2018.

European Commission (2013). *European Health Interview Survey (EHIS wave 2) – Methodological manual.* Luxembourg: Publications Office of the European Union. doi: https://doi.org/10.2785/43280

Jagger, C., Gillies, C., Cambois, E., Van Oyen, H., Nusselder, W., Robine, J.M. (2010). The Global Activity Limitation Index measured function and disability similarly across European countries. *Journal of Clinical Epidemiology*, 63, 892–899. doi:https://doi.org/10.1016/j.jclinepi.2009.11.002.

Mazziotta, M., & Pareto, A. (2016). On a Generalized Non-compensatory Composite Index for Measuring Socio-economic Phenomena. *Social Indicators Research*, 127, 983–1003. doi: https://doi.org/10.1007/s11205-015-0998-2

Mazziotta, M., & Pareto, A. (2017). Synthesis of indicators: the composite indicators approach. In: F. Maggino (Ed.), *Complexity in Society: From Indicators Construction to their Synthesis* (pp.159–191). *Social Indicators Research Series*, vol. 70. Springer. doi: https://doi.org/10.1007/978-3-319-60595-1_7

OECD (2008). *Handbook on constructing composite indicators. Methodology and user guide.* Paris: OECD Publications.

Sebastiani, G., & Solipaca, A. (2014). Disabilità. In: G. Costa, S. Salmaso, C. Cislaghi (Eds.). *Misurare in sanità pubblica: registri e sorveglianza. Situazione attuale e prospettive* (pp. 159–167). *Rapporti ISTISAN*, 14/23. Roma: Istituto Superiore di Sanità.

Sen, A. K. (1993). *Capability and well-being.* In: M.C. Nussbaum & A. Sen, (Eds) *The Quality of Life* (pp. 30–53). Oxford University Press, Oxford.

Sen, A. K. (1999). *Development as freedom.* New York: Knopf.

Simplican, S. C., Leader, G., Kosciulek, J., & Leahy, M. (2015). Defining social inclusion of people with intellectual and developmental disabilities: An ecological model of social networks and community participation. *Research in Developmental Disabilities*, 38, 18–29. doi: https://doi.org/10.1016/j.ridd.2014.10.008.

United Nations, (2007). Convention on the Rights of Persons with Disabilities. New York: United Nations. http://www.un.org/disabilities/documents/convention/convoptprot-e.pdf. Accessed 8 June 2018.

United Nations, (2010) *Analysing and measuring social inclusion in a global context.* New York, United Nations. http://www.un.org/esa/socdev/publications/measuring-social-inclusion.pdf. Accessed 8 June 2018.

United Nations, (2015). *Transforming our world: the 2030 Agenda for Sustainable Development.* Resolution A/RES/70/1 of the General Assembly. New York, United Nations. http://undocs.org/A/RES/70/1. Accessed 8 June 2018.

Whiteneck, G., & Dijkers, M.P. (2009). Difficult to measure constructs: conceptual and methodological issues concerning participation and environmental factors. *Arch. Phys. Med. Rehabil.*, 90 (11), S22–S35. doi: https://doi.org/10.1016/j.apmr.2009.06.009.

WHO (2001). *The International Classification of Functioning. Disability and Health.* Geneva: World Health Organization.

Measurement of Well-being in Territories: An Application for Italian Provinces

Roberto Costa, Carlo Declich, Elena Marchesich, and Susi Osti

Abstract This contribution intends to present a comparison between well-being levels of Italian Provinces, thanks to the synthesis of the 2014 territorial well-being indicators "BES delle Province" (ISTAT-CUSPI). The Mazziotta-Pareto Index (MPI) was used, pursuant to the methodology ISTAT has been using since 2015 for the calculation of composite country-wide well-being indicators. Herein, we report the main steps for the constitution of the global indicator and the domain-based indicators. Additionally, we present alternative indicators to highlight their differences compared with the MPI and motivating the choice of the latter thanks to influence analysis. Finally, we report results with province-based rankings and maps that allow identification of distinctive characteristics of well-being in various territories for comparative purposes, both within single domains and globally. The snapshot of Italy that emerges from this may not always be consistent with the stereotype of the rich North vs. poor South.

Introduction

> What you measure affects what you do. If you don't measure the right thing, you don't do the right thing. (J. E. Stiglitz)

Measurement of well-being of individuals and society has long been a discussion topic. Recently, this topic has overstepped Academia to be tackled by decision makers, official statistics, international organizations and civil society. Part of the debate concerns the necessity to evaluate progress in our society not only by conventional economic measurements such as the GDP, which many – based on

R. Costa · E. Marchesich (✉)
ISTAT, Trieste, Italy
e-mail: rocosta@istat.it; elmarche@istat.it

C. Declich · S. Osti
ISTAT, Venezia, Italy
e-mail: declich@istat.it; osti@istat.it

A. Bianco et al. (eds.), *Italian Studies on Quality of Life*, Social Indicators Research Series 77, https://doi.org/10.1007/978-3-030-06022-0_4

an alleged equivalence between well-being and economic progress – consider the main tool for the measurement of development.

Starting from 2001, the Organisation for Economic Co-operation and Development (OECD) promoted several initiatives to support measurement and fostering of social progress. The 2008 economic crisis further accelerated the research for new reference measurements for policies to be paired with purely economic measurements. The most significant work in this field is the final Report of the Commission for measurement of economic performance and social progress, known as the Stiglitz-Sen-Fitoussi Commission (2009). The Commission set forth 12 recommendations that, among the other aspects, promoted: a multileveled approach to well-being measurement that also takes into account subjective elements; the usage of sustainability indicators not merely for environmental aspects but to include economic and social sustainability; the development of a single synthesis indicator for the evaluation of quality of life.

Part of the debate shifted on the opportunity to conceive synthesis indicators that would simplify the immediate understanding of the real depth of a phenomenon and would not give raise to misleading or twisted interpretations. On one side, the usage of composite indicators over batteries of elementary indicators allows for a more straightforward representation and interpretation of multilayered realties with no loss of base information, thus promoting communication to the public and usage of data by decision-makers. On the other side, when ill-conceived or misinterpreted, these composite indicators may convey misleading messages, uphold simplistic conclusions or, in worst case scenario, endorse biased or inadequate political choices. These shortcomings may be overcome when the composite indicator is based on a solid theoretical framework, relies on solid data and is steered by a consistent methodology (OECD 2008).

Measurement of Equitable and Sustainable Well-being in Italy

The project to measure equitable and sustainable well-being – born of a joint initiative of Italian National Council for Economics and Labour (CNEL) and National Institute of Statistics (ISTAT) – is part of the international debate on "Beyond GDP". The central idea is that economic parameters alone are inadequate to evaluate the progress of societies and should be complemented by social and environmental information and by measures of inequality and sustainability (Giovannini et al. 2012). Starting from a multi-dimensional approach to the concept of well-being, this project shall provide an ample array of indicators as a tool to monitor the condition of population and territory, inform citizens and steer political decisions.

They selected 130 indicators, combined into 12 domains. These indicators have been elaborated and analyzed in five BES Reports,[1] starting from 2013. In the third

[1] BES stands for *Benessere Equo e Sostenibile*, Equitable and Sustainable Well-being.

Report (ISTAT 2015) composite indicators at regional level have been published for the first time, as a synthesis of elementary indicators in each of the nine outcome[2] domains.

The "BES delle Province" project[3] was fostered by the need for an additional depth of study at the local level. It has the twofold objective of analyzing the well-being structure in large areas whilst evaluating the importance and accuracy of actions of local administrations to improve the well-being of their communities. Currently 82 indicators are available (ISTAT and CUSPI 2015). They have been calculated for the entirety of Italian territory at the province, regional and country levels.[4]

The availability of such an articulate dashboard of indicators has the advantage of pinpointing the leading distinctive traits of the well-being structure in the province area, highlighting strengths and weaknesses, risks and opportunities, bringing together BES measurement on an area with the information requirements that are necessary for the governance to foster its development (Taralli 2013). Conversely, however, reading the entirety of the dashboard may be a daunting task. It is therefore necessary to provide a synthesis of indicators for each domain as well as globally. These two approaches – *i.e.* composite indicators vs. sets of indicators – should not be seen as mutually exclusive. They should be considered jointly: the first indicator presents a simple and immediate assessment of the phenomenon whilst the second provides in depth analysis.

Main Steps to Build a Composite Province BES Indicator

In constituting a global composite indicator, the multi-dimensional aspects of the phenomenon require overcoming of certain conceptual and definition hindrances, including the choice of the system of elementary indicators within each domain, the adoption of the synthesis method within each domain and the calculation of a composite overall indicator that allows ranking of well-being at provincial level.

---

[2]We define as "outcome" the domains that have direct effects on well-being, while other domains that measure elements that are functional to improvement of well-being are called "instrumental".

[3]The "BES delle Province" project is a collaboration between ISTAT and the Coordination of Statistics Offices of Italian Provinces (CUSPI). In the project, the term "Province" indicates both types of local institution for territorial areas introduced with Law 56/2014 (so-called "Delrio Law"): the Extended Province Areas (AVP) and Metropolitan Cities (CM). The latter as of 1 January 2015 have taken over the previous Provinces of the same name.

[4]For a full list of indicators and documentation of the "BES delle Province" project, please refer to website www.besdelleprovince.it

Selection of Domains and Indicators

We carried out the analysis on the entirety of 110 Italian Provinces in 2014. In this first experimentation, we focused on eight outcome domains.

The measurement model for BES is based on a "formative" approach (Diamantopoulos and Winklhofer 2001): the group of indicators that were selected to define the latent BES variable defines the variable itself. In other words, all selected indicators contribute to the definition of the concept of well-being. Therefore, we decided to include in the calculation of the composite domain indicators the highest number of indicators that were present in the "BES delle Province" database (Table 1), only striking out the following:

- Indicators with a polarity that was not well defined or that did not have an immediate interpretation, for which there was no clear connection with the investigated phenomenon;
- Indicators highly correlated ($r \geq 0.9$) with other descriptive indicators of the same theme, as their information content would have ended up weighting several times in the constitution of the indicator;
- Indicators eliminated in 2015, following considerations regarding their significance in the BES.

In a few instances and due to technical requirements, we operated a transformation of indicators and subsequently we created a new indicator derived from the previous one(s). For instance, this is what occurred for the two indicators pertaining the Level of literacy proficiency of students and the Level of arithmetical proficiency. These two indicators were highly correlated and have been substituted by a single indicator, called Level of student proficiency, which was the result of the simple arithmetic mean of the two previous ones.[5]

Table 1 Number of indicators available in 2014 for the BES of provinces and used in this work

Domain	Available	Used
Health	8	8
Education and training	8	6
Work and life balance	9	5
Economic well-being	11	9
Social relationships	8	6
Security	6	5
Landscape and cultural heritage	5	3
Environment	8	7
Politics and institutions	11	0
Research and innovation	7	0
Quality of services	7	0
TOTAL	88	49

[5]For a full list of used indicators, please consult the Table 3 in the Appendix.

Within each domain and for the selected indicators, some values are missing. Missing values are less than 10% and often limited to newly created Provinces. In these instances the missing value has been substituted with the datum of the previously existing Province from which the new Province was created.

Calculation of the Composite Domain Indicators

We followed the ISTAT methodology to construct the composite Province-BES indicators, taking into account the following set of theoretical and practical requirements:

- Spatial comparability
- Non substitutability of simple indicators
- Simplicity of computation
- Easy comprehension and use
- Robustness of the results.

We have experimented with multiple synthesis methods, thanks to ISTAT-developed COMIC (COMposite Indices Creator) software, which enables:

- Calculation of composite indicators with different methodologies (0–1 Indices Mean, Z-scores Mean, Jevons Index, Geometric Mean Index (GMI), Mazziotta-Pareto Index (MPI)).[6] All these methods fulfilled most of the expected properties of a composite indicator, whilst maintaining an adequate level of simplicity for fruition by laypersons;
- Creation of rankings for each synthesis method;
- Comparison between the various synthesis methods, specifically through influence analysis, which evaluates if rankings by geographic units change by eliminating one elementary indicator from the starting group and if so, to what degree;
- Reporting of results.

The comparison between the domain indicators calculated with the various methods eventually led to the choice of MPI. This index fulfilled all the requisites of spatial comparability, allowed only partial substitution of components and ensured robust results (De Muro et al. 2011). Specifically, the syntheses calculated with 0–1 Indices Mean and with Z-scores Mean, whilst ensuring a good degree of robustness, relied on a compensative approach that was inadequate to the “formative” approach of the BES framework (non-substitutability of indicators within the domains). The

[6]The first two methods are based on aggregation, via arithmetic mean, of elementary indicators transformed with the min-max method and standardized deviations. Jevons Index and GMI aggregate, via geometric mean, elementary indicators transformed into index numbers and with the min-max method.

Jevons Index and GMI provided results that were less robust compared to the MPI. Additionally, Jevons Index proved problematic during calculation when dealing with null value data.

In calculating the MPI, elementary indicators were first standardized and then aggregated with an "adjusted" arithmetic mean with a penalty coefficient (Mazziotta and Pareto 2015). This coefficient depends, for each unit (Province), on the variability of the indicators compared to the mean value. Thus, we penalized the score of the units that, having the same arithmetic mean, possessed a higher unbalance of values between the indicators ("horizontal" variability).

Formally, given a matrix $X = \{x_{ij}\}$ of n lines (statistical units) and m columns (indicators) the result is $Z = \{z_{ij}\}$ where:

$$z_{ij} = 100 \pm \frac{x_{ij} - \mathrm{M}_{x_j}}{\mathrm{S}_{x_j}} 10$$

M_{x_j} and S_{x_j} being respectively mean and standard deviation of the j-th indicator, x_{ij} the value of the j-th indicator in the i-th unit and $\pm$ representing the sign of the relation (polarity) between the j-th indicator and the phenomenon that we intend to measure.

The composite indicator of the i-th unit is calculated with this general formula:

$$\mathrm{MPI}_i^{+/-} = \mathrm{M}_{z_i} \pm \mathrm{S}_{z_i} cv_i$$

where M_{z_i} and S_{z_i} are the normalized mean and the standard deviation of the i-th unit, $cv_i = \mathrm{S}_{z_i}/\mathrm{M}_{z_i}$ is the coefficient of variation of the i-th unit and sign $\pm$ depends on the type of phenomenon that is being considered. In this analysis, we used MPI with a negative penalty, as positive variation in the indicator correspond to increasing values of well-being.

The formula may be easily broken down into two parts: the "mean" effect given by the mean of standardized indicators (addictive component) and the "penalty" effect. The indicator provides values that are approximately included in the 70–130 interval, allowing quick distinction between the units with a well-being level above the average (values higher than 100) and those below average. So the higher is the indicator, the more is the well-being of the geographical area and the indicator assumes high value when the mean is high and the standard deviation is low. In this way, starting from a simple approach like linear aggregation, MPI assumes imperfect substitutability between different domains of well-being (De Muro et al. 2011).

From Domain Indicators to Global Well-being Indicator

For each domain, we created a ranking of 110 Provinces that asserts their positioning regarding each component of well-being. For the calculation of the global BES

Table 2 Influence analysis for MPI and GMI

	MPI		GMI	
Removed domain indicator	mean	S.D.	mean	S.D.
Health	5.180	4.890	7.490	7.980
Education and training	5.360	5.840	6.150	6.820
Work and life balance	4.890	4.740	4.400	4.670
Economic well-being	4.050	4.310	4.850	5.190
Social relationships	4.040	3.750	2.890	3.630
Security	5.160	5.080	3.760	4.560
Landscape and cultural heritage	3.960	3.950	3.800	3.940
Environment	5.470	5.160	3.640	5.360
Mean	4.770	4.710	4.620	5.270
S.D.	0.601	0.643	1.417	1.372

indicator, or "superindicator", the same synthesis methodology was replicated, this time starting from the composite domain indicators and ultimately creating a Province-based ranking for the global well-being level on the territory (for full ranking see Table 4 in the Appendix).

In order to test sensitivity of results according to the approach used, we applied two alternate methods, both of which are only partially compensative: the MPI with negative adjustment and the GMI. The latter requires a lower degree of substitutability between the indicators compared to the MPI. This characteristic would make it preferable for calculation of a global well-being indicator, as it would penalize units with higher variability in their domain indicators, *i.e.* units that highlight uneven levels in the various aspects of well-being. However, MPI seems to ensure a higher degree of robustness compared to the GMI (Table 2): influence analysis shows that the average shift in rankings, following the removal of a domain indicator from the global indicator, is very similar with both methods (4.77 with MPI *vs* 4.62 with GMI). However, variability of said shifts is much higher in GMI compared to MPI (standard deviation respectively 5.27 and 4.71), and the means of the shifts for each domain are also more variable in GMI (from 2.89 to 7.49) compared to MPI (from 3.96 to 5.47).

Results: The Maps of Well-being

Figures 1 and 2 represent the scores obtained by the BES global indicator with the two methods. The scale is set in deciles that determine the color hue of Italian Provinces. One may notice that the MPI generated map does not highlight the traditional dualism between the North and South of the country: Provinces with the highest values are located in the Alpine region (in particular in the North-East), and in Central areas (Tuscany, Marche and Umbria). Conversely, some Provinces of

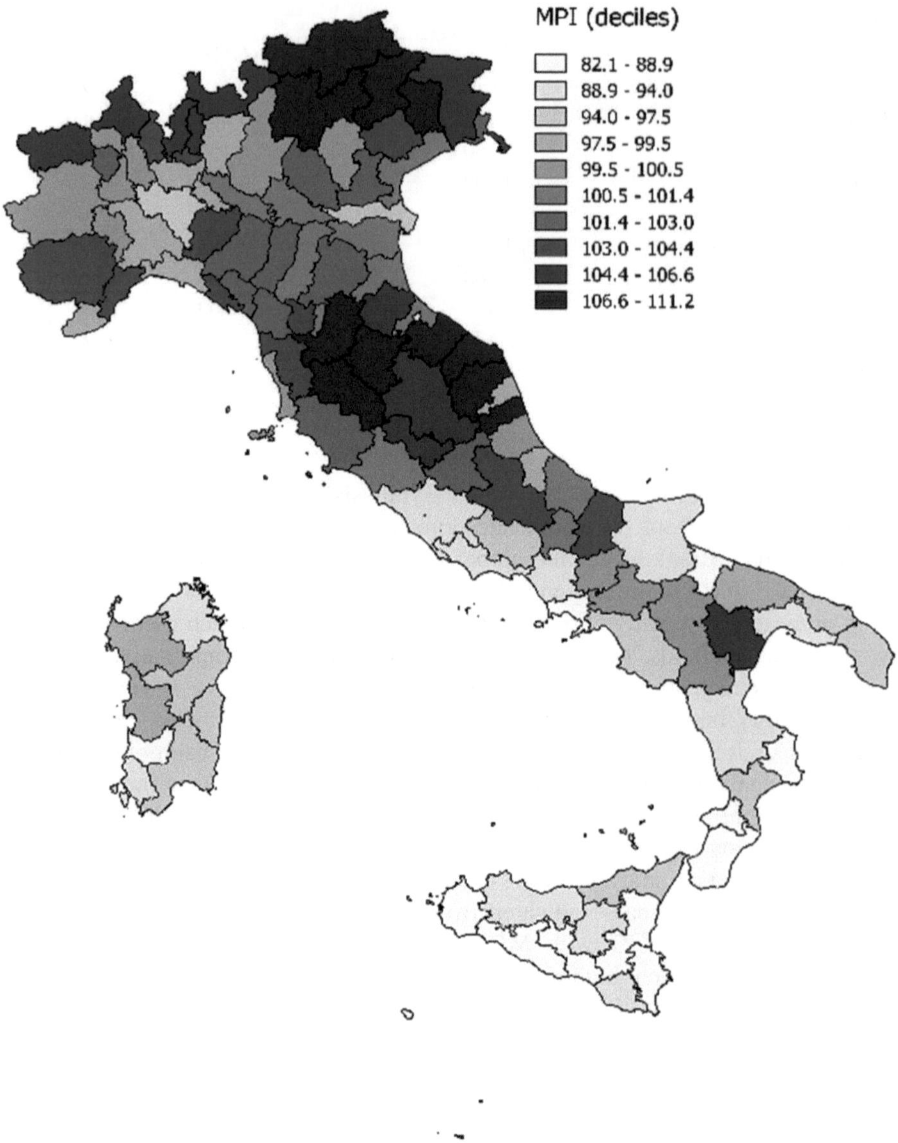

Fig. 1 Global wellbeing indicator – MPI

the Po Valley and the Tyrrhenian Sea display lower values. The GMI generated map does not highlight substantial discrepancies.

The examination of single domains allows for in-depth analysis of the predominant elements that feature and influence the global well-being level.

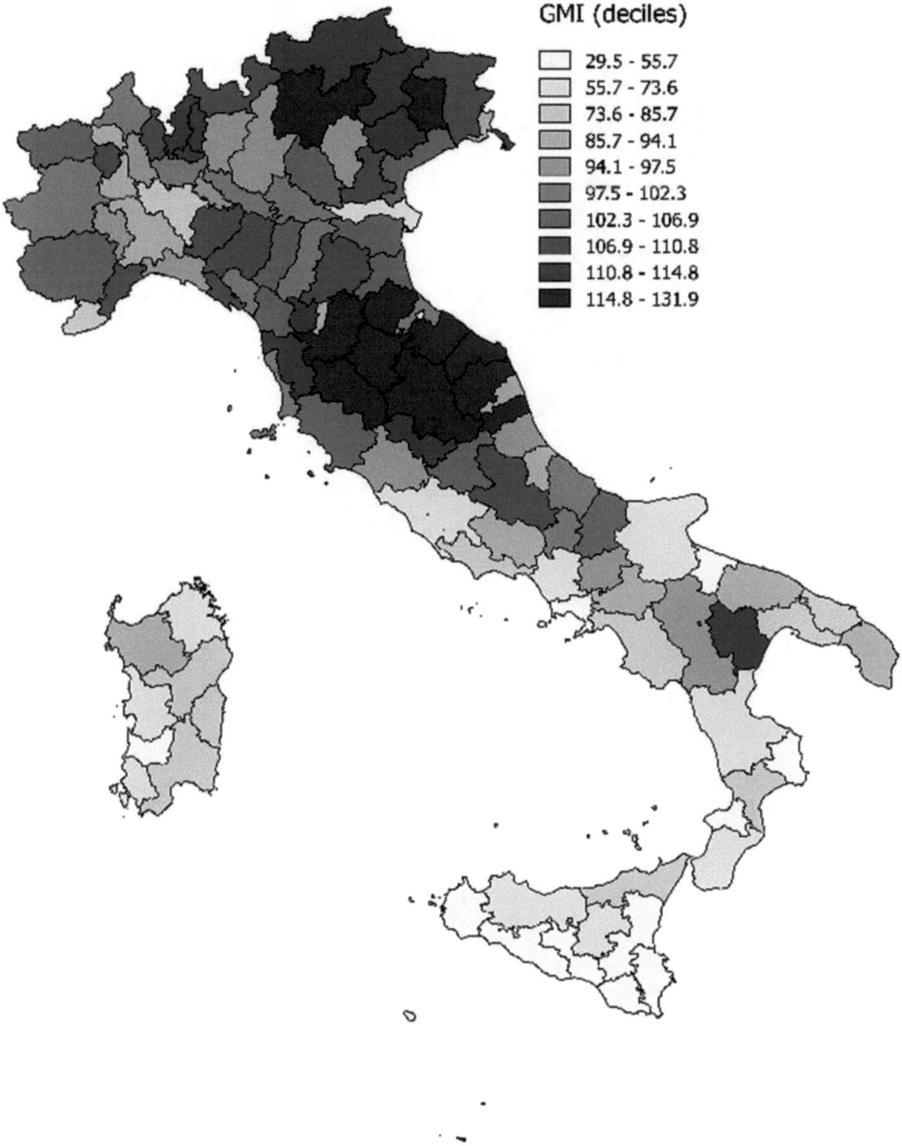

Fig. 2 Global wellbeing indicator – GMI

In Figs. 3 and 4, we mapped the composite indicators for Health and Education. In the first map, mortality and life expectancy play a crucial role in the creation of the ranking. At the provincial level, the outcome is more homogeneous overall compared to the global indicator. Provinces with the highest values are located in

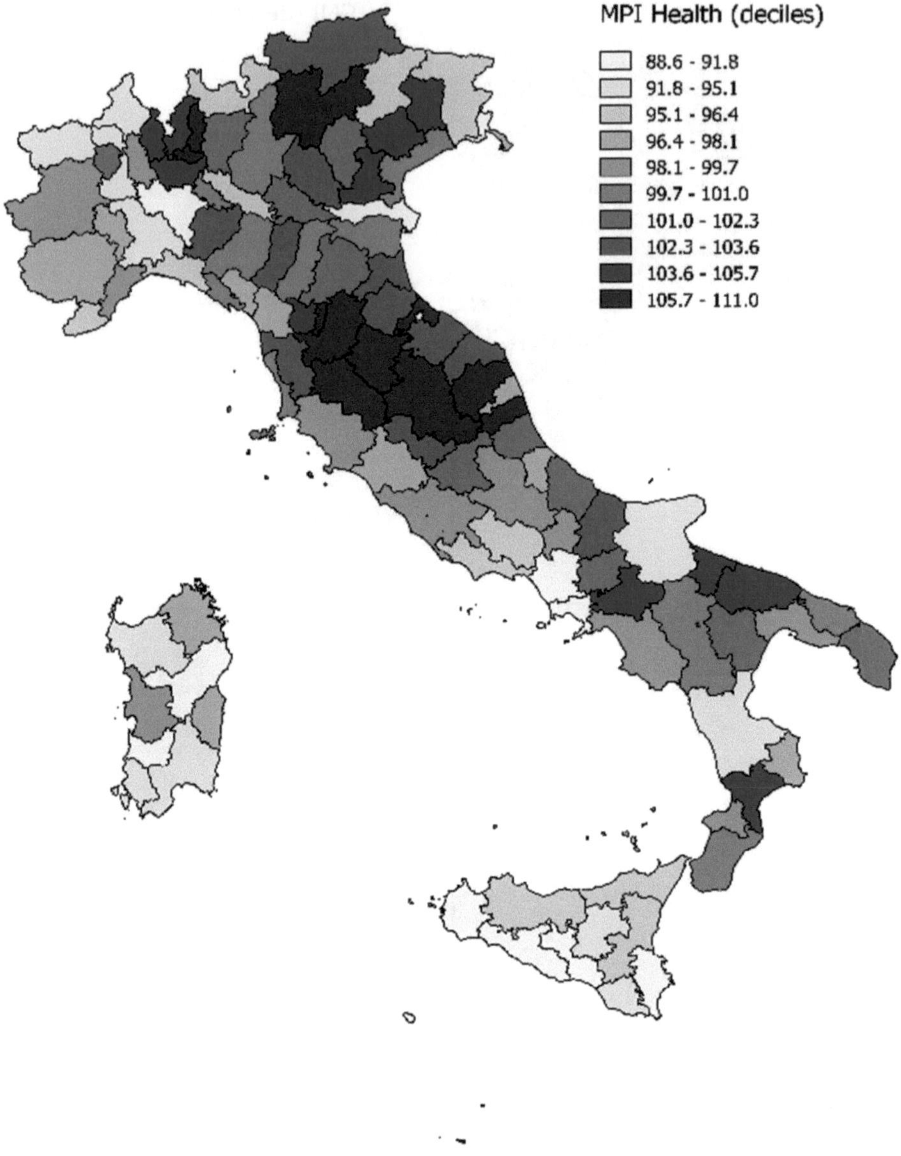

Fig. 3 Health indicator – MPI

Tuscany (Siena, Arezzo, Florence). Naples sits at the bottom of the ranking, with the lowest life expectancy for both men and women.

As far as Education is concerned, the Island Regions (Sardinia and Sicily), Apulia and Calabria report the lowest values, while the Adriatic and Tyrrhenian coastline provinces ranked high. The Tuscany and Marche Provinces, compared to other

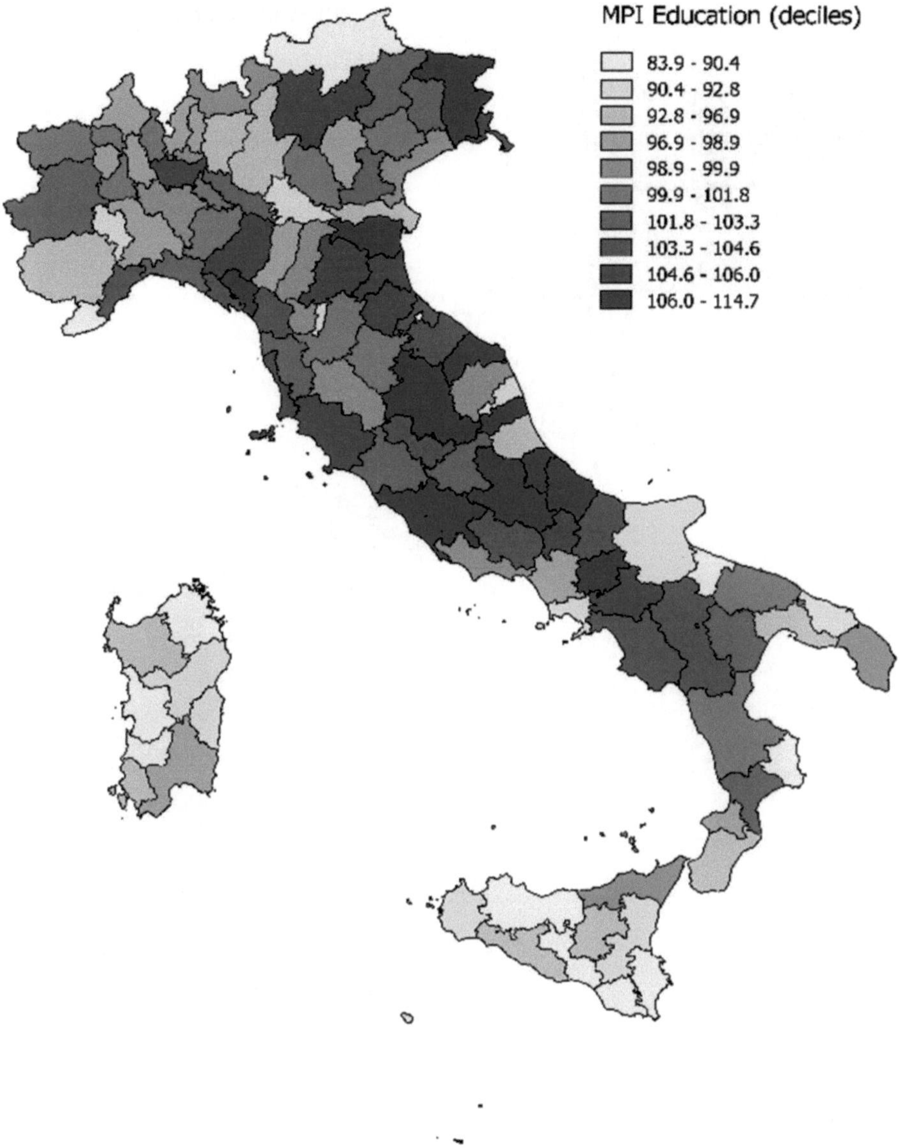

Fig. 4 Education indicator – MPI

domains, scored lower in Education. We note that the Autonomous Province of Bolzano is located in the first decile, because it was negatively affected by the very low values of indicators regarding participation in secondary and tertiary education.

Figures 5 and 6 report the maps that concern the main economic aspects of well-being. Here once again the discrepancy between the South, the Islands and part

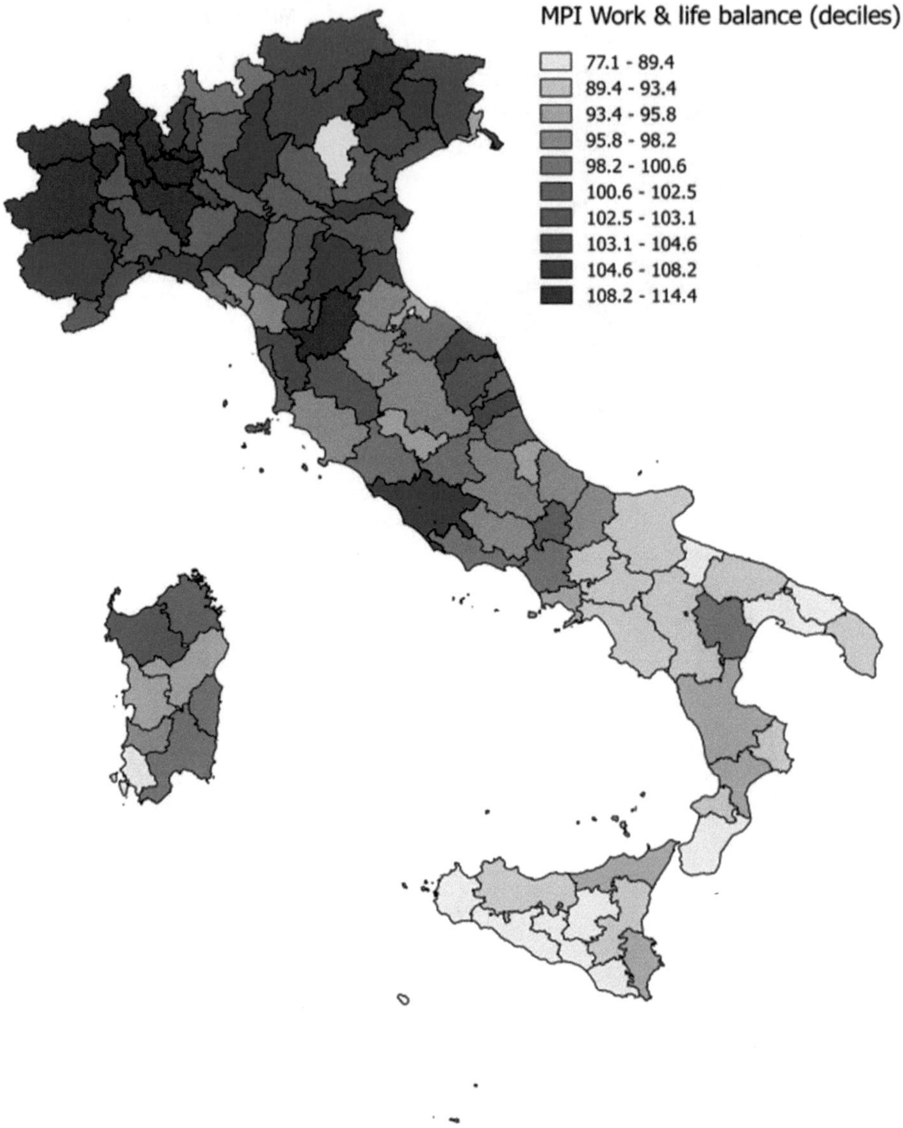

Fig. 5 Work & life balance indicator – MPI

of Central Italy compared to the rest of the Country is clearly visible. This bears witness to a net fracture between Provinces: almost all the Center-North Provinces have values of the composite indicator in the Work indicator that exceed median value, whilst the Southern Provinces are much lower. Provinces with the highest values in this indicator are in Piedmont and Lombardy (Biella, Milan, Monza and

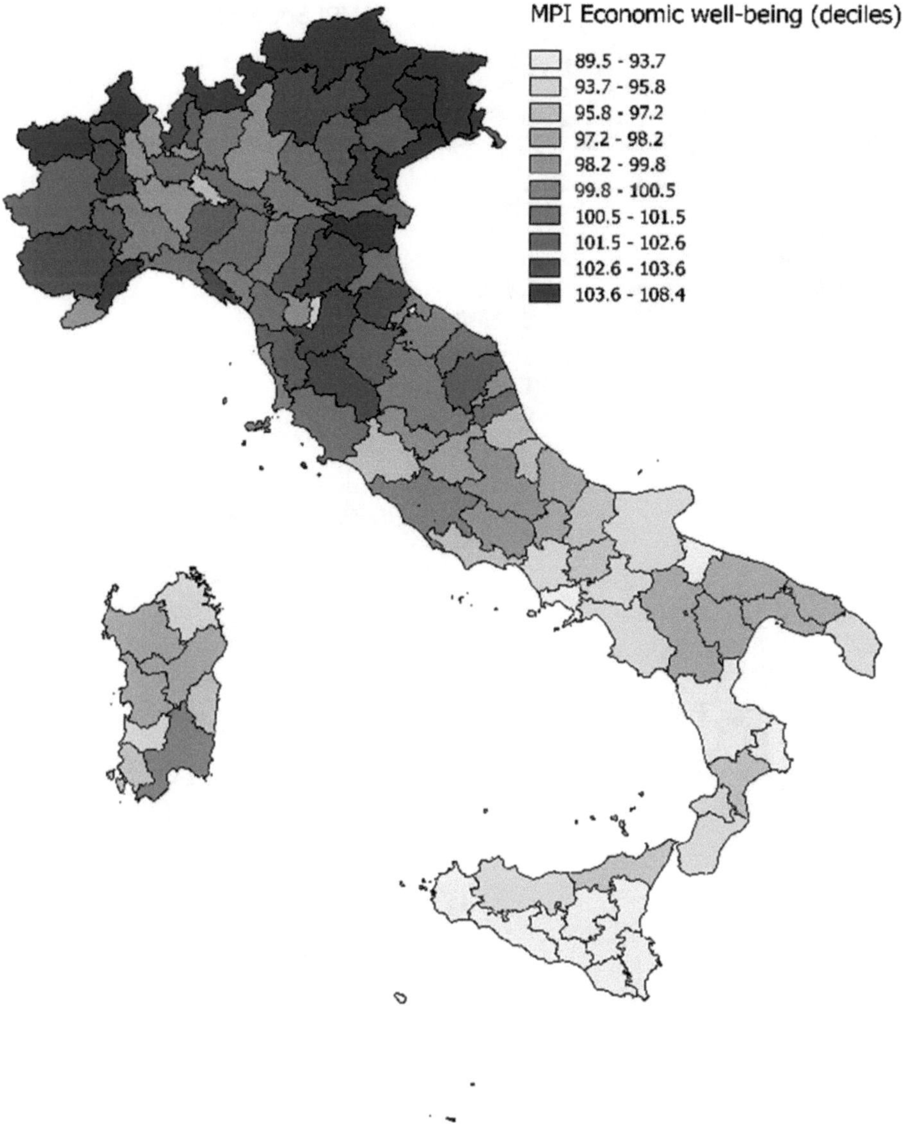

Fig. 6 Economic well-being indicator – MPI

Brianza), while the lowest ones are located in Sicily and Apulia. Finally, Vicenza ranks in the first decile due to the highest level of work-related accidents.

Regarding Economic Well-being (Fig. 6), the North-South dichotomy is even more apparent, clearly showing the economic distress of the South of the Country. It should be noted that, in the North, the lowest values are located in the traditionally

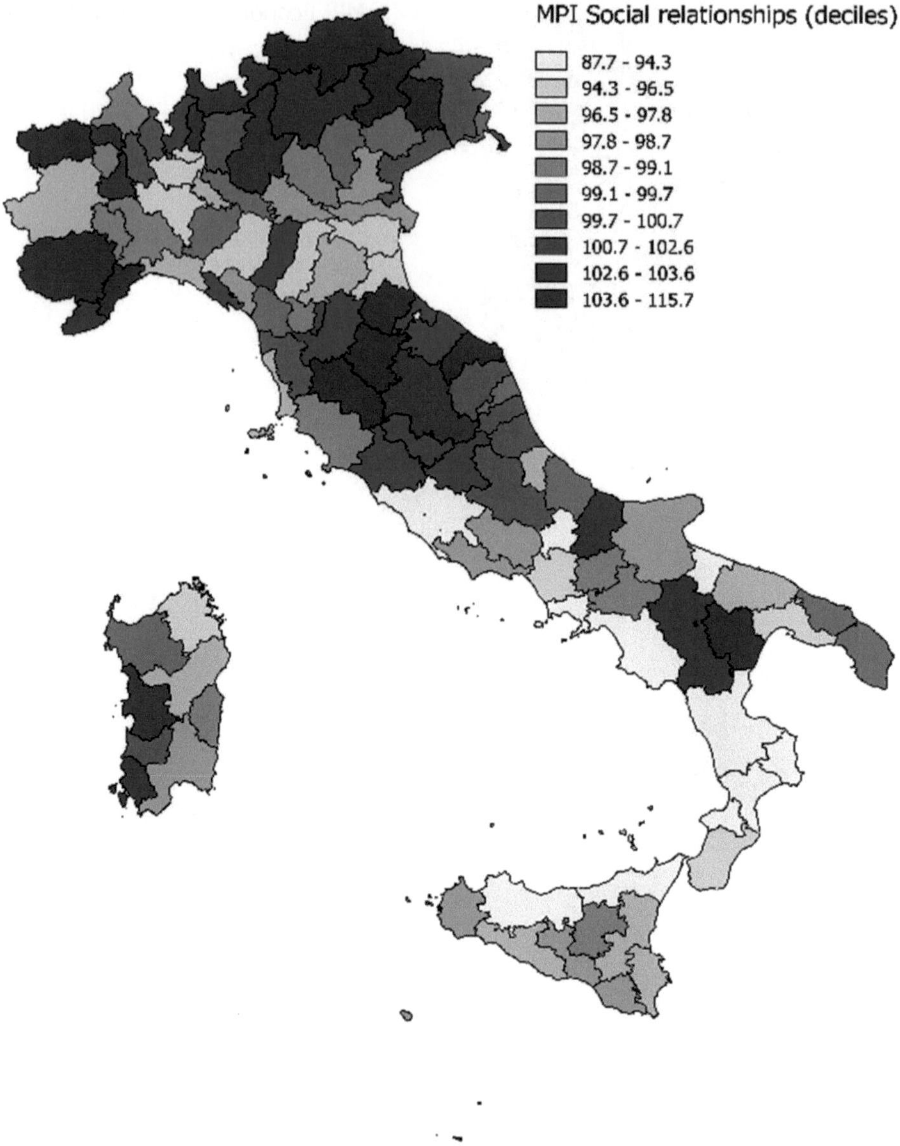

Fig. 7 Social relationship indicator – MPI

very productive Po Valley. Here we can assume that perhaps the economic crisis struck the well-being levels the hardest.

The Social relationship indicators (Fig. 7) present elevated values in the Alpine area, Central Italy and the Provinces on the Adriatic Coast. As with previous domains, the Po Valley area is overall lower compared to the nearby area.

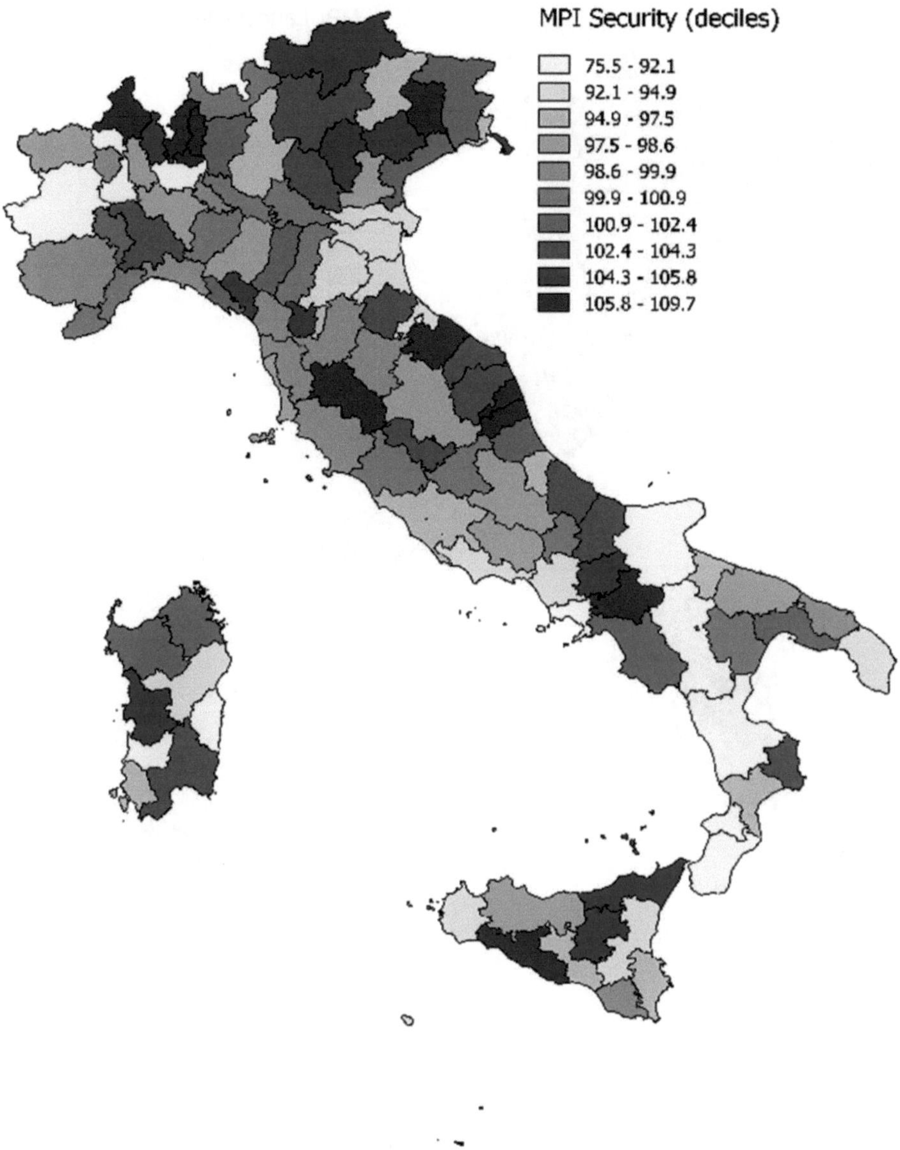

Fig. 8 Security indicator – MPI

Regarding the composite indicator of the Security domain (Fig. 8), the most secure regions are scattered across the map. Generically, the least densely populated areas rank the highest. Specifically, for both maps in Figs. 7 and 8, we can observe that all Metropolitan Cities ranked poorly, proving that the social distress in these areas makes relations difficult and worsens the security level.

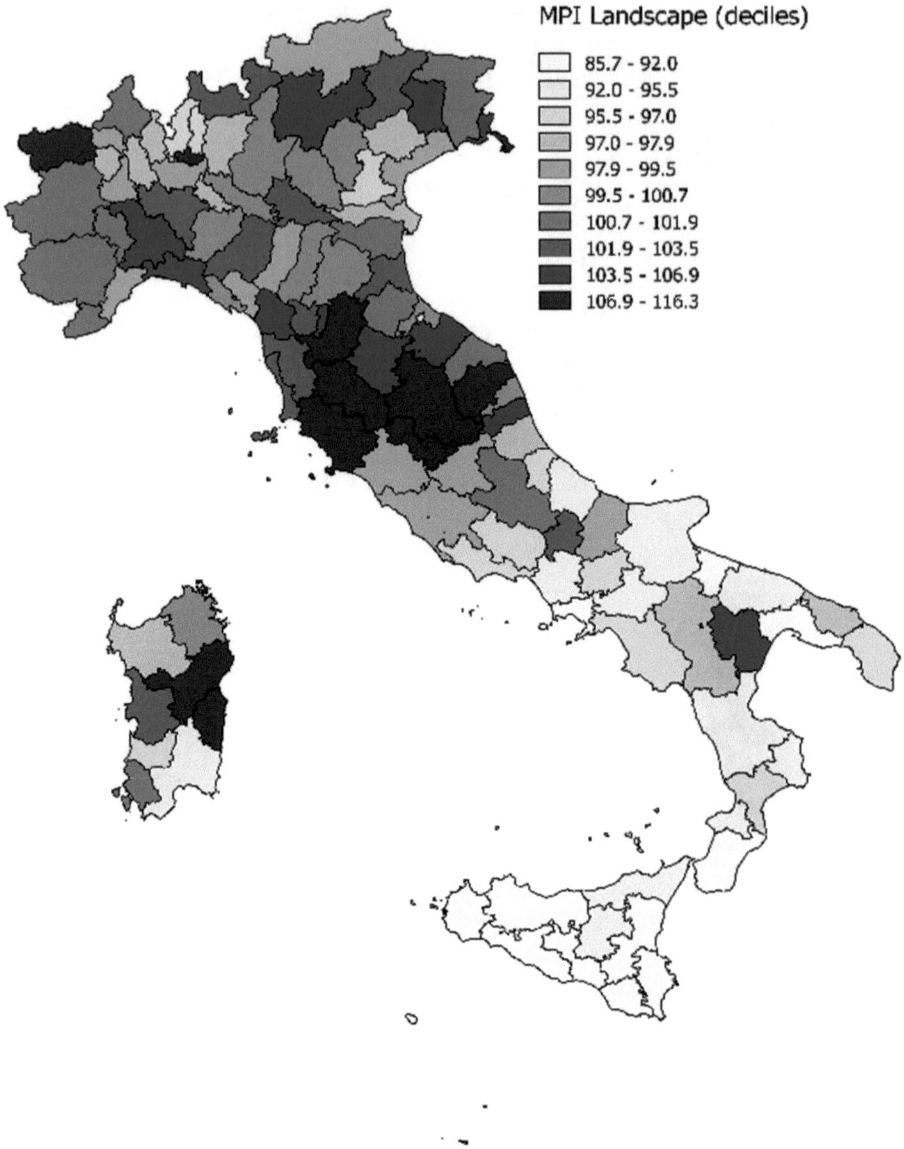

Fig. 9 Landscape and cultural heritage indicator – MPI

Once again, in the Landscape and Cultural Heritage domain the South is set apart from the rest of the Country. Provinces of Central Italy reported the highest levels, with a higher number of museums and larger historical gardens and parks (Fig. 9).

The analysis of the Environment domain indicators (Fig. 10) reports large discrepancies between the areas of the Country as well as among the factors that

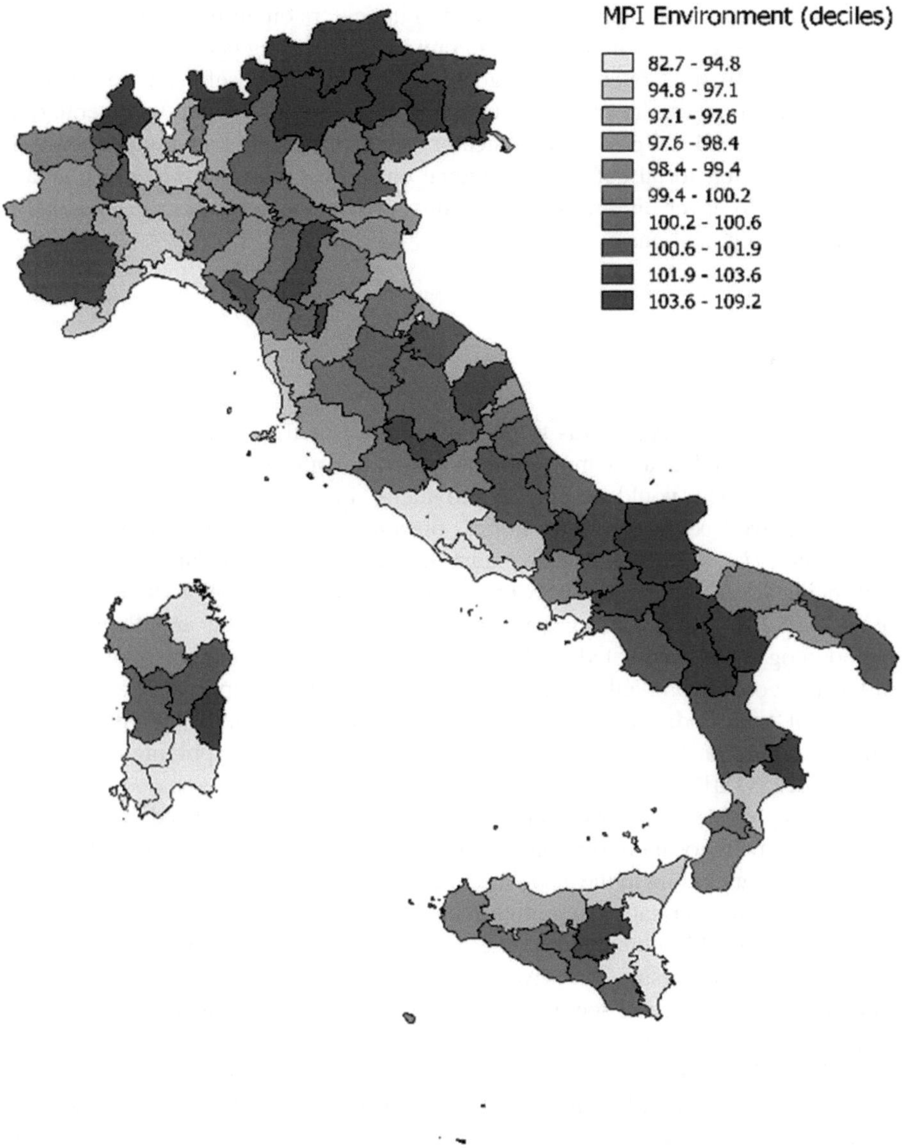

Fig. 10 Environment indicator – MPI

influence the complex theme of Environment. The map of the composite indicator ranks the Alpine Provinces the highest, with very high results specifically as far as availability of city parks and non-exceedance of air pollution levels are concerned. Provinces of the Po Valley, Tyrrhenian Coast, North East Sicily and South Sardinia all sit at the bottom of the list, mainly due to indicators on air pollution, percentage of waste that is disposed in landfills and presence of cycling paths.

Although this was not among the goals of the paper, it is useful, anyhow, with all due caution, compare the provincial results with the regional ones. In general, only for possible domains,[7] provincial indicators are less variable than regional ones. In fact, for their territorial detail, the regional ones must take into account a greater variability. Moreover, in almost all domains, provincial indicators are included in the range of regional ones.

Conclusions

The purpose of this paper was to present a robust methodology for measurement well-being, intended as a multi-dimensional phenomenon, in Italian Provinces. This methodology would be able to provide a simple and immediate reading of the overall well-being of the territories, preventing loss of information on single phenomena (*i.e.* on a single elementary indicator) that contribute to the overall well-being level. Taking the previously mentioned ISTAT "BES delle Province" project of 2014 as a starting point and following Mazziotta and Pareto (MPI) methodology, we calculated eight composite domain indicators (one for each pillar that constitutes well-being, consistently with ISTAT approach) as well as a provincial "superindicator" of well-being. The latter was obtained by replicating the MPI procedure on domain indicators and, as comparison, by applying a geometric mean index (GMI).

Results provide ample inspiration for analysis. As it was expected, if we include additional layers to the traditional categories associated with well-being (revenue, work etc.) by including in the analysis indicators regarding the health of individuals, environment, social relationships and so on, the outlook of Italy is much more varied and less predictable compared to the traditional North-South dichotomy. It may or may not be surprising that several Center-North Provinces (Tuscany, Umbria, Marche) rank high in well-being, along with the Alpine area and even some South areas, even higher than the traditionally "rich" areas of the Country (such as the Po Valley). Other dichotomies are also relevant, such as the discrepancy between the mountain and plain Provinces or between Metropolitan Cities (where security, environment and social relationships – among the others – all rank as critical aspects) and smaller sized Provinces.

The MPI methodology provides encouraging performances in terms of robustness, varying results by relatively not much if single indicators are removed, which is made even more evident during the calculation of the comparison "superindicator" with the alternative GMI method.

[7]The domains are Economic well-being, Education, Environment, Health, Social relationship and Work. The regional data used are the AMPI 2014 indicators, the same year of the data of the paper.

Analyses like this may be a very valuable tool in pinpointing the distinctive elements of the well-being fabric between territories, in order to implement actions that aim at promoting well-being and overcoming differences.

Appendix

Table 3 Indicators used for the constitution of the composite indicator by domain (number of indicator within its domain, polarity, minimum and maximum value)

N.	Indicator	Polarity	Minimum value	Maximum value
Health (themes: life expectancy, mortality)				
I.1	Life expectancy at birth (M)	+	77.5	81.0
I.2	Life expectancy at birth (F)	+	82.3	85.9
I.3	Infant mortality rate	−	0.6	6.9
I.4	Traffic accidents (15–34 years old)	−	0.0	3.2
I.5	Cancer mortality rate (20–64 years old)	−	7.1	11.9
I.6	Cancer mortality rate (65 and older)	−	17.8	36.4
I.7	Suicide mortality rate	−	0.1	1.5
I.8	Preventable mortality	−	3.9	7.6
Education and training (themes: school attendance, education level, competences, lifelong learning)				
II.1	Early leavers from education and training	−	4.1	33.4
II.2	Working age people with lower rates of education	−	27.9	57.4
II.3	Attendance secondary education	+	73.9	118.5
II.4	Attendance tertiary education (19–25 years old)	+	14.1	64.4
II.6_5	Level of student proficiency	+	166.5	222
II.8	Working age people in life-long education	+	3.2	10.9
Work and life balance (themes: participation, commitment, security)				
III.2bis	Gender differences in non-participation rates |F-M|	−	1.0	24.6
III.3	Employment rate (20–64 years old)	+	38.5	76.6
III.4bis	Gender differences in employment rates |F-M|	−	9.9	32.6
III.8	Rate of occupational injuries	−	13.7	52.3
III.9	Rate of dire occupational injuries	−	0.7	4.6
Economic well-being (themes: revenue, richness, inequalities, economic struggle)				
IV.1	Per household gross disposable income	+	26,222.6	56,588.7
IV.2	Average yearly revenue for employees	+	11,923.9	28,818.3

(continued)

Table 3 (continued)

N.	Indicator	Polarity	Minimum value	Maximum value
IV.4	Yearly annual pension amount	+	12,510.6	20,306.6
IV.5	Retired people with lower pensions	–	6.2	19.7
IV.6	Average household capital	+	188.2	522.5
IV.7bis	Gender differences in average revenue from employment |F-M|	–	3439.8	10,716.8
IV.8	Age differences in average revenue from employment	–	4185	14,197.8
IV.9	Issued eviction notices	–	0.0	7.3
IV.10	Rate of non-performance in household loan	–	0.5	2.3
Social relationships (themes: disability, civil society)				
V.1	Schools without architectural barriers (internal and external)	+	16.2	63.1
V.2	Schools without internal architectural barriers	+	0.9	14.3
V.3	Schools without external architectural barriers	+	0.0	11.1
V.6	Social cooperatives presence	+	0.9	5.0
V.7	Non-profit organizations presence	+	18.2	104.0
V.8	Number of volunteers older than 14 per 100 people	+	3.0	41.0
Security (themes: criminality and physical integrity)				
VII.1	Homicide rates	–	0.0	7.4
VII.2	Reported crimes	–	59.8	848.2
VII.3	Reported violent crimes	–	3.0	41.1
VII.5	Deaths per 100 vehicular accidents	–	0.5	7.6
VII.6	Deaths per 100 vehicular accidents on country streets (excluding highway)	–	0.0	11.5
Landscape and cultural heritage (themes: heritage)				
VIII.1	Existence of well-preserved historic urban areas	+	35.7	79.1
VIII.2	Density of historic gardens and parks of public interest	+	0.0	34.7
VIII.3	Open museums	+	0.1	5.8
Environment (themes: environmental quality, use of resources, environmental sustainability)				
IX.1	Availability of city parks	+	1.8	978.2
IX.3	Exceedance of air pollution levels – PM10 (maximum no.)	–	1.0	123.0
IX.4	Household energy consumption	–	895.7	1604.1
IX.5	Issued drinkable water per day	–	150.3	404.5
IX.6	Cycling pathway density	+	0.0	157.2
IX.7	Energy by renewable sources	+	2.0	574.3
IX.8	Urban waste disposed in landfills	–	0.0	330.6

Table 4 MPI values and its breakdown in mean effects and penalty effects

Rank	Province	MPI	Mean effect	Penalty effect	Rank	Province	MPI	Mean effect	Penalty effect
1	Pordenone	111.19	111.29	0.099	56	Brescia	100.46	100.83	0.375
2	Siena	110.95	111.57	0.618	57	Vicenza	100.37	100.90	0.528
3	Aut. Prov. Trento	110.44	110.57	0.128	58	Benevento	100.37	101.12	0.754
4	Aut. Prov. Bolzano /Bozen	108.69	110.88	2.196	59	Leghorn	100.31	100.61	0.303
5	Ascoli Piceno	108.53	108.87	0.344	60	Asti	100.24	100.66	0.422
6	Florence	108.15	108.66	0.509	61	Turin	100.09	100.92	0.830
7	Macerata	107.23	107.40	0.173	62	Avellino	99.81	100.90	1.090
8	Ancona	107.04	107.46	0.420	63	Teramo	99.74	99.96	0.222
9	Belluno	107.01	107.71	0.696	64	Novara	99.71	100.07	0.354
10	Pesaro and Urbino	106.61	106.73	0.120	65	Potenza	99.70	100.81	1.107
11	Arezzo	106.60	107.02	0.413	66	Vercelli	99.51	100.35	0.840
12	Perugia	106.57	107.08	0.510	67	Bergamo	99.39	99.63	0.239
13	Forlì-Cesena	106.44	106.80	0.365	68	Genoa	99.34	100.07	0.729
14	Aosta	106.25	107.91	1.665	69	Fermo	99.22	99.68	0.452
15	Matera	106.13	106.56	0.431	70	Alessandria	99.19	99.63	0.447
16	Trieste	105.55	106.06	0.512	71	Milan	99.02	100.55	1.533
17	Terni	105.53	105.84	0.309	72	Lodi	98.61	98.79	0.180
18	Lecco	105.37	105.95	0.584	73	Sassari	98.12	98.29	0.171
19	Udine	105.13	105.50	0.370	74	Imperia	98.10	98.71	0.607
20	Verbano-Cusio-Ossola	104.90	106.25	1.350	75	Pescara	97.83	98.52	0.687
21	Sondrio	104.70	105.31	0.607	76	Bari	97.67	98.18	0.507
22	Como	104.48	105.08	0.598	77	Oristano	97.61	98.83	1.219
23	Monza and Brianza	104.44	105.73	1.299	78	Pavia	97.41	98.30	0.890
24	Pistoia	104.23	104.37	0.138	79	Frosinone	96.96	97.14	0.186
25	Treviso	104.15	104.38	0.226	80	Ogliastra	96.69	98.22	1.527
26	La Spezia	104.14	104.30	0.160	81	Lecce	96.46	96.84	0.379
27	Cuneo	103.88	104.44	0.559	82	Nuoro	95.86	97.29	1.437
28	Varese	103.84	104.27	0.434	83	Salerno	95.67	96.40	0.727
29	Pisa	103.82	103.99	0.171	84	Brindisi	95.61	96.13	0.521
30	Savona	103.53	103.93	0.403	85	Cagliari	95.18	95.83	0.644
31	Campobasso	103.38	103.72	0.333	86	Rovigo	95.14	95.80	0.663
32	Piacenza	103.30	103.40	0.103	87	Catanzaro	94.52	95.14	0.617
33	L'Aquila	103.10	103.77	0.672	88	Messina	94.20	94.76	0.567

(continued)

Table 4 (continued)

Rank	Province	MPI	Mean effect	Penalty effect	Rank	Province	MPI	Mean effect	Penalty effect
34	Biella	102.96	103.56	0.599	89	Enna	93.34	94.28	0.940
35	Bologna	102.55	103.10	0.557	90	Olbia-Tempio	93.24	93.89	0.649
36	Grosseto	102.50	102.91	0.415	91	Taranto	92.84	93.32	0.473
37	Padua	102.43	102.70	0.274	92	Latina	92.83	93.37	0.535
38	Reggio Emilia	102.14	102.27	0.132	93	Rome	92.22	95.33	3.114
39	Verona	102.13	102.20	0.075	94	Carbonia-Iglesias	92.15	93.04	0.894
40	Parma	102.07	102.39	0.319	95	Caserta	91.07	91.38	0.305
41	Massa-Carrara	101.92	102.30	0.378	96	Foggia	90.95	92.05	1.099
42	Lucca	101.68	102.00	0.319	97	Cosenza	90.76	91.52	0.768
43	Gorizia	101.61	102.60	0.986	98	Palermo	88.92	89.25	0.337
44	Rieti	101.60	101.70	0.098	99	Ragusa	88.89	89.71	0.819
45	Venice	101.30	101.88	0.586	100	Crotone	88.89	90.87	1.986
46	Ferrara	101.24	101.94	0.699	101	Reggio Calabria	88.60	89.45	0.850
47	Modena	101.21	101.48	0.270	102	Medio Campidano	88.15	88.85	0.704
48	Chieti	101.18	101.56	0.376	103	Agrigento	88.05	90.24	2.194
49	Ravenna	101.02	101.52	0.501	104	Barletta-Andria-Trani	87.35	88.47	1.120
50	Cremona	100.72	100.86	0.139	105	Trapani	87.30	87.82	0.522
51	Mantua	100.69	100.96	0.274	106	Caltanissetta	87.23	88.03	0.800
52	Isernia	100.66	101.26	0.601	107	Syracuse	86.49	86.90	0.409
53	Prato	100.65	101.64	0.988	108	Vibo Valentia	86.15	87.93	1.782
54	Viterbo	100.51	100.64	0.126	109	Catania	86.10	86.39	0.292
55	Rimini	100.50	101.17	0.669	110	Naples	82.13	82.61	0.483
	ITALY	100.42	100.47	0.043					

References

De Muro P, Mazziotta M, Pareto A (2011) Composite Indices of Development and Poverty: An Application to MDGs. Social Indicator Research 104: 1–18

Diamantopoulos A, Winklhofer HM (2001) Index Construction with Formative Indicators: An Alternative to Scale Development. Journal of Marketing Research 38(2): 269–277

Giovannini E, Morrone A, Rondinella T, Sabbadini LL (2012) L'iniziativa Cnel-Istat per la misurazione del Benessere equo e sostenibile in Italia. Autonomie locali e servizi sociali 1/2012: 125–136

ISTAT (2015) Bes 2015. Il Benessere equo e sostenibile in Italia. http://www.istat.it/it/files/2015/12/Rapporto_BES_2015.pdf. Accessed 05 Jun 2018

ISTAT and CUSPI (2015) Il Benessere equo e sostenibile delle province. http://www.besdelleprovince.it/fileadmin/grpmnt/1225/pubblicazione_nazionale.pdf. Accessed 05 Jun 2018

Mazziotta M, Pareto A (2015) On a Generalized Non-compensatory Composite Index for Measuring Socio-economic Phenomena. Social Indicator Research. doi: https://doi.org/10.1007/s11205-015-0998-2

OECD (2008) Handbook on Constructing Composite Indicators. Methodology and User Guide, OECD Publications, Paris

Stiglitz J, Sen A, Fitoussi J (2009) Report by the Commission on the Measurement of Economic Performance and Social Progress, https://www.insee.fr/en/information/2662494. Accessed 05 Jun 2018

Taralli S (2013) Indicatori del Benessere Equo e Sostenibile delle Province: informazioni statistiche a supporto del policy-cycle e della valutazione a livello locale. Rassegna Italiana di valutazione XVI(55)

Corruption Indicators and Prevention Policies

Enrico Carloni

Abstract In the panorama of Italian corruption prevention policies, the importance of relying on corruption indicators is central, in particular for the development of prevention plans, introduced by the Italian law, by each authority. The central issue is not as much quantifying the amount of corruption, as understanding where it comes from, and under what conditions it is possible to turn on an alert. In this context, there is a need to rely not only on robust indicators of "corruption", but also on indicators capable of "alerting" the system in the presence of risk factors. This is a field in which Italy is developing a leading experience since the development of "abnormal indicators" by the National Anti-Corruption Authorities (ANAC) in the field of public contracts. "Contrast" indicators developed by ANAC are a further new group of interesting indicators aimed at assessing the effectiveness of prevention policies with respect to controlling corruption.

Administrative Corruption and Corruption Indicators

The necessity to "measure corruption" in the Italian system has become a matter of great interest in recent years. This requirement is associated with widespread dissatisfaction in the public debate with the most frequently referenced indicators (Galli 2015) and the consequent "impressionistic" reading of the phenomenon. In particular, this need is increasingly pressing at the institutional level. The issue is tied to the specific functions entrusted to The National Anti-Corruption Authority (ANAC), which pursuant to Article 1, paragraph 1, letter c of the law no. 190/2012 "analyses the causes and factors of corruption and identifies responses that can favour prevention and enforcement". According to another important provision, the corruption prevention plan "provides an assessment of the different levels of

E. Carloni (✉)
Department of Political Science, University of Perugia, Perugia, Italy
e-mail: enrico.carloni@unipg.it

A. Bianco et al. (eds.), *Italian Studies on Quality of Life*, Social Indicators Research Series 77, https://doi.org/10.1007/978-3-030-06022-0_5

exposure public offices have to the risk of corruption", and consequently, "indicates organizational measures aimed at preventing this risk".

In the shift from an essentially repressive enforcement approach to a broader, preventative approach, in which good conduct and social practices are emphasized (without necessarily corresponding with specific offenses against the public administration), the issue of the definition and demarcation of the phenomenon takes on greater significance: it is no longer just a question of understanding the dynamics of corruption, beyond the central core of criminally relevant conduct, but rather to frame those behaviours that, while not necessarily relevant for the purposes of criminal law, need to be addressed in terms of the prevention and combatting of corruption, and thus, in some way, "measured" for this purpose.

A corresponding approach can be found in recent national policies to prevent and combat corruption. This process began with law no. 190 of 2012, which introduced a new conception of administrative corruption (Clarich and Mattarella 2013). This includes (but is not limited to) criminally liable conduct, so as to "include not only the full range of crimes against the public administration regulated by Title II, Chapter I of the criminal code, but also situations in which – regardless of criminal relevance – a malfunction in the administration emerges, due to the use of assigned functions for private ends, namely the pollution of administrative action *ab externo*, whether the action proves successful or remains at the level of an attempt" (ANAC 2013b).

This approach is therefore broadly "comprehensive of the various situations in which, in the course of administrative activity, there is evidence of the abuse by an individual of the power entrusted to him, in order to obtain private benefits" (Comitato interministeriale 2013; GRECO 2008). This results in a broad concept of corruption (ANAC 2015b), which essentially emerges as a consequence of a shift of emphasis from "enforcement" (of actions that constitute a crime) to "prevention" (Cantone and Carloni 2017). This entails the need to anticipate enforcement measures, and embrace a broader group of phenomena that can determine the emergence of episodes of corruption.

The theme of the "measurement of corruption" is closely linked to the Italian corruption prevention system, and constitutes something of a necessary prerequisite for a system that aims to develop "targeted" solutions to counter the phenomenon in its effective consistency (Carloni 2017).

As part of a broad interpretation of the phenomenon, and an equally extensive and pervasive strategy to prevent and combat corruption, which is designed to be as "systemic" as the phenomenon it is intended to combat (Corte dei Conti 2009), administrations are called upon to develop their own anti-corruption policy, according to the guidelines defined by legislation and the National Anti-Corruption Authority, following the National Plan. It is important that individual administrations are not left to proceed "in the dark" when preparing a prevention plan, hence the necessity to provide indicators that can guide leaders and managers in the preparation of appropriate measures for the context, both inside and outside the administration.

A prevention strategy that is based on an approach that involves the assessment of the risk of corruption, and the preparation of appropriate measures to contain it, requires not only access to a specific set of skills, but also "instruments" that can serve as a guide when estimating the level of risk: the issue of the measurement of corruption thus becomes a requirement that affects the entire anti-corruption system, not only the "centre" that is called upon to develop the fundamental strategies.

In this light, it is clear how the inadequacy of the prevalently used corruption indicators also results from their failure to act as a benchmark for decentralized strategies. This is particularly true in the Italian context, which is characterized by extraordinary regional variability, in terms of the quality of administration, and requires more data and calibrated and adaptable indicators for specific local contexts and the various sectors of public intervention.

While it is important for a region (and a country) to have a clearer and fairer perception of the level of corruption, as is the case for citizens and stakeholders (starting from investors), the measurement of the "stock of corruption" does not necessarily constitute the most significant problem, or at least the most useful aspect, in the development of a strategy to prevent and combat corruption.

Indicators of Abnormality and Risk

A slightly different approach, which is certainly relevant from the perspective of law enforcement policies, is associated with access to useful indicators that can highlight a specific "risk" of corruption, known as *alarm bells* or *red-flags*: such indicators are capable of "alerting" the system in the presence of abnormalities that may signal a risk of corruption.

As the National Anti-Corruption Authority has stated, with regard to the debate on corruption indicators, "it is not as important to measure corruption, as much as to understand where it emerges from, and to issue an alert when such conditions arise, a warning light that can help prevention" (ANAC Advisory Board 2017).

This is not the only context in which there is a need to develop abnormality or anomaly indicators, however. Similar measures are required in the anti-money laundering field (Banca d'Italia 2013) and anti-terrorism, and the related rules that apply to the public administration. This model, which could potentially be closely connected with that of anti-corruption (such as the anomaly measures issued by the Ministry of the Interior, with the decree of September 25, 2015) is interesting for both the wealth of anomaly indicators employed, and the distinction made between the types of indicators: those regarding anomalies relating to objective and subjective aspects, involving those who perform the operation. In any case, these are indicators that work as "alarm bells", and as such are addressed to the administration, which should not issue an alert in the event of the mere presence of one or more indicators, but rather take action should such eventualities arise for a specific evaluation.

The National Anti-Corruption Authority has not only analyzed this outlook, but has also developed it, above all in the field of public contracts. Numerous abnormality indicators have been established, which are not necessarily symptomatic of maladministration, but operate by highlighting elements that deserve to be brought to the attention of those subjects deputised to perform control functions, and above all the administrations themselves (ANAC 2017).

This approach can also be found in European Commission documentation. A number of suitable corruption indicators were proposed in a 2013 study, as part of a survey conducted in eight countries, including Italy, and five areas of public intervention (ANAC 2017). Also at the European level, the need to develop indicators for the fight against illicit conduct has been developed in the context of anti-fraud policies, firstly with the definition of a series of indices regarding risk factors to be taken into consideration, and then with the development of *alert* indicators, to be produced automatically from the data available in administrative databases for the purposes of both self-assessment and supervision by European institutions (ANAC 2017).

The fundamental idea is that the use of an array of abnormality indicators, if calibrated for a geographical context, can allow the level of risk to be represented in effective terms. This is made possible by concentrating on a specific territorial area, in particular if this set of indicators is in turn supported by other objective or perceptive elements and indicators.

Evidently the opportunity to process such indicators depends on access to data, and therefore the availability of databases containing useful information, also pertaining to different action and organization profiles, among which it is possible to identify a correspondence.

In particular, the public contracts database has the greatest and most direct potential for use and development for these purposes. This is not only true in the Italian context, as equally significant databases exist on the use of the European Cohesion Fund: significant abnormalities, especially if cross-referenced with other significant aspects that can confirm specific risk conditions, can act as useful *red-flags* for prevention policies.

An early experience, in the field of public contracts, took place in the field of the regulation of the traceability of financial flows for the purpose of combating mafia infiltration in public tenders (law no. 136 of 13 August 2010): in this context indicators of anomalies and distortion of competition have been developed, as a result of which initiatives to prevent and combat corruption have been presented (Racca 2013).

Some examples which involve the indicators developed by ANAC in the field of public contracts include: the use of closed procedures (negotiated procedures, direct assignments, fiduciary piecework) with reference to the total number of procedures used by the same contracting authority, calculated in terms of both the number of procedures and the amount involved, the use of fractionation strategies, or the number of contracts awarded and modified as a result of variants (ANAC 2013a). Each of these indices can result from elements that depend on factors from different contexts, or from statistically less probable, but absolutely natural events: therefore, this is not simply a matter of corruption indicators, and furthermore, not necessarily of indicators which show a higher risk of corruption, as long as adequate grounds are found to justify the "abnormalities".

However, the National Anti-Corruption Authority interprets some "abnormalities" as manifestations of a possible risk of corruption, and therefore interprets certain abnormality indicators as risk indicators, with regard to "significant anomalies". According to the national anti-corruption plan (ANAC 2015a), "delay or failure to approve planning instruments, the excessive use of emergency procedures or contract extensions, the recurrence of small assignments with the same object, or the reiteration of the insertion of specific interventions in planning actions, which do not lead to the phase of awarding and the execution of tenders awarded with frequency to the same subjects, or tenders with a single valid offer, are all elements that reveal a lack of planning and, in the final analysis, signs of a distorted or improper use of discretionary powers".

It is true, however, that certain studies demonstrate how "abnormalities" often correlate with a high level of "perceived" corruption, or "objective" corruption indexes, often as an indicator of criminal activity or other evidence of corruption (such as the shutting down of municipalities as a result of mafia infiltration), corroborating the idea of a correspondence between abnormalities and risk, at least in statistical terms.

In any case, these points illustrate how the most productive approach in operational terms is to establish of indicators, which integrate the different models and make it possible to "clean up" the results, compensating for the limits of each approach and indicator if taken individually. This is a theme that has been central to the most recent studies on corruption, which reflect on the creation of more reliable and robust indicators from different angles and with different scientific and methodological approaches (Sequeira 2012).

In the framework of Italian anti-corruption policies, the theme is closely intertwined with the characteristics of the prevention approach, which is based on national guidelines, but with a centrality of strategies and decentralized solutions, at the level of each administration that characterizes the model (Merloni 2013; Di Cristina 2013; Fabrizio 2015). Therefore, in risk assessment and, in particular, in the process of external and internal risk analysis that has to be developed, the availability of appropriate instruments to "alert" individual administrations and, conversely, to notify the Anti-Corruption Authority about the need to pay particular attention to appropriate prevention measures, takes on a strategic value.

Starting from the ISO risk management regulations, and the "possibility of a corruption event occurring" (ISO 31000, 2010), through the interpretation of this approach in the National Anti-Corruption Plan, the risk assessment process (the identification, analysis and weighting of risk) has involved a delicate and complex transition (GRECO 2011), which has been a decisive precondition for the establishment of prevention measures.

With reference to the data that emerged from the first systematic evaluation, albeit of a sample, of the quality of prevention plans conducted by the National Anti-Corruption Authority (ANAC 2015a), it is clear that the analysis of the (external and internal) context and the process of *risk assessment* (which results, in particular, from the provision of Article 1, paragraph 9, of the law 190/2012, according to which the Anti-Corruption Plan responds, inter alia, to the need to "identify the activities ... in which there is a higher risk of corruption"), which is associated with the effectiveness of *risk management*, are the main problematic areas with a view to developing an adequate prevention system (OECD 2009).

From this point of view, "there emerges a general inadequacy of the risk management process". In particular, "the most critical phase is the analysis of the external context, which is insufficient or inadequate" (ANAC 2015a). In other terms, "the ability of administrations to read and interpret socio-territorial dynamics, and to take them into account in the drafting of the plan proved inadequate" (ANAC 2015a). This conclusion, while inevitably provisional and interim, given the structurally mobile and "work in progress" nature of the plans, confirms the need for indicators capable of guiding administrations in understanding their level of risk.

It is clear that the attention paid to the issue by the Authority, combined with the need to elaborate not only indicators capable of showing existing corruption (albeit at a greater level of territorial or sectorial detail), but also indicators of "risk", serves to develop more targeted strategies of administrative prevention.

Indicators of Administrative Anti-corruption Efforts

A contiguous, yet still diverse theme, regards the indicators of the fight against corruption, which in turn is connected with the utility/need to have access to indicators capable of effectively demonstrating the capacity of institutions to fight the spread of deviant behaviour and corrupt practices. This has traditionally involved the use of data to demonstrate the action of prosecutors and the efforts of the criminal justice system to combat illicit conduct, which is clearly a different matter from the more comprehensive measurement of the status of a territory, or the country as a whole, in terms of real or perceived corruption.

The development of indicators in the field of combatting "administrative" corruption involves a reliance on data held by different administrations, primarily with respect to decisions and proceedings concerning (administrative, financial, and disciplinary) liability for relevant events in the fight against corruption: such data are currently available in a fragmented form, as they are provided, checked and processed with variable methods and systematic approaches (GRECO 2008).

This leads to a question that is central in the detection of the phenomenon of corruption, and, as previously observed, no less important in terms of risk assessment and enforcement activity: the availability of access to databases that are updated with quality information. This clearly no longer applies to the judicial databases alone, and involves the need for integration and communication between the various databases involved in anti-corruption monitoring.

The development of a broader approach, in terms of both the definition of the phenomenon of corruption, and the articulation of the remedies intended to contain it, brings with it the need to develop an extensive capability in the monitoring of anti-corruption activity, in terms of both the effective adoption and implementation of specific measures and instruments (ANAC 2016b), and the effectiveness of these mechanisms. For the purposes of this discussion, this is principally relevant in terms of the verification, on the part of the Anti-Corruption Authority, of the adoption of prevention mechanisms, and therefore the overall quality of prevention plans.

While the risk indicators primarily involve local administrations, the indicators of measures to combat corruption regard the exercise of supervisory and monitoring tasks, and the adaptation and updating of the national plan, which are the responsibility of the Anti-Corruption Authority. However, the question can also be relevant for other subjects: for example, for the same government service, with regard to the evaluation of the activation and effectiveness of measures relating to disciplinary responsibility, or the functionality of the performance cycle.

The question lends itself, evidently, to different levels, to the incisiveness of indicators, and the complexity of data processing: it is one thing, in fact, to develop indicators, even summary indicators, capable of representing the effective adoption and "execution" of preventative measures, for example (with reference to the measures envisaged in the anti-corruption system, and therefore entrusted by legislation and the National Plan to the plans of the individual administrations), drawing on the wealth of information provided annually in reports published by the authorities responsible for prevention (ANAC 2016a). An analysis of these databases could provide a prospective, not dissimilar to the "transparency compass" that was produced in the context of transparency obligations (see www.magellanopa.it/bussola), and therefore generate one or more indicators capable of representing the level of (at least formal) *compliance* (ANAC 2016b) of the individual administrations (Del Sarto and Gnaldi 2018).

This theme is connected, in the system of preventive measures, with the powers of supervision and sanction attributed to the National Anti-Corruption Authority (Article 9 Paragraph 5 of Decree Law no. 90 of June 24, 2014), as stipulated by the same authority within its own guidelines (ANAC regulations of 9 September 2014), and the consequent penalties for "failure to adopt" obligatory plans and measures required by legislation and the National Anti-Corruption Plan. It is worth noting, in this regard, that the following are considered equivalent to omitted adoption: the approval of provisions that merely acknowledge the measures required by law, the approval of measures which "mimic" those of other administrations, and provisions that merely reproduce national indications and forecasts (as in the case of the code of conduct). Essentially, the demonstration of the adoption and activation of preventative measures requires a more sophisticated analysis than the simple verification of the presence, in the administrative plan and the "transparent administration" section of the website, of compulsory measures.

A more complex prospect involves the establishment of suitable indicators to represent the *effectiveness* (or "quality") of enforcement measures, which will involve the cross-referencing of a large amount of data, from different sources:

such as, for example, measures regarding the adoption of differentiated codes of conduct, the effectiveness of which can be evaluated by comparing data regarding the adoption of the measure with data relating to the disciplinary sanctions imposed (all of which can be referenced in the reports of the responsible bodies), obtainable from the Court of Audit, or criminal records, such as indictments for crimes against the public administration.

In conclusion, for the Italian state it appears that the path leading to the preparation of indicators of anti-corruption activity, which could act as a guideline in the evaluation of the effectiveness of preventative measures, remains to be developed (ANAC 2017). This is a particularly significant challenge, as it involves the establishment of an administrative system capable of progressive improvement, in terms of its integrity and capacity to combat corruption, defined by President Mattarella as an "evil that pollutes civil life" (9 December 2015), against which it is important to strengthen the effectiveness of the "antibodies" present in the system.

References

ANAC (2013a). Corruzione sommersa e corruzione emersa in Italia: modalità di misurazione e prime evidenze empiriche. www.anticorruzione.it

ANAC (2013b). Rapporto sul primo anno di attuazione della legge n. 190/2012. www.anticorruzione.it

ANAC (2015a). Rapporto sullo stato di attuazione e la qualità dei piani triennali di prevenzione della corruzione nelle amministrazioni pubbliche 2015–2017. in www.anticorruzione.it;

ANAC (2015b). Aggiornamento 2015 al Piano nazionale anticorruzione, Determinazione n. 12 del 28 ottobre 2015. www.anticorruzione.it

ANAC (2016a). Scheda per la predisposizione, entro il 16 gennaio 2017, della relazione annuale del Responsabile della prevenzione della corruzione. www.anticorruzione.it

ANAC (2016b). Piano triennale di prevenzione della corruzione relativo al triennio 2016–2018. www.anticorruzione.it

ANAC (2017). Analisi istruttoria per l'individuazione di indicatori di rischio corruzione e di prevenzione e contrasto nelle amministrazioni pubbliche coinvolte nella politica di coesione.

ANAC Advisory Board (2017). Lettera dei consiglieri dell'ANAC al quotidiano il Foglio. www.anticorruzione.it.

Banca D'Italia (2013). Indicatori di anomalia per le società di revisione e revisori legali con incarichi di revisione su enti di interesse pubblico, provvedimento del 30 gennaio 2013.

Cantone, R., Carloni, E. (2017). La prevenzione della corruzione e la sua Autorità. *Diritto pubblico*, 3, 903–944.

Carloni, E. (2017). Misurare la corruzione? Indicatori di corruzione e politiche di prevenzione. *Politica del diritto*, 3, 445–466.

Clarich, M., Mattarella, B.G. (2013). La prevenzione della corruzione. In Mattarella, B.G., Pelissero, M. (Eds.), *La legge anticorruzione* (pp. 59–70). Torino: Giappichelli.

Comitato interministeriale (2013). Linee di indirizzo del Comitato interministeriale (d.p.c.m. 16 gennaio 2013) per la predisposizione, da parte del Dipartimento della funzione pubblica, del Piano nazionale anticorruzione di cui alla legge 6 novembre 2012, n. 190. www.anticorruzione.it.

Corte dei Conti (2009). Giudizio sul rendiconto generale dello Stato 2008, Memoria del Procuratore generale, Corte dei Conti, Roma, 2009, p. 237.

Del Sarto, S., Gnaldi, M. (2018). Considerazioni sull'efficacia delle relazioni del Responsabile della Prevenzione della Corruzione come strumento di prevenzione. In Gnaldi, M., Ponti, B. (eds.): *Misurare la corruzione oggi: obiettivi, metodi, esperienze* (pp. 154–172). Milano: Franco Angeli.

Di Cristina, F. (2013). I piani per la prevenzione della corruzione. In Mattarella, B.G., Pelissero, M. (Eds.), *La legge anticorruzione* (pp. 91–111). Torino: Giappichelli.

Fabrizio, F. (2015). L'impatto delle misure anticorruzione e della trasparenza sull'organizzazione amministrativa. *Il Diritto dell'economia*, 3, 483–506.

Galli, G. (2015, May 25). Quegli indici poco credibili che penalizzano l'Italia. *Il Sole 24 ore.*

GRECO - Group of States against corruption (2008). Evaluation report on Italy. Council of Europe, Strasburgo.

GRECO - Group of States against Corruption (2011). Lessons learnt from the three Evaluation Rounds (2000-2010). www.coe.int

ISO (2010). ISO 31000 – Risk management. https://www.iso.org

Merloni, F. (2013). I piani anticorruzione e i codici di comportamento. *Diritto penale e processo*, 8S, 4–14.

OECD (2009). Towards a sound integrity framework: instruments, processes, structures and conditions for implementation. Parigi, 2009.

Racca, G.M. (2013). La prevenzione e il contrasto della corruzione nei contratti pubblici. In Mattarella, B.G., Pelissero, M. (Eds.), *La legge anticorruzione* (pp. 125–152). Torino: Giappichelli.

Sequeira S. (2012). Advances in measuring corruption in the field. In Serra, D., Wantchekon, L. (Eds.), *New advances in experimental research on corruption* (pp. 145–175). Emerald Group Publishing Limited.

Corruption Prevention: First Evidences from the 2015 RPC Survey for Italian Municipalities

Michela Gnaldi and Simone Del Sarto

Abstract Corruption prevention is noticeably interwoven with the social integrity and overall quality of life of a Country. The Italian "anti-corruption law" of 2012 introduces a new figure, the prevention-of-corruption supervisor, who yearly reports, through a pre-specified questionnaire (named the RPC form), if and how prevention measures are implemented within the public institution he/she represents. We use the response pattern to the questionnaire provided by a sample of Italian municipalities for a twofold purpose: (i) providing a summary measure of corruption prevention accomplished by the sample at issue; (ii) classifying and qualifying the municipalities according to their behaviour in terms of corruption prevention using a latent class model. Results show that municipalities can be partitioned into two groups, according to their virtuosity. Moreover, we observe that virtuous municipalities are the biggest ones (i.e., on account of the resident population), which experienced at least one corruptive event over the past year.

Introduction

Monitoring corruption – by both fighting it through penal sanctions and preventing it through administrative measures – is a crucial condition for raising the integrity system and the overall quality of life of a Country. Corruption can be broadly defined as the misuse of power in the interests of illicit gain (Andersson and Heywood 2009). The World Bank sees corruption as the single greatest obstacle to economic and social development (World Bank 2006a) and fighting corruption, together with establishing good governance, as necessary parts of supporting sustainable

M. Gnaldi
Department of Political Sciences, University of Perugia, Perugia, Italy
e-mail: michela.gnaldi@unipg.it

S. Del Sarto (✉)
Italian National Institute for the Evaluation of the Education System (INVALSI), Rome, Italy
e-mail: simone.delsarto@email.com

A. Bianco et al. (eds.), *Italian Studies on Quality of Life*, Social Indicators Research Series 77, https://doi.org/10.1007/978-3-030-06022-0_6

development (World Bank 2006b). The World Economic Forum further estimates the cost of corruption to be more than 5 per cent of global GDP.

Yet, despite the widespread agreement that corruption is one of the key challenges for policy makers, there is still a rather weak consensus on how best to measure it. Indeed, the most commonly used measurement means of corruption – the so-called perception-based and non-perceptual or objective measures – are affected by conceptual, methodological or political problems (Heywood and Rose 2014; Carloni 2017) that limit their utility as a guide for developing effective anti-corruption policies. In particular, as it will be better specified in the next section, perception-based measures based on subjective perceptions of corruption mostly expressed by experts, may not mirror actual experiences of corruption and might be driven by general sentiment reflecting, for example, media coverage (Andersson and Heywood 2009; Mancini 2016). On the other side, objective measures using statistical and market proxies and judicial measures pose other constraints linked both to their partial usability in cross-country studies and to their limited utility for preventing corruption (i.e., a conviction for a corruption crime may occur many years after the corruptive event took place).

In order to address the lack of reliable indicators of corruption, further measures of corruption have been proposed and developed, such as measures of risk-of-corruption and indicators of administrative-contrast and prevention of corruption. These latest indicators imply a shift from an essentially penal and repressive focus, typical of traditional measures of corruption, to a broader preventive approach for fighting corruption, in which not only illegal and criminal conducts come into play, but also, most generally, any social malpractice which, even if not framed in a specific type of penal offence against public administration, requires nonetheless special attention in order to prevent corruption (Carloni 2018).

In the Italian context, the annual report filled in by the prevention-of-corruption supervisor – "Responsabile per la Prevenzione della Corruzione" (RPC) within the "Piano Triennale per la Prevenzione della Corruzione" (PTPC) – which is the object of analysis of the present contribution, has to be considered one of such latest measures. Specifically, with the recent law n.190 of 2012, named "Provisions for the prevention and repression of corruption and lawlessness in the public administration", each public institution has to adopt a three-year plan for corruption prevention (the PTPC), which provides an assessment of the different exposure levels of offices to the risk of corruption and specifies the organisational changes designed to prevent such risk. To this general aim, each institution selects a supervisor, called prevention-of-corruption supervisor (the RPC): among his/her tasks, the supervisor has to fill in an annual report about the efficacy of the prevention measures defined by the PTPC. Such report is filled in through a questionnaire, made available in spreadsheet format by the Italian National Anti-Corruption Authority (ANAC) and has to be uploaded in the "transparent administration" section of the public institution website.

The purpose of the present work is twofold: (i) we provide a first synthetic measure of corruption prevention of a sample of 232 Italian municipalities, by aggregating the answers provided by RPCs to the opening questions of the RPC form sections; (ii) we classify and qualify our sample of municipalities according to what stated in the RPC form. Since the RPC form summarises what each municipality has accomplished to prevent and contrast corruption, according to the annual program defined in the PTPC, our second purpose is to cluster municipalities into homogeneous groups as regards to the adopted anti-corruption measures. To this aim, we rely on the latent class model (Lazarsfeld 1950; Lazarsfeld and Henry 1968), which allows us to cluster units with a similar behaviour on account of a latent and unobserved characteristic (i.e., corruption).

This contribution is organised as follows: in section "Measures of Corruption Prevention in the Context of Existing Corruption Indicators" a literature review specifying details of available measures to fight and prevent corruption is provided, while section "The Prevention-of-Corruption Supervisor (RPC) Form Data" presents a description of the Italian prevention-of-corruption supervisor (RPC) questionnaire and data. Section "Results" shows the overall results of our analyses and section "Conclusions" discusses the main results.

Measures of Corruption Prevention in the Context of Existing Corruption Indicators

The necessary premise to what will be discussed in the following sections is that corruption is very difficult to measure. Indeed, corruption is a black, latent box: it cannot be directly observed and analysed as people involved in corruptive activities to the aim of illicit gains have interest to hide them. What is more, corruption is inherently complex as it encompasses several activities at different levels of gravity, from trivial to much more severe activities (i.e., a bribe to avoid prosecution for a traffic transgression; a falsification of public decisions for illicit private interests). Moreover, there exist many different types of corruption varying according to (i) the sectors where they happen (public or private, political or administrative); (ii) the involved actors (public officials, private citizens, politicians); (iii) the degree to which they are formalised (systemic or occasional) (Andersson and Heywood 2009). Such a complexity translates in an overall difficulty to develop a single comprehensive definition of corruption, and this in turn yields to validity issues of measurement tools designed to measure corruption. In fact, corruption measurement is at risk of being invalid anytime it lacks a clear operational definition of what is the object of measurement and what is exactly meant for corruption.

And yet, there are a number of measures of corruption, commonly referred to as "perception-based" measures, objective measures and judicial measures. Perception-based measures are founded on the subjective perception of corruption provided by experts and non-experts and are generally expressed at a country-level. The two most widely known perception-based measures are the World Bank's Control of Corruption (Kaufmann et al. 2011) and Transparency International's Corruption Perceptions Index (Transparency International 2012). Despite their widespread use in comparative studies, such measures are highly criticised. Critics point out that because they are based on perceptions, they are inherently prone to bias and serve as imperfect proxies for actual levels of corruption (Kurtz and Schrank 2007; Razafindrakoto and Roubaud 2010). Others (Rose and Peiffer 2012) underline that perceptions may not be related to actual experiences of corruption, and they can be driven by general sentiment reflecting prior economic growth (Kurtz and Schrank 2007) or media coverage of important cases of corruption (Mancini et al. 2017). What is more, rankings of countries based on surveys on corruption perception are obtained through composite indicators and are liable to their typical limits, that is: (i) the judgements made during the process of construction of a composite measure introduce sources of uncertainty in the measurement so that, for instance, choosing to adopt a certain criterion for aggregating simple indices (summative or multiplicative) or a certain weighting system (subjective or objective) will impact on the final ranking (Saisana et al. 2005; Munda et al. 2009); (ii) through the aggregation of simple indices, the final synthetic indicator will result unable to provide information on the very nature of the underlying phenomenon. Further, Donchev and Ujhelyi (2014) show that while perceptions and experiences can be highly correlated overall, the relationship between them is non-linear, meaning that such measures are better able to discriminate between countries in which corruption perception is low and worse at discriminating between those in which corruption perception is high.

On the other side, non-perception-based measures are objective indexes based on proxies, that is, market or statistical indicators tied with corruption, such as the price of input purchased by a public administration, the rate of criminal convictions to public officials for crimes related to corruption, and so on. One of such measures is that developed by Golden and Picci (2005), who propose a new measure of corruption based on the difference between the quantity of infrastructure and public spending on it among 20 regions in Italy. Despite having less statistical criticalities of perception-based measures, also objective measures are prone to criticisms linked to (i) their limited usability in cross-country studies, because different countries adopt different judicial systems; (ii) their partial utility for preventing corruption (i.e., a conviction for a corruption crime may occur many years after the corruptive event took place); their misleading information potential as, for instance, an increase in the number of convictions for corruption might depend on an increased level of efficacy of the underlying judicial system, rather than on an increased level of corruption.

In order to address the lack of reliable indicators of corruption, further measures of corruption have been developed, such as measures of risk-of-corruption and indicators of administrative-contrast and prevention of corruption. Corruption prevention seeks to identify potential weaknesses in a public organisation, its structure, processes and staff in order to highlight red flags capable to uncover its vulnerabilities and opportunities for malpractices, and make corresponding recommendations for their reduction and minimization. Thus, corruption prevention consists in the detection and minimisation of the causes and conditions for corruptive activities, through the development and implementation of a system of appropriate ex ante controls, as well as deterrence of persons from the commission of crimes of corruption and malpractices (Li 2014). Preventive measures of corruption imply a shift from an essentially penal and repressive focus, typical of traditional measures of corruption, to a broader preventive approach to fighting corruption, in which not only illegal and criminal conducts come into play, but also, most generally, any social behaviour and malpractice which, even if not framed in a specific type of penal offence against public administration, requires nonetheless special attention in order to prevent corruption Carloni (2018).

The tasks of corruption prevention are addressed by implementing a number of corruption prevention measures, such as (i) anti-corruption national programmes and their subsequent assessment through surveys; (ii) provision of information about a person holding an office at a public level; (iii) corruption risk analysis; (iv) anti-corruption assessment of legal acts; (v) education and public awareness. In Italy, the annual report filled in by the prevention-of-corruption supervisor (RPC) within the "Piano Triennale per la Prevenzione della Corruzione" (PTPC), which is the object of analysis of the present paper discussed at length in the next section, is the measurement instrument chosen by the Italian National Anti-Corruption Authority (ANAC) to assess the efficacy of the prevention measures defined by the PTPC.

The Prevention-of-Corruption Supervisor (RPC) Form Data

The new system introduced by the Italian ANAC is unique and does not have equals in the international panorama. The rationale behind the logic of the law n. 190 of 2012 is that dealing with corruption needs not only to develop indicators measuring, ex-post, the incidence of corruption events and their counter effects in terms of economic, social, cultural development, but also, ex-ante, indicators to alert the so-called "red-flags", that is, the presence of risk factors, even before the corruption event has taken place.

The data considered in this work refer to the RPC forms filled in 2015. Each of them has been individually downloaded from the "transparent administration" section of the municipality institutional website. The RPC form has several sections reflecting different aspects about the efficacy of prevention measures, defined in the PTPC adopted by each institution. In this work, we consider the responses to the opening questions of each section, requiring the institution at issue to state whether it has accomplished the required activities. The questions are related to the following contents (in square brackets it is reported the original label within the RPC form):

1. monitoring of the sustainability of all measures, including mandatory (general) and additional (specific) measures, identified in the PTPC [2A]. This question belongs to the "Risk management" section, which is the cornerstone of the PTPC, since it defines the areas, hence the specific measures, to be accomplished by any single administration;

2. fulfilment of additional measures, in addition to mandatory ones [3A];
3. computerising the flaw to fuel data publication in the “transparent administration” website section [4A];
4. monitoring of the data publication processes [4C];
5. training of employees, specifically devoted to prevention of corruption [5A];
6. staff turnover, as a risk prevention measure [6B]. According to the PTPC, turnover reduces the risk of privileged relations between administrations and users. As such, turnover removes the privilege, and all those routine practices, which may illegitimately advantage someone at the expenses of someone else, damaging the principles and conditions of impartiality and fairness;
7. checking the truthfulness of statements made by parties concerned with unfitness for office causes [7A]. Indeed, when a public employee accepts the role, he/she must grant a declaration of non-existence of unfitness for office causes;
8. implementation of measures to verify the existence of incompatibility conditions [8A]. At the moment of the acceptance of the role, a public employee must also declare the non-existence of incompatibility conditions;
9. adoption of prearranged procedures for issuing permits for assignment performance [9A];
10. development of a standard procedure for the collection of misconducts information by public employees (whistleblowing) [10A]. The whistleblower is in fact the employee who glimpses a potential swindle, a danger or any other potential risk, which may damage citizens, colleagues, stakeholders, the institution itself and its reputation, and for this reason decides to inform the public institution.

Three possible answers can be provided to these questions: “Yes”, “No, but expected by the PTPC” and “No, not expected by the PTPC”, labelled with “1”, “2” and “3”, respectively. As it can be noted, responses “1” and “3” correspond to actions in line with the PTPC, while the second is the least virtuous one.

The sample analysed in this contribution refers to the RPC forms of 232 Italian municipalities, individually downloaded from the “transparent administration” section of the municipality institutional website. The sample comprises all Italian province municipalities, all the other municipalities with at least 40,000 inhabitants and particular “advised” municipalities, as stated by ANAC act n.71 of 2013.

Moreover, three covariates are included in the dataset: the geographic location, the municipality dimension and the occurrence of a corruptive event. The first is a categorical variable with three levels, according to the geographic position of the municipality (“North”, “Centre” and “South and islands”). The dimension of a municipality is considered categorical as well, and obtained according to the resident population within municipality, divided in quartiles. Finally, the variable “occurrence of a corruptive event” is dichotomous and is directly obtained from the RPC form (question 2B).

Results

In this section, results are reported as regards the analyses on the RPC data described in the previous section. In particular, in section "A First Synthetic Measure of Corruption Prevention in Italian Municipalities" a first exercise to build a composite indicator on corruption prevention is presented, with the description of the ways such index is computed and some first evidences from the sample at issue. Furthermore, section "Latent Class Analysis: Model and Results" illustrates a Latent Class analysis of the data and shows, together with some necessary methodological premises, the resulting clustering of municipalities in similar groups, according to what stated in the RPC forms.

A First Synthetic Measure of Corruption Prevention in Italian Municipalities

Considering the questions of the RPC form introduced in section "The Prevention-of-Corruption Supervisor (RPC) Form Data", a possible indicator that allows for a synthetic description of the public administration behaviour in terms of adoption of corruption prevention measures can be the following:

$$\text{CICP}_i = \sum_j w_{ij},$$

where CICP is the acronym of Composite Indicator for Corruption Prevention. Index i refers to the statistical unit (i.e., the municipality, in this case), while the items are indexed with $j = 1, \ldots, 10$. As such, this indicator is a weighted sum of the responses to the ten selected items of the RPC form. Each answer is then weighted considering the following weights:

- $w_{ij} = 1$ if municipality i answers "Yes" to item j (most virtuous behaviour), corresponding to the response modality labelled as "1";
- $w_{ij} = 0$ if municipality i answers "No, not expected by the PTPC" to item j, labelled as "3";
- $w_{ij} = -1$ if municipality i answers "No, but expected by the PTPC" to item j (least virtuous behaviour), labelled as "2".

Variable weighting is a crucial phase in the composite indicator building process, as different weights potentially lead to different results. However, the effects of using several weighting techniques in obtaining a composite indicator of corruption prevention are out of the scope of this work; rather, the aim is to provide a first synthetic insight about what has been accomplished by the selected sample of municipalities in terms of corruption prevention. As ten questions are used for building the CICP at issue, and considering the weighting system defined above,

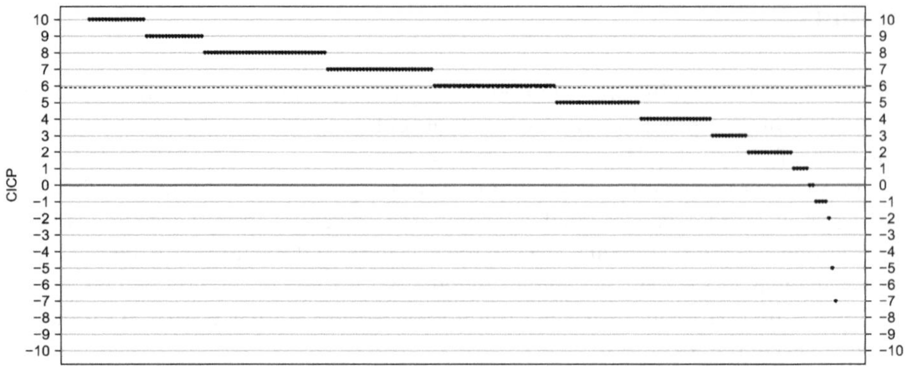

Fig. 1 Graphical representation of the Composite Indicator for Corruption Prevention (CICP), computed for the sample of the 232 municipalities. The dashed line represents the mean of the indicator, equal to 5.91

CICP ranges between -10 and 10. Figure 1 shows the CICP values obtained from the selected sample of 232 municipalities and reported in a decreasing way, from left to right.

In this graph, each point identifies a municipality and the average of the CICP over the sample (equal to 5.91) is reported with a dashed line. As it can be seen, very different behaviours can be highlighted within the sample. Eighteen administrations obtain a CICP equal to 10, that is, the maximum possible value of the indicator, and can be considered the most virtuous ones. In fact, such municipalities have accomplished all the measures expected by the PTPC. On the contrary, in the bottom of Fig. 1, it can be observed other institutions with a value of the CICP around 0, or even negative. Fourteen municipalities show values of the indicator below 1: this is the group of the least virtuous administrations.

In Table 1a we report some descriptive measures of the CICP distribution, according to the geographic location (North, Centre, and South and Islands) and the Region the municipalities belong to. It is possible to appreciate a slight difference in the distribution of the indicator in the three geographic areas. Specifically, municipalities in the North reveal an average CICP equal to 6.48, with a standard deviation (SD) of 2.56. A similar performance is obtained by Central Italy administrations (mean CICP $= 6.28$, SD $= 2.38$). Differently, Southern municipalities of Italy reveal the lowest average for CICP, equal to 5.28 (SD $= 3.07$), one point lower than in the other areas of Italy. Moreover, in the South we can observe a larger CICP variability, since the coefficient of variation (CV) – obtained by the ratio between the standard deviation and the mean – is equal to 0.58 versus 0.38 in the other two areas. Figure 2 (left panel) depicts the differences in the distribution of the CICP with respect to the geographic area through a boxplot. As we can see, boxplots of Northern and Central Italy are very similar, while that of Southern Italy presents, with respect to the other two areas, a lower median (marked horizontal line) and a higher variability, deducible from the greater distance between the "whiskers" (dotted lines coming out of the box), which represents the difference between the third and first quartile of the distribution.

Similarly, in Table 1b a summary of the CIPC distribution according to the municipality dimension is reported. As already outlined above, the variable referred to the municipality dimension is considered categorical, with four levels according

Table 1 Summary of the distribution of the Composite Indicator for Corruption Prevention by Region and geographic location (a) and municipality dimension (b): *n* is the absolute frequency of municipalities belonging to the strata, while the dimension is considered categorical with four levels according to the quartiles of the population distribution within municipality (Q1, Q2, Q3 and Q4)

(a)

Region	*n*	Min	Max	Mean	Median	Std. dev.
Valle d'Aosta	1	9	9	9.00	9.0	–
Piemonte	13	0	10	6.23	6.0	2.83
Liguria	4	4	6	5.00	5.0	0.82
Lombardia	27	−1	9	6.00	7.0	2.69
Trentino-Alto Adige	1	10	10	10.00	10.0	–
Friuli-Venezia Giulia	4	7	10	8.25	8.0	1.50
Veneto	14	2	9	6.07	6.5	2.09
Emilia-Romagna	13	3	10	7.62	8.0	2.60
North	*77*	*−1*	*10*	*6.48*	*7.0*	*2.56*
Toscana	18	2	10	6.39	6.5	2.45
Marche	12	2	10	6.00	6.0	2.37
Umbria	3	6	9	8.00	9.0	1.73
Lazio	20	1	10	6.10	7.0	2.45
Centre	*53*	*−1*	*10*	*6.28*	*7.0*	*2.38*
Abruzzo	7	5	8	6.57	7.0	0.98
Molise	2	2	5	3.50	3.5	2.12
Campania	28	−1	10	4.75	5.0	2.95
Puglia	22	−5	10	4.91	5.5	3.78
Basilicata	2	1	6	3.50	3.5	3.54
Calabria	6	4	8	6.50	7.0	1.38
Sicilia	20	−7	10	5.80	6.0	3.66
Sardegna	15	1	9	5.53	6.0	2.39
South and islands	*102*	*−7*	*10*	*5.28*	*6.0*	*3.07*
Total	*232*	*−7*	*10*	*5.91*	*6.0*	*2.80*

(b)

Quartiles	*n*	Min	Max	Mean	Median	Std. dev.
Q1	58	−7	10	4.83	5	3.12
Q2	58	−1	10	5.76	6	2.80
Q3	58	−2	10	5.76	6	2.54
Q4	58	2	10	7.29	7	2.16
Total	*232*	*−7*	*10*	*5.91*	*6*	*2.80*

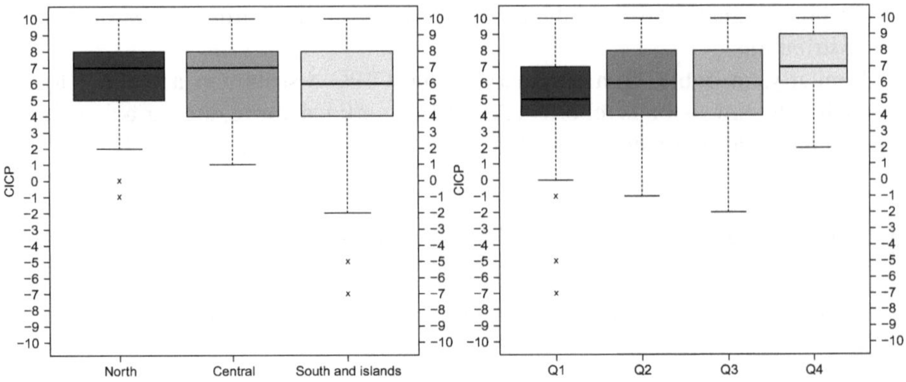

Fig. 2 Boxplots of the Composite Indicator for Corruption Prevention (CICP), stratified by geographic location (left panel) and municipality resident population (right panel), divided in quartiles (Q1, Q2, Q3 and Q4)

to the quartiles of the population distribution within each municipality, labelled as Q1, Q2, Q3 and Q4, respectively. We can note that the distribution of the indicator moves to higher values as dimension increases (hence, gradually moving from Q1 to Q4), as the mean of the CIPC passes from 4.83 in the smallest municipalities, belonging to the first quartile, to 5.76 (for Q2 and Q3), to 7.29 in the biggest municipalities (Q4). Moreover, the standard deviation of the CIPC decreases as dimension increases, leading to a reduction of the CV, hence of the variability. Such differences can be clearly observed in the boxplots reported in Fig. 2 (right panel).

Latent Class Analysis: Model and Results

When the objective is to cluster units of a sample into homogeneous groups, a very useful statistical methodology is the latent class (LC) model, one of the most well-known latent variable model. The classification of the units is made according to several categorical variables – such as the responses to some questionnaire items – which can be considered as the observable manifestation of an underlying latent (i.e., unobservable) variable which, in our case, is corruption.

Let $\boldsymbol{Y}_i = [Y_{i1}, \ldots, Y_{ir}]^\top$ denote the random vector of the responses of unit i to the r items of a questionnaire, $i = 1, \ldots, n$, where n is the sample size. Each Y_{ij} is a categorical variable with m_j categories: in this work we consider $m_j = 3$ for each item j, since three different responses can be provided to the selected items (see section "The Prevention-of-Corruption Supervisor (RPC) Form Data"). Moreover, it is assumed the existence of one discrete latent variable C with k support points, corresponding to the latent classes in the population. Each support point has a prior probability, denoted with π_c, $c = 1, \ldots, k$. Hence, the (conditional) probability of a response equal to y provided by a unit belonging to latent class c is the following:

$$\lambda_{j|c}(y) = P(Y_{ij} = y|C_i = c), \quad j = 1, \ldots, r, \quad y = 1, \ldots, m_j, \quad c = 1, \ldots, k.$$

Assuming local independence (i.e., the responses to the items are independent given the latent class), the probability of observing response pattern $\boldsymbol{y}_i = [y_{i1}, \ldots, y_{ir}]^\top$ given that unit i belongs to class c, can be obtained as the product of the single $\lambda_{j|c}$ over the r items:

$$P(\boldsymbol{y}_i|c) = \prod_{j=1}^{r} \lambda_{j|c}(y_{ij}).$$

Furthermore, it is possible to assign the sample units (i.e., any single municipality, in our case) to one of the k latent classes, according to the response pattern, using the posterior probability that unit i belongs to latent class c, obtained as follows:

$$P(c|\boldsymbol{y}_i) = \frac{P(\boldsymbol{y}_i|c)\pi_c}{\sum_{c=1}^{k} P(\boldsymbol{y}_i|c)\pi_c}, \quad c = 1, \ldots, k. \tag{1}$$

Specifically, each unit is classified into the latent class with the largest posterior probability.

The LC model is applied to the sample at issue and the following results are attained. First of all, the number of latent classes k is chosen according to the model showing the minimum BIC index (Schwarz 1978). Using this criterion, we can select $k = 2$ latent classes, for which we obtain the following estimates of the prior probabilities: $\pi_1 = 0.482$ and $\pi_2 = 0.518$.

Moreover, the estimates of the conditional probabilities of response, $\lambda_{j|c}$, are reported in Table 2. As we can see, the answers labelled as "1" (i.e., a positive response) is the most frequent in our sample for almost all ten items, since the relative conditional probabilities are often high (>60%). Nevertheless, units in the first latent class have larger conditional probabilities of response category "1" than units in the second. Instead, a higher probability of response modalities "2" and "3" can be observed for units belonging to the second latent class: for this reason, this class is characterised by municipalities with a higher probability to not accomplish the activities reported in the form, mainly because such activities are not expected by the national plan (PTPC); in fact, the conditional probabilities of modality "3" are greater than those for modality "2". Overall, these two groups of municipalities particularly differ in the outcomes of items 7 and 8, since the most likely response to these two items is "1" for administrations in the first latent class, while the response modality with the highest probability is "3" for the second.

Finally, using Eq. (1), the posterior latent class classification of each unit is crossed with the covariates described at the end of section "The Prevention-of–Corruption Supervisor (RPC) Form Data", with the aim of further qualify each latent class. Specifically, the occurrence of a corruptive event and the municipality dimension show an interesting relation with the latent class membership (results are reported in Table 3). As far as the municipality dimension is concerned – see

Table 2 Estimated conditional response probabilities for the ten items of the RPC form

Item	Latent class	Response 1	2	3
1	1	0.875	0.036	0.089
	2	0.660	0.059	0.281
2	1	0.815	0.000	0.185
	2	0.615	0.075	0.311
3	1	0.811	0.055	0.134
	2	0.582	0.069	0.348
4	1	0.909	0.000	0.091
	2	0.886	0.052	0.062
5	1	0.926	0.051	0.023
	2	0.860	0.119	0.020
6	1	0.549	0.185	0.266
	2	0.387	0.204	0.409
7	1	0.724	0.042	0.234
	2	0.077	0.187	0.736
8	1	0.817	0.001	0.181
	2	0.031	0.187	0.782
9	1	0.906	0.045	0.049
	2	0.804	0.033	0.163
10	1	0.850	0.092	0.058
	2	0.645	0.133	0.222

Table 3 Two-way tables between latent class classification and municipality dimension, divided in quartiles, according to the distribution of the municipality resident population (a) and occurrence of corruptive events (b). Row-percentages are reported within parenthesis

(a)

	Latent class		
Quartiles	1	2	Total
Q1	20 (34.5%)	38 (65.5%)	58
Q2	27 (46.6%)	31 (53.4%)	58
Q3	29 (50.0%)	29 (50.0%)	58
Q4	33 (56.9%)	25 (43.1%)	58
Total	109	123	232

(b)

	Latent class		
Corruptive events	1	2	Total
None	79 (43.9%)	101 (56.1%)	180
At least one	23 (69.7%)	10 (30.3%)	33
Total	102	111	213[a]

[a] 19 units have missing response in the occurrence of corruptive events

Table 3a – it can be observed that only one unit over three (34.5%) in the least populated (or smallest) municipalities (i.e., Q1) belongs to the first latent class: such proportion clearly increases as the municipality dimension increases (i.e., moving toward Q4). Hence, the first latent class is mostly characterised by the most populated municipalities. Looking at the occurrence of a corruptive event in Table 3b, we can observe that almost 70% of the municipalities admitting the occurrence of at least one corruptive event, belongs to the first latent class, while such proportion decreases to around 44% within the institutions with no corruptive events. Then, a further characteristic of the first latent class is a prevalence of institutions experiencing corruptive events.

Conclusions

This contribution deals with corruption prevention, whose purpose is to minimise, as much as possible, corruption damaging effects on economy, democracy, promotion of social welfare, consolidating national security and improving the quality of provision of public services. In the Italian context, the annual report filled in by the prevention-of-corruption supervisor – “Responsabile per la Prevenzione della Corruzione” (RPC) – is a measure of corruption prevention and represents the object of our interest in this work.

The purpose of our work is twofold: (i) providing a synthetic measure of corruption prevention – the Composite Indicator of Corruption Prevention (CICP) – of our sample of 232 Italian municipalities, by aggregating the answers provided by RPCs to the opening questions of the RPC form sections; (ii) classifying and qualifying our sample of municipalities into homogeneous groups as regards to the adopted anti-corruption measures, relying on a latent class approach, which allows us to cluster units with a similar behaviour on account of a latent and unobserved characteristic (i.e., corruption).

Our results show that, despite a general tendency to fulfil the corruption prevention law, it is also possible to identify a group of least virtuous municipalities showing very low values for the CICP, meaning that these municipalities did not even accomplish many of the mandatory anticorruption measures, expected by the anticorruption law n.190 of 2012. These municipalities, in particular, deserve the special attention of the Italian Anticorruption Authority (ANAC).

The subsequent analyses of the CICP distribution per municipality geographic area and dimension further highlight that (i) municipalities belonging to Southern Italy display, with respect to the other two areas (North and Centre of Italy), a lower value for the CICP and a higher variability, that is, a generally worse and more spread level of completion of mandatory anti-corruption measures; (ii) big municipalities (on account of their resident population) show, overall, better and less variable behaviours in terms of mandatory anti-corruption measures accomplishment than small municipalities.

The consequent latent class analysis additionally shows that municipalities can be partitioned into two latent groups, characterised by similar behaviours: the first collects municipalities showing a high probability of implementing measures to prevent corruption (i.e., the most virtuous municipalities), while the second class includes less virtuous municipalities. Moreover, by accounting for covariates, we further qualify the ascertained latent classes. Specifically, we observe that the latent class made by virtuous municipalities is composed by the biggest municipalities experiencing at least one corruptive event over the past year. The big dimension of a municipality seems thus to be a good condition for the alignment to the anticorruption law. On the contrary, the southern location of a municipality seems to play a negative role on the adoption of the best practices in terms of corruption prevention.

The new system introduced by the ANAC is unique, does not have equals in the international panorama, and it is becoming a model to reproduce by other Governments at national level anytime the attention is focused on corruption prevention (ex-ante) other than repression (ex-post). Dealing with corruption needs not only to develop indicators measuring the incidence of corruption once such events have already occurred, but also ex-ante indicators to alert red-flags and control the phenomenon. Clearly, being able to control and prevent corruption based on composite indicators derived from data "declared" by the same public administrator has also downsides, whose severity is very variable and still unexplored.

References

Andersson S, Heywood PM (2009) The politics of perception: use and abuse of Transparency International's approach to measuring corruption. Political studies 57(4):746–767

Carloni E (2017) Misurare la corruzione? Indicatori di corruzione e politiche di prevenzione. Politica del diritto 48(3):445–465

Carloni E (2018) Italian anti-corruption and transparency policies. In: Grasse A, Grimm M, Labitzke J (eds) Italien zwischen Krise und Aufbruch: Reformen und Reformversuche der Regierung Renzi, Springer Fachmedien Wiesbaden, Wiesbaden, pp 365–386, DOI 10.1007/978-3-658-16092-0_14

Donchev D, Ujhelyi G (2014) What do corruption indices measure? Economics & Politics 26(2):309–331

Golden MA, Picci L (2005) Proposal for a new measure of corruption, illustrated with Italian data. Econ Polit 17(1):37–75

Heywood PM, Rose J (2014) "Close but no Cigar": the measurement of corruption. Journal of Public Policy 34(3):507–529

Kaufmann D, Kraay A, Mastruzzi M (2011) The worldwide governance indicators: methodology and analytical issues. Hague Journal on the Rule of Law 3(2):220–246

Kurtz MJ, Schrank A (2007) Growth and governance: Models, measures, and mechanisms. Journal of politics 69(2):538–554

Lazarsfeld PF (1950) The logical and mathematical foundation of latent structure analysis, Princeton University Press, New York, pp 362–412

Lazarsfeld PF, Henry NW (1968) Latent structure analysis. Houghton Mifflin, Boston

Li RBL (2014) Measures to prevent corruption and to encourage cooperation between all sectors of society. Work product of the 16th UNAFEI UNCAC training programme. Resource

material series no. 92, part two. Available at http://www.unafei.or.jp/english/pdf/RS_No92/No92_13VE_Li2.pdf
Mancini P (2016) A comparative research on the print press coverage of corruption. URL http://anticorrp.eu/wp-content/uploads/2016/09/D6.1.2.pdf
Mancini P, Mazzoni M, Cornia A, Marchetti R (2017) Representations of corruption in the British, French, and Italian press: Audience segmentation and the lack of unanimously shared indignation. The International Journal of Press/Politics 22(1):67–91
Munda G, Nardo M, Saisana M, Srebotnjak T (2009) Measuring uncertainties in composite indicators of sustainability. International Journal of Environmental Technology and Management 11(1–3):7–26
Razafindrakoto M, Roubaud F (2010) Are international databases on corruption reliable? A comparison of expert opinion surveys and household surveys in sub-Saharan Africa. World development 38(8):1057–1069
Rose R, Peiffer C (2012) Paying bribes to get public services: A comparative guide to concepts and measures. CSPP Studies in Public Policy (494), URL https://ssrn.com/abstract=2180793
Saisana M, Saltelli A, Tarantola S (2005) Uncertainty and sensitivity analysis techniques as tools for the quality assessment of composite indicators. Journal of the Royal Statistical Society: Series A (Statistics in Society) 168(2):307–323
Schwarz G (1978) Estimating the dimension of a model. The annals of statistics 6(2):461–464
Transparency International (2012) Corruption perceptions index 2012. Berlin: Transparency International
World Bank (2006a) Combating corruption. URL http://www.worldbank.org/en/topic/governance/brief/anti-corruption
World Bank (2006b) Governance and anti-corruption. ways to enhance the World Bank's impact. URL http://siteresources.worldbank.org/INTOED/Resources/governance_anticorruption.pdf

Transparency and Socio-political Environment in Italy

Emma Galli, Ilde Rizzo, and Carla Scaglioni

Abstract Transparency of public administration may contribute to the quality of citizens' life and affect trust in government because of its informative value and monitoring function. Notwithstanding the legislative and administrative efforts undertaken at every level of public administration in Italy, apart from Galli et al. (Transparency, quality of institutions and performance in the Italian municipalities. WP11/2017/DE/UECE, ISEG, University of Lisbon, 2017), not much attention has been given to measuring the degree of transparency. Additionally, even though transparency is also considered an important aspect of social capital affecting the so-called "Equitable and Sustainable Well-being" (BES), none of the indicators proposed within the BES approach aims at assessing transparency itself.

Our paper proposes an integrated analysis of transparency and BES indicators, specifically the digital, social and political dimensions, and provides evidence that in large Italian municipalities there is a correlation between transparency and the intensity of Internet use, trust in institutions, social participation and, to a lower extent, civic and informal political participation.

Ilde Rizzo – Former President of the National Anticorruption Authority (ANAC, 2012—April 2014).

E. Galli (✉)
Department of Social and Economic Sciences, University of Rome Sapienza, Rome, Italy
e-mail: emma.galli@uniroma1.it

I. Rizzo
Department of Economics and Business, University of Catania, Catania, Italy

C. Scaglioni
University of Reggio Calabria "Mediterranea", DiGiEs, Reggio Calabria, Italy

A. Bianco et al. (eds.), *Italian Studies on Quality of Life*, Social Indicators Research Series 77, https://doi.org/10.1007/978-3-030-06022-0_7

Introduction

Recently, the definition of welfare has evolved considerably, including equity and sustainability as its fundamental elements, thus leading to searching well-being measures different from GDP. In line with the several international initiatives that have been carried out over the past decade (e.g., Stiglitz et al. 2009; OECD 2011), in Italy, the so-called "Equitable and Sustainable Well-Being" (BES)[1] approach has been developed to provide a multi-dimensional measurement of well-being. Institutional transparency may play a crucial role in increasing the level of trust in the institutions, thus affecting people's well-being by monitoring the use of public resources and the achievement of institutional goals. However, none of the indicators proposed within the BES approach has hitherto aimed at capturing transparency. It is also worth noting that transparency has brought about significant legislative and administrative efforts at all levels of public administration in Italy but, apart from Galli et al. (2017), no attention has been paid so far to providing a detailed measure of the degree of transparency and exploring its economic implications.

In this context, our paper aims at filling this gap and bridging the analyses of BES and transparency to propose the first integrated investigation of transparency and BES indicators at regional level. Based on four different dimensions, that is, transparency, digital, social, and political, we assess whether the transparency of public administration is correlated with the quality of the socio-political environment.

The remainder of this chapter is organized as follows: section "Transparency within the equitable and sustainable well-being approach" describes the conceptual and institutional framework of both the well-being and transparency dimensions; section "Transparency and well-being: empirical evidence" presents the data and discusses the empirical evidence at regional level in Italy; and section "Conclusions" offers concluding remarks.

Transparency Within the Equitable and Sustainable Well-Being Approach

Equitable and Sustainable Well-Being Approach: Definitions and Measures

Recently, the definition of welfare has evolved considerably, moving towards a broader meaning that includes several aspects. Undoubtedly, the introduction of two additional elements—equity and sustainability—has helped to enrich substantially

[1]This is the label used for the Italian well-being measurement project (see section "Degree of transparency").

this definition. The former element states that welfare must be spread equitably among citizens and territories, as inequality creates social conflicts. The latter affirms that well-being must be also sustainable, limiting the exploitation of social and natural resources to ensure welfare for future generations (Stiglitz et al. 2009). Social science research has witnessed an increasing interest in the analysis and measurement of subjective well-being, complementary to the traditional GDP and production measures.[2] In this respect, an important role has been played by the Commission on the Measurement of Economic Performance and Social Progress (CMPEPS),[3] which has identified the limits of GDP as an indicator of economic performance and social development and promoted alternative measures of people's well-being. Defining the well-being of individuals and territories is a complex concept, which is multidimensional and multi-causes. It also covers numerous different aspects of human being and refers to the quality of life of every person, not only to economic features. To this end, the following eight dimensions should be considered simultaneously: (i) material living standards (income, consumption, and wealth); (ii) health; (iii) education; (iv) personal activities, including work; (v) political voice and governance; (vi) social connections and relationships; (vii) environment (present and future conditions); and (viii) insecurity (economic, as well as physical) (Stiglitz et al. 2009).

Following this approach, since 2011, OECD has led a project called "Better Life Index", based on the "Compendium of OECD well-being indicators" (OECD 2011), which includes 11 dimensions of well-being: housing (housing conditions and spending, e.g., real estate pricing); income (household income and financial wealth); jobs (earnings, job security, and unemployment); community (quality of social support network); education (education and returns of the investment in education); environment (quality of the environment); governance (involvement in democracy); health; life satisfaction (level of happiness); safety (murder and assault rates); and work-life balance. Later, in 2014, the OECD provided a common framework for measuring people's well-being at the regional level by considering nine dimensions of their material conditions (income, jobs, and housing) and quality of life (health, education, environment, safety, access to services, and civic engagements) (OECD 2014).

In line with these international initiatives, in 2010, Italy formed a joint Committee composed by ISTAT (the Italian Institute of Statistics) and CNEL (the Italian Council for Economics and Labour) and developed a project for measuring well-being. The measurement consists of a dashboard of 134 individual indicators, distributed over 12 domains, which cover cultural heritage, education, economic and subjective welfare, environment, health, innovation, jobs, politics and institutions, social relations, quality of service, and safety at national and local levels.

[2]See, among others, Frey and Stutzer (2000) and Gasper (2010).

[3]CMPEPS was established in 2008 by the President of the French Republic, Nicholas Sarkozy, and was composed by Joseph Stiglitz, Amartya Sen, and Jean-Paul Fitoussi.

It is worth noting that such a multidimensional approach can ease and inspire policy makers in shaping priorities and policy actions. From this perspective, policies are no longer and not only aimed at increasing the wealth of a country/area but at improving the conditions that foster a better quality of life. This has led the Italian Parliament to approve, in 2016, a reform of the Budget Law, in which some BES indicators, selected by an *ad hoc* Committee, had to be included in the Document of Economics and Finance (DEF).[4] The new procedures also state that, by February 15 of each year, the Minister of Economy would report to the Parliament on the progress of BES indicators. If properly implemented, this reform, based on the connection between ISTAT well-being indicators and policy measures in the socio-economic field, might provide all involved stakeholders in public governance a tool for policy evaluation.

Transparency and Well-Being

The capability of public administrations to become transparent and allow citizens to properly monitor administrative activities is one of the parameters for the proper functioning of a public institution and strengthens both institutional and interpersonal trust (Kumlin and Rothstein 2005). In other words, transparency may contribute to the quality of citizens' lives, both for its informative value and monitoring function, and is also likely to affect the domain of governance and trust in the government. Additionally, the CNEL-ISTAT BES Report (2013) clearly states: "[. . .] the transparent relationship with public and private institutions, operating in the political, economic and social fields, their efficiency and the level of satisfaction for their functioning strengthen institutional and interpersonal confidence. On the contrary, widespread discretion in rules, low transparency and corruption negatively affect trust in the ability to create an equal society where everyone can feel guaranteed" (p. 133).

Although the issue of public transparency has not been explicitly considered in all the above-mentioned measurement projects, it represents an additional strategic element that affects well-being. Indeed, there is a growing literature on transparency, which addresses the different definitions of transparency, as well as measurement issues.[5] Some contributions have empirically investigated the impact of demographic (population size and density, age, gender), economic (unemployment, public debt), political (parties' competition, ideology, electoral turnout, presence of women in political institutions), and social (education, social capital, Internet diffusion) dimensions on transparency in several countries (see, among others,

[4]Among the 12 selected indicators, four are included in the DEF 2017 for the first time: average disposable income per capita, index of disposable income distribution, non-participation rate to the job market and CO2 emissions.

[5]For a recent and extensive review on transparency see Cucciniello et al. (2016).

Swamy et al. 2001; Alt et al. 2006; Esteller and Polo-Otero 2010; Alatas et al. 2009; Bertelli and Piotrowsky 2010; Caamaño-Alegre et al. 2011; Bastida et al. 2011; Jorge et al. 2011; Albalate 2013; Navarro Galera et al. 2015; Alcaraz-Quile et al. 2015; Ferraz Esteves de Araújo and Tejedo-Romero 2016). Other researchers have recently explored the connections between transparency and other aspects of well-being, such as trust in public institutions, political participation and quality of government, perception of legitimacy, civic satisfaction (see, among others, Islam 2004; Welch et al. 2005; Park and Blenkinsopp 2011; Piotrowski and Van Ryzin 2007; Piotrowski 2008; Benito and Bastida 2009; Worthy 2010; de Fine Licht et al. 2014; Grimmelikhuijsen and Meijer 2012). The findings of this literature stream show these connections are mostly positive and context dependent.

Transparency Rules in Italy

Major reforms to favor transparency in public administrations and improve integrity and performance in OECD countries, including Italy, have been introduced. A complete review of Italian regulation on these topics is outside the scope of this paper. However, we recall that, since 2009, transparency has received increasing and systematic attention.[6] A renewed effort occurred in 2012: the Anticorruption Bill,[7] which among the other things, focuses on transparency as a tool to foster integrity and accountability and puts the basis for new rules[8]on publication requirements, transparency, and disclosure of information. These rules have enlarged the scope of transparency in terms of both the public offices involved (almost 10,000) and number of obligations (around 270). The detailed definition of transparency obligations and monitoring of its fulfilment stems from the National Anticorruption Authority (Autorità Nazionale Anticorruzione, ANAC). At a decentralized level, the fulfilment of the transparency obligation is certified by the Independent Evaluation Unit (Organismo Indipendente di Valutazione, OIV),[9] and the related information is published on each public administration's website.

Transparency obligations are quite diversified, ranging from information on political-administrative bodies and top public managers and officers of each public organization to information on the private-public companies that provide local public services, about external consulting and collaboration, public procurement, management of property and assets, timing of payments, provision of public ser-

[6]Legislative Decree no. 150/2009 containing "*Provision on optimization of the productivity of public employees and efficiency and transparency of public administrations.*"

[7]Law no. 190/2012 containing "*Provisions for the prevention and repression of corruption and illegality in public administration.*"

[8]Legislative decree no. 33/2013 containing "*Rules about publicity, transparency and information provision of public administrations.*"

[9]OIV is appointed in each administration by the political decision-maker. It has many tasks, including the evaluation of performance.

vices, and civic access to information. The information is made accessible through the compulsory adoption of a standardized format for publication on websites (*Amministrazione trasparente*), and the right to access information is widened (*accesso civico*) to favor the public opinion monitoring of public organizations activities.[10]

While over the past decade significant attention has been paid to both BES and transparency individually, the relationship between transparency and BES is almost unexplored.

Transparency and Well-Being: Empirical Evidence

Degree of Transparency

We investigate the relationship between transparency and BES at regional level in Italy. First, we look at the transparency of local governments. Several motivations underlie such a choice. The municipal level of government, being closer to citizens, is the natural candidate for any analysis on accountability and trust in public institutions. Indeed, decentralization represents the institutional framework, which should favor citizens' political participation, governments' political accountability and responsiveness to people's preferences, and effectiveness in the provision of public services (Daughters and Harper 2007; Oates 2008).

For transparency, we use a new measure, that is the Composite Transparency Index (CTI) constructed and computed by Galli et al. (2017) for 2013. CTI aggregates "official" information on several aspects concerning the integrity and management of municipality activity, which is published on the municipality website (in the section *Amministrazione Trasparente)* and validated by the OIV.[11] We aggregate, at regional level, the CTIs calculated for a sample of 114 main municipalities (province capitals), located in different areas of the country and differently populated, which are also heterogeneous in terms of social and political features.

[10] Legislative decree no. 97/2016, containing "*revision and simplification of rules on the prevention of corruption, publicity and transparency,*" has enlarged the access to information further by allowing the generalized dissemination of information upon request.

[11] The CTI is constructed as a simple average of two sub-indicators referring to *Integrity* (CTI *Integrity*) and *Performance* (CTI *Performance*). The value of the items included in each sub-indicator is based on the OIV evaluation (according to criteria established by ANAC) in terms of information existence, completeness, updating and openness. Values are normalized and the average for all indices is set equal to unity. The values for each item are recalculated in relation to the average and given equal weights, consistent with the ANAC methodology. For further details, see Galli et al. (2017).

Fig. 1 Transparency dimension. CTI. (*Source:* Elaborated by the authors)

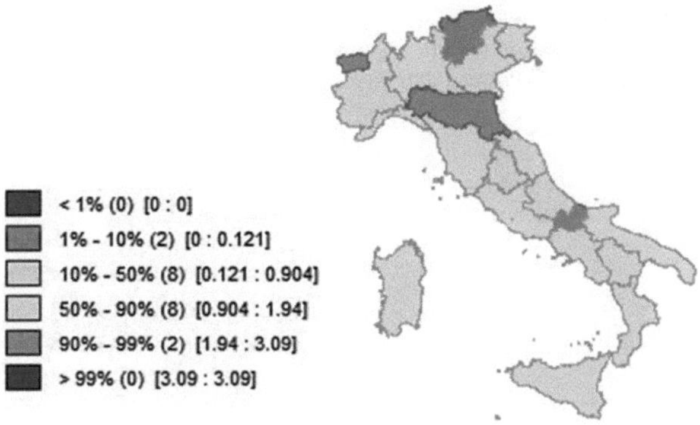

Regarding well-being measures, for 2013, our year of interest, a complete BES dataset is available only at regional level.[12] Therefore, because of data constraints, we consider both transparency and well-being at the regional level.

For simplicity, we provide a map of Italy for each dimension, where the Italian regions[13] are clustered into percentiles according to the geographical distribution of each indicator. Black shades indicate higher values, while gray shades refer to a lower performance.

As per Fig. 1, CTI exhibits marked differences across regions, ranging from 3.09 in Valle d'Aosta to 0.04 Molise.[14] With respect to the national average of 1.06, southern regions seem to have lower values in terms of degree of fulfillment of transparency obligations. However, it is worth noting that no clear cut geographical pattern emerges for the traditional divide north–center–south, since differences among regions also occur within each macro-area. However, none of the southern regions belong to the highest percentile, where we can find Valle d'Aosta (3.09) and Emilia-Romagna (2.23). Two values are worth nothing, as they are not in line with

[12]Only recently the BES framework has been applied at municipal level, under a project called "UrBes" (Istat 2014).

[13]Italy is politically and administratively divided in 20 regions. Five enjoy a special statute and wide autonomy (*Regioni a Statuto Speciale*) because of their multilingual status, border-line position, or historical reasons, such as the risk of secessionism (Friuli-Venezia-Giulia, Sicilia, Sardegna, Trentino Alto Adige consisting of the two Autonomous Provinces of Trento and Bolzano, Valle d'Aosta). Fifteen regions (Piemonte, Lombardia, Veneto, Emilia-Romagna, Toscana, Liguria, Marche, Umbria, Abruzzo, Lazio, Molise, Basilicata, Campania, Puglia, Calabria) are characterized by an ordinary statute (*Regioni a Statuto Ordinario*).

[14]Trentino-Alto Adige Region shows a value equal to 0, because it has not introduced transparency regulations immediately after their issuance by the central government. This is due to its status of special statute region (*Regione a Statuto Speciale),* which has allowed it not to adhere to the national transparency obligations and establish its own regulations. Therefore, we can consider the value of Trentino-Alto Adige an outlier.

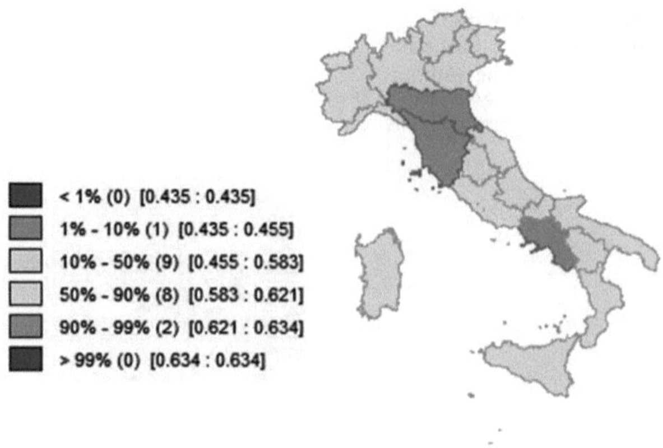

Fig. 2 Digital and demographic dimension. Internet use. (*Source:* Istat 2014)

their macro-areas: Puglia (1.01) and Piemonte (0.77); the former shows a higher value than the neighboring regions, while the latter is the opposite.

Selected BES Indicators

Regarding BES, recalling the main conclusions reached in the literature[15] on the determinants of transparency, we focus on several indicators representing the digital, social, and politico-institutional dimensions, which are relevant for transparency: intensity of Internet use, trust in public institutions, social participation, voter turnout, civic and political participation, and women's participation in the municipal councils to capture the quality of the digital, politico-institutional, and social environments (Istat 2014). Overall, it appears BES indicators have a more clearly defined geographical pattern than CTI.

As far as the digital dimension is concerned, Fig. 2 represents the intensity of Internet use, measured by the percentage of people aged 16–74 years who have used internet at least once a week during the 3 months before the interview. Digital innovation and its use can both be seen as indirect determinants of well-being but also pre-conditions for the diffusion and access to knowledge and public information. Overall, in 2013, the use of the Internet was above 58% in the center and north, although it is still behind the rest of Europe, where the average is around 72%. A technological disadvantage emerges in the south of Italy and in the islands.

As aforementioned,[16] it is well-established that citizens' trust in institutions as well as civic and political participation increase individual and social wellbeing, encouraging social cohesion and greater efficiency of public policies (Nannicini et al. 2013). The presence of transparent relationships among all stakeholders involved

---

[15]See section "Equitable and sustainable well-being approach: definitions and measures".

[16]See section "Equitable and sustainable well-being approach: definitions and measures".

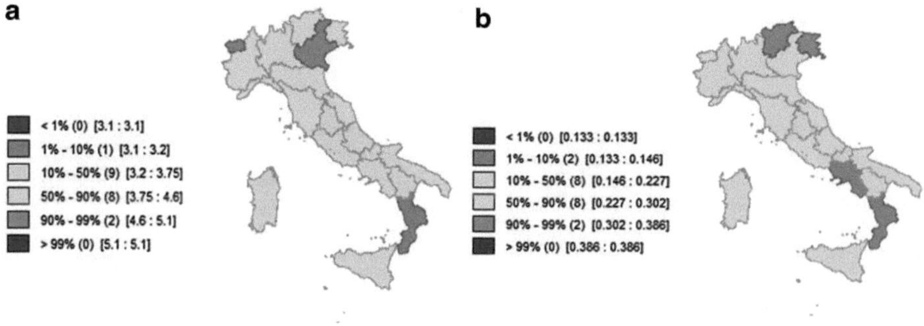

Fig. 3 Social dimension. (**a**) Trust in institutions. (**b**) Social participation (*Source:* Istat (2014))

(public and private institutions, citizens, etc.) is a pre-condition to boost all these aspects.

Figure 3 shows two dimensions of social capital, respectively, the vertical *trust in institutions* (Fig. 3a) and the horizontal *social participation* (Fig. 3b). Trust in institutions is measured as the average score of trust in regional, provincial, and municipal governments, expressed by people aged 14 and over, on a scale from 0 to 10, and social participations is measured by the percentage of people aged 14 and over that have performed at least one social activity over the past 12 months.[17]

From the map presenting trust in institutions (Fig. 3a), the center regions are closer to the southern ones and the islands have quite low values, being behind the north. Instead, with respect to social relations (Fig. 3b), the center and-north show an overall high horizontal trust and a gap with the south and islands.

The politico-institutional dimension that drives well-being is measured through three different indicators: *voter turnout,* which is the traditional channel of political participation, measured as percentage of eligible voters who cast a ballot in the last election for the European Parliament (Fig. 4a); a more informal channel, the *civic and political participation*, measured by the percentage of people aged 14 and over who performed at least one of the activities of civic and political participation)[18] (Fig. 4b); and *women's participation in local councils,* measured as the percentage of women elected in municipal councils in the total number of people elected, aggregated per Region (Fig. 4c).

[17]The relevant activities are: participation in meetings of associations (cultural/recreational, ecological, civil rights, peace); participation in meetings of trade union organizations, professional, or trade associations; meetings of political parties and/or performance of free activities for a party; payment of a monthly or quarterly fee for a sports club.

[18]Relevant activities are to speak about politics at least once a week; to get informed about politics at least once a week; to attend online consultation or voting on social (civic) or political (e.g., urban planning, petitions) issues at least once in the 3 months prior to the interview; or to read and post opinions on social or political issues on the web at least once in the 3 months prior to the interview.

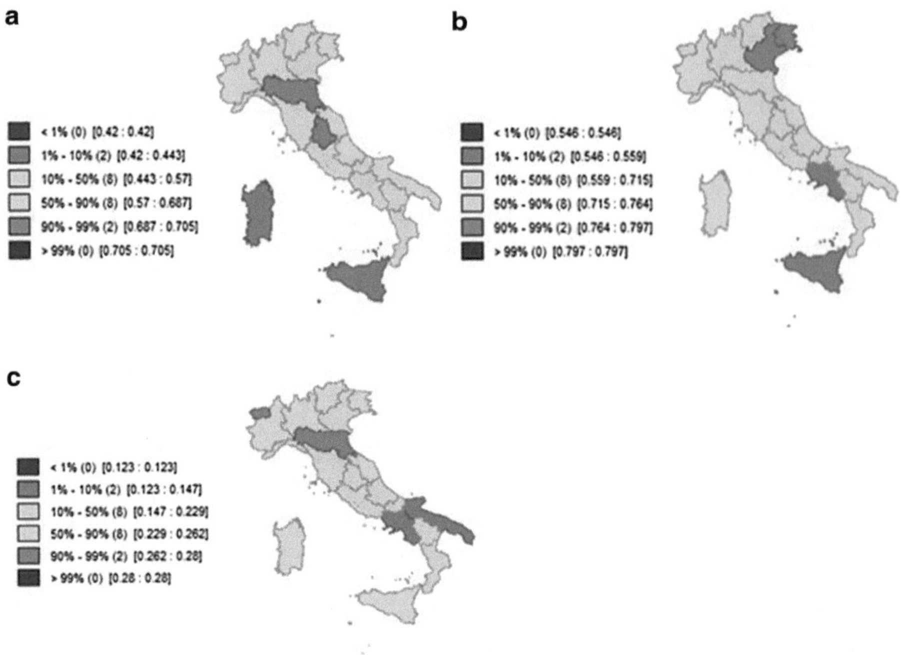

Fig. 4 Political dimension. (**a**) Voter turnout. (**b**) Civic and political participation. (**c**) Women's participation in municipal councils. (*Source:* Istat 2014)

While in the southern regions, the percentage of voters' turnout is 57% and below, in the north and center, the value increases to 70% (with the exception of Veneto).

Civic and political participation has the highest values (between 71% and 76%) in the central regions, while the North appears more scattered (between a minimum of 56% and maximum of 80%). Women's participation in municipal councils is overall quite low, from a minimum of 12% in two southern regions (Campania and Puglia) to a maximum of 28% in two center-northern regions (Emilia-Romagna and Valle d'Aosta). However, the intermediate values are unevenly distributed across the country.

Correlations Between Transparency and BES

The above graphical analysis allows us to identify existing patterns in transparency, as well as in the analyzed areas of well-being. As a further step, we perform a simple correlation between the CTI and each of the BES indicators. Table 1 shows the Pearson's product moment correlation coefficient.

Table 1 Correlations between CTI and BES indicators ($\alpha = 0.05$)

Dimensions	Indicators	Correlation CTI
Digital	Internet use intensity	0.66
Social	Trust in institutions	0.66
	Social participation	0.52
Political	Voters' turnout	0.16
	Civic and political participation	0.46
	Women's participation in municipal councils	0.50

Source: Elaborated by the authors

CTI is highly correlated with both Internet use intensity and trust in institutions (0.66), as well as with social participation and women's participation in municipal councils, although slightly less (0.52 and 0.50, respectively). Public administrations require an adequate digital infrastructure to implement transparency and guarantee information access to stakeholders on the web. Moreover, virtuous institutions tend to be more transparent. Therefore, it is not that surprising transparency is high, especially where digital education and trust in institutions are high. At the same time, the presence of women in political institutions, generally considered more pro-social and less inclined to corruption, may favor transparency. Conversely, the correlation between transparency and the other two dimensions of political participation is rather weak: 0.46 when considering civic and political participation and decreases to 0.15 when considering voter turnout. This evidence suggests transparency is somehow linked with informal channels of political information and participation, while the traditional channel of voting does not seem to play any role. This latter result might be explained by the fact that voter turnout is measured for European elections, which are traditionally less participative than national ones. However, it is worth noting that Italy generally has a higher turnout in European elections than other European countries (Fiorino et al. 2016). Moreover, the low correlation between voting and transparency is also confirmed when we use local voting turnout.[19]

Therefore, the above correlations are overall in line with the main conclusions of the literature on transparency, and seem to suggest CTI is a suitable indicator to measure transparency in Italy.

Conclusions

This paper addresses an issue that has not received attention so far in the literature, that is, whether there exists a relationship between transparency and equitable and sustainable well-being in Italy. To investigate such a relationship, we use a

[19]Data refer to 2014 (Istat 2014).

new indicator by Galli et al. (2017) to measure transparency. Considering the main conclusions reached in the literature on the determinants of transparency, we also use BES indicators representing digital, social, and politico-institutional dimensions. We provide evidence that, at regional level, there is correlation between transparency and some BES indicators in Italy, namely the intensity of Internet use, trust in institutions, social participation, and, to a lower extent, civic and informal political participation and women's participation in municipal councils. Overall, our results are in line with the conclusions reached in the literature on transparency and seem to confirm CTI appears to be a suitable indicator to measure transparency in Italy. Although caution is advised, this preliminary evidence suggests transparency can be a component of well-being, and such a relation is worth exploring. As such, further analysis is needed to investigate the determinants of transparency.

References

Albalate, D. (2013). The institutional, economic and social determinants of local government transparency. *Journal of Economic Policy Reform,* 16 (1), 90–107. doi: https://doi.org/10.1080/17487870.2012.759422.

Alcaraz-Quile, F.J., Navarro-Galera, A., Ortiz-Rodríguez, D. (2015). The influence of Administrative culture on sustainability transparency in European local governments. *Administration & Society,* 50 (4), 555–594. doi: https://doi.org/10.1177/0095399715616838.

Alt, J.E., Lassen, D.D., Rose, S. (2006). The causes of fiscal transparency: Evidence from the US States. *IMF Staff Papers* 30, 30–57.

Alatas V., Cameron, L., Chaudhuri, A., Erkal, N., Gangadharan, L. (2009). Gender, culture, and corruption: Insights from an experimental analysis. *Southern Economic Journal* 75(3), 663–680.

Bastida, F., Benito, B., Guillamón, M. (2011). The determinants of local governments' financial transparency. *Local Government Studies* 37(4), 391–406. doi: https://doi.org/10.1080/03003930.2011.588704.

Benito, B., Bastida, F. (2009). Budget transparency, fiscal performance, and political turnout: An international approach. *Public Administration Review* 69 (3), 403–417. doi:https://doi.org/10.1111/j.1540-6210.2009.01988.x.

Bertelli, A., Piotrowsky, S.J. (2010). *Measuring municipal transparency.* Unpublished paper prepared and presented at 14th IRSPM conference Bern. Switzerland on April 1.

CNEL-ISTAT, (2013). Comitato sulla misura del progresso in Italia. *La misurazione del Benessere equo e sostenibile*, Roma.

Caamaño-Alegre, J., Lago-Peñas, S., Reyes-Santias, F., Santiago-Boubeta, A. (2011). Budget transparency in local governments: An empirical analysis. *International Studies Program Working Paper* 11-02. Andrew Young School of Policy Studies. Georgia State University.

Cucciniello, M., Porumbescu, G.A., Grimmelikhuijsen, S. (2016). 25 years of transparency research: Evidence and future directions. *Public Administration Review,* 77(1), 32–44. doi: https://doi.org/10.1111/puar.12685.

Daughters, R., Harper L. (2007). Fiscal and Political Decentralization Reforms. In E. Lora (Ed.), *The State of State Reform in Latin America*, Inter-American Development Bank.Washington, D. C.

de Fine Licht, J., Naurin, D., Esaiasson, P., Gilljam, M. (2014). When does transparency generate legitimacy? Experimenting on a context-bound relationship. *Governance* 27(1), 111–134. doi:https://doi.org/10.1111/gove.12021.

Esteller, A., Polo-Otero, J. (2010). Análisis de losdeterminantes de la transparencia fiscal: Evidenciaempírica para losmunicipioscatalanes. *Documentos de Trabajo FUNCAS*. 560/2010.
Ferraz Esteves de Araujo, J.F., Tejedo-Romero, F. (2016). *Political and Economics Determinant of Information Transparency in Spanish Local Governments*. mimeo.
Fiorino, N., Ricciuti, R., Pontarollo. N. (2016). Voter turnout in the European Parliament Elections: A spatial analysis. *CESifo n. 5910.*
Frey, B.S., Stutzer, A. (2000). Happiness, economy and institutions. *The Economic Journal* 110(466), 918–938. doi: https://doi.org/10.1111/1468-0297.00570.
Galli, E., Rizzo, I., Scaglioni, C. (2017). Transparency, quality of institutions and performance in the Italian municipalities. *WP11/2017/DE/UECE*, ISEG, University of Lisbon.
Gasper, D. (2010). Understanding the diversity of conceptions of well-being and quality of life. *Journal of Socio-Economics*,39(3), 351–360.doi: https://doi.org/10.1016/j.socec.2009.11.006.
Grimmelikhuijsen, S.G, Meijer A.J. (2012). The effects of transparency on the perceived trustworthiness of a government organization: Evidence from an online experiment. *Journal of Public Administration Research and Theory*, 24 (1), 137–157. doi:https://doi.org/10.1093/jopart/mus048.
Islam, R. (2004). Do more transparent governments govern better?. *Policy Research Working Paper 3077,* World Bank.
Istat (2014). *Rapporto Bes 2014: il benessere equo e sostenibile in Italia*. Roma.
Jorge, S.M., Moura, P.S, Pattaro, A.F., Lourenço, P.R. (2011). *Local government financial transparency in Portugal and Italy: A comparative exploratory study on its determinants*. Paper presented at the 13th Biennial CIGAR conference held in Ghent (Belgium) on June 9–10.
Kumlin, S., Rothstein, B. (2005). Making and breaking social capital: The impact of the welfare state institutions. *Comparative Political Studies* 38(4), 339–365. doi: https://doi.org/10.1177/0010414004273203.
Nannicini, T., Stella, A., Tabellini, G., Troiano, U. (2013). Social Capital and Political Accountability. *American Economic Journal: Economic Policy*, 5 (2), 222–50. doi: https://doi.org/10.1257/pol.5.2.222.
Navarro Galera, A., de los Rios Berjillos, A. Lozano Ruiz M., Tirado Valencia, P. (2015). Identifying motivation of the local governments to improve the sustainability transparency. *Transylvanian Review of Administrative Sciences* 45(E), 149–167.
Park, H., Blenkinsopp, J. (2011). The roles of transparency and trust in the relationship between corruption and citizen satisfaction. *International Review of Administrative Sciences,* 77(2), 254–274. doi: https://doi.org/10.1177/0020852311399230.
Oates, W.E. (2008). On the evolution of fiscal federalism: Theory and institutions. *National Tax Journal*, 61(2), 313–334.
OECD (2011). *Compendium of OECD well-being indicators*. Paris.
OECD (2014). *How's Life in Your Region?: Measuring Regional and Local Well-being for Policy Making*. OECD Publishing, Paris. doi: https://doi.org/10.1787/9789264217416-en.
Piotrowski, S. J. (2008). *Governmental Transparency in the Path of Administrative Reform.* Albany. NY State: University of New York Press.
Piotrowski, S.J., Van Ryzin, G.G. (2007). Citizen attitudes towards transparency in local government. *The American Review of Public Administration,* 37(3), 306–323. doi: https://doi.org/10.1177/0275074006296777.
Stiglitz, J., Sen, A., Fitoussi, J.P. (2009). *Report by the Commission on Measurement of Economic and Social Progress*. Paris.
Swamy, A., Knack, S., Lee, Y.,Azfar, O. (2001). Gender and corruption. *Journal of Development Economics* 64(1), 25–55. doi: https://doi.org/10.1016/S0304-3878(00)00123-1.
Welch, E., Hinnant, C., Moon, C. (2005). Linking citizen satisfaction with e-government and trust in government. *Journal of Public Administration Research and Theory,* 15(3), 371–391. doi: https://doi.org/10.1093/jopart/mui021.
Worthy, B. (2010). More open but not more trusted? The effect of the freedom of information act 2000 on the United Kingdom central government. *Governance,* 23(4), 561–582. doi: https://doi.org/10.1111/j.1468-0491.2010.01498.x.

The Quality of Life in the Historic Centre of Naples: the use of PLS-PM Models to measure the Well-Being of the Citizens of Naples

Rosanna Cataldo, Fabio Corbisiero, Luigi Delle Cave, Maria Gabriella Grassia, Marina Marino, and Emma Zavarrone

Abstract How do the citizens of the historic centre of a city perceive the quality of their living conditions? The objective of this research has been to identify a series of indicators focused on the crucial aspects that, directly or indirectly, influence and determine the level of well-being of individuals and local communities in the city of Naples, describing and measuring specific social and local phenomena. In the survey, the same dimensions of the BES (Benessere Equo Sostenibile – Equitable and Sustainable Well-being) have been considered, together with others added ad hoc, relating to topics such as tourism and district, factors closely related to the character of the city's historic centre. In this paper we propose the use of Structural Equation Models, estimated using the Partial Least Squares-Path Modeling method, to measure the perception of the quality of life and to identify the weights of its dimensions and items.

R. Cataldo (✉)
Department of Economics and Statistical Science, University of Naples Federico II – Complesso di Monte S. Angelo, Naples, Italy
e-mail: rosanna.cataldo2@unina.it

F. Corbisiero · L. Delle Cave · M. G. Grassia · M. Marino
Department of Social Science, University of Naples Federico II – vico Monte della Pietà, Napoli, Italy
e-mail: fabio.corbisiero@unina.it; luigi.dellecave@unina.it; mgrassia@unina.it; mari@unina.it

E. Zavarrone
Department of Business, Law, Economics and Consumer Behaviour – "Carlo A. Ricciardi", University IULM - Via Carlo Bo, 1, Milan, Italy
e-mail: emma.zavarrone@iulm.it

A. Bianco et al. (eds.), *Italian Studies on Quality of Life*, Social Indicators Research Series 77, https://doi.org/10.1007/978-3-030-06022-0_8

Quality of Life in the Urban Context

Over the last few decades, the concept of quality of life has changed contextually with the changes in the needs of the population and in the cultural, social and value models of reference. The theoretical framework of the concept – developed from philosophical reflections on the primary and secondary needs of the individual (Inglehart 1983) – has gradually grown more complex in order to embrace a multitude of factors that situate the concept of quality of life at the heart of many disciplines (from economic to ecological, from psychological to sociological). National and international studies on this topic have contributed to the establishment of a research tradition that, starting from the results of the Movimento degli indicatori sociali (Social Movement Index) in the 1960s, has placed the state of the material and immaterial well-being of the citizens at the centre of the debate, with different undertones. As Nuvolati recalls (Nuvolati 2009, 2010), after the first important studies carried out in the 1970s and 1980s (Baldwin et al. 2002; Campbell et al. 1976; Szalai and Andrews 1980; Stull 1987), the number of research studies has been increasing, with theoretical insights into the concept of quality of life which have also involved several Italian scholars (Cicerchia 1996; Gadotti 1986; Graziosi 1979; Schifini 1988; Spanò 1989; Vergati 1985). In general, the close relationship between the dimensions of "quality of life" and "well-being" often makes the use of both terms in literature interchangeable, but what is important to emphasize in relation to the theoretical and methodological reflections on the quality of life is the constant reference to a multidimensional set of domains: economy, health, social relationships, environment, and security (Hajiran 2006). There is a widespread agreement among scholars of different disciplines in defining the quality of life as a broad concept, which includes the whole range of factors that affect our everyday life, beyond the strictly material aspects (Stiglitz et al. 2010). In the field of social sciences, the concept of quality of life represents a theoretical point of view through which to observe the changes related to lifestyles and to identify a series of problems that are assuming particular significance in post-industrial societies. These changes regard, in general, a multiplicity of dimensions (material and immaterial) that can be associated to (and can involve) the state of well-being of the individuals. Poverty, pollution, security, social isolation, the availability of services, for example, are just some of the factors that contribute to define the concept of quality of life and that are particularly evident when we analyse the "urban context". During the last years, the empirical research has paid particular attention to the study of the quality of life in urban contexts with the aim to estimate how liveable a city is in its multiple aspects. In this sense, talking about quality of life in the urban context means to analyse in depth the places where these phenomena are most striking and are able to affect the populations emerging needs, lifestyles and expectations. Such considerations lead us to analyse a context – the city – where economic and cultural factors, material and immaterial elements, intertwine and determine the quality of life as a result of a process that does not depend on the mere presence of an infrastructure but rather on the real use of the city itself. The urban space, in the physical and social sense, is the "boundary" in which the living conditions, accessibility and usability of services can affect the well-being of citizens. Although the quality of life in cities remains a phenomenon which is not simple to be read (Martinotti 1988), conditioned by the same complexity and size as the urban contexts (Gasparini 2000), analyzing the phenomenon is crucial in order to respond to the social needs of the citizens and is one of the main objectives of local government policies, also linked to the ability of the public actor to respond to the local needs.

The Survey: Objectives and Methodology

The objective of this research has been to identify a series of indicators focused on the crucial aspects that, directly or indirectly, influence and determine the level of well-being of individuals and local communities in the city of Naples, describing and measuring specific social and local phenomena. The historic centre of Naples represents an example of an urban settlement as an international historic layering of cultural, natural and social values. In 1995 the historic centre of Naples was recognized by UNESCO as a "world heritage site of humanity". It is the location of memories of the past, a geographical area in which a large part of the national cultural heritage is concentrated, in terms of both buildings and the wider urban fabric, consisting of streets, gardens and squares. It is an architectural heritage characterized by its intrinsic value, art as a historical message, with extremely productive yet not fully effective cultural districts. However, it is also characterized by certain peculiarities that often compromise the quality of life of its citizens, having a significant impact on the well-being of the individuals living in the area on a daily basis. In particular, the research has focused on the identification of subjective social indicators for the evaluation and perception of whether and how far the citizen is satisfied with his/her living conditions.[1] When we examine the concept of quality of life at the urban level and try to measure it and evaluate it, we are faced with a difficult challenge, both methodologically and theoretically, as structured initiatives in this direction are not yet widespread. The data are not easily accessible, and, above all, they have been collected and systematized little, badly and unevenly. For this reason, the questionnaire was designed in order to analyze the perceptions expressed by the respondents with respect to a list of issues that affect the individual and collective well-being. In this research we considered as the starting point one of the most articulate and well-constructed achievements in the research of an alternative measurement of well-being: the BES, an indicator of Equitable and Sustainable Well-being. This project was stimulated by the belief that the parameters against which to evaluate the progress of a society should not be only economic,

[1] While objective social indicators are statistics which represent social facts independent of personal evaluation, subjective social indicators are measures of individual perceptions and evaluations of social conditions (Noll 2004).

but also social and environmental, accompanied by measurements of inequality and sustainability. The BES has been taken as a reference point. Our questionnaire is making use of some of its dimensions and related items; other dimensions have been added ad hoc. In detail, out of the twelve dimensions of the BES, nine dimensions have been chosen to build the questionnaire because they have been considered to be dimensions closely linked to the concept of perceived quality of life in the historic centre contest. They are: "Environment", "Economic Well-Being", "Social Relations", "Personal Safety", "Subjective Well-Being", "Landscape and Cultural Heritage", "Quality of Services", "Work and Reconciliation of Life Time" and "Education and Training". In particular these last two dimensions have merged into a single block "Personal data". Three dimensions have not been considered in building the questionnaire: "Health", "Research and Innovation", "Politics and Institutions", because they are mainly quantitative in size and, for matters pertaining to the METRICS project, they have been considered to be topics not strictly related to the concept of perceived quality of life of the citizens of Naples historic centre. Two dimensions have been added ad hoc such as "Tourism" and "District", factors closely related to the city's historic centre. In particular tourism in recent years has become activity that enables the influx of tourists throughout the year, and therefore the citizens of the historic center must live daily with the constant presence of tourists. This situation on the one hand can be positive for the local economy but on the other hand it can negatively affect the quality of life of citizens. All of these dimensions have been taken into account in the measurement of the quality of life of the citizens of Naples historic centre, combining dimensions that directly or indirectly affect and determine the level of well-being of individuals and local communities. The questionnaire consists of 7 thematic sections:

- *The District* (7 questions)
  This dimension concerns the level of satisfaction of the respondents with respect to their living conditions and their level of knowledge of the neighbourhood;
- *Environment and Tourism* (5 questions)
  The environment in which the citizens live strongly affects their well-being. From the resources that feed the production and the economy, to the pleasure that the contact with nature gives us, human well-being is inextricably linked and dependent on the environment. Tourism is not always a positive resource for the quality of life of citizens, and therefore it is useful to analyze the impact that it exerts on the local population;
- *Quality of Services* (11 questions)
  The analysis of well-being and of the opportunities of progress requires an assessment of the infrastructure and the provision of services, reinterpreting them in light of their functionality and efficiency, the degree of use, measures of accessibility, the quality of the service generated and any possible congestion;
- *Networks and Social Relations* (5 questions)
  The intensity of the social relationships that are maintained and the social network in which they are placed not only affects the psycho-physical well-being

of the individual, but represents a form of "investment" that can strengthen the effects of human and social capital;

- *Safety* (5 questions)

  Personal security is a fundamental element in the well-being of individuals. The most important impact of crime on the well-being of people is the sense of vulnerability that it determines. The fear of being a victim of criminal acts can greatly affect your personal freedom, your quality of life, and the development of the area. The issue of violence is also closely related to personal safety and quality of life;
- *Subjective well-being* (3 questions)

  The assessment of subjective well-being is considered by citizens as one of the most important elements in the evaluation of general well-being; and
- *Personal data* (10 questions)

  Professional status, type of contract and income are crucial determinants that strongly affect the perception of an individual's quality of life.

Most of the dimensions were detected by using measurement scales that connect the degree of "agreement" or "disagreement" with specific statements, in order to understand the opinions of respondents with respect to the different thematic sections. In other cases, multiple choice questions were formulated. The statistical population forming the subject of this study consists in the population of the residents of the historic centre of Naples. The unit of analysis in this case is represented by the individual resident. As a sampling list, it was decided to use the electoral lists, made available by the Municipal Election Office. From this list, a simple random sample was chosen. The quality of life is considered in this work as a Composite Indicator (CI). CIs, in the social sciences, are used increasingly frequently for the measurement of very complex phenomena, such as poverty, progress and well-being (Mazziotta and Pareto 2011; Salzman 2003). The goal of much research in the social, economic and political fields is to obtain a whole description of the various facets of a complex phenomenon, through a suitable synthesis of the associated elementary indicators (EIs) (Lauro et al. 2017). Accordingly, a CI can be considered as a latent concept, not directly measurable, whose estimation can be obtained through the values of the Manifest Variables (MVs). The existing literature offers different alternative methods in order to obtain a CI. The Structural Equation Models (SEMs) (Wold 1985), estimated using the Partial Least Squares-Path Modeling method (PLS-PM) (Tenenhaus et al. 2005), can be used to compute a system of CIs. According to this methodology, it is possible to define a CI as a multidimensional Latent Variable (LV) not measurable directly and related to its single indicators or MVs by either a reflective or formative relationship or by both (this defines the measurement or outer model). Each CI is related to other CIs, in a systemic vision, by linear regression equations specifying the so called Structural Model (or Inner Model). So, we use the PLS-PM to measure the perception of the quality of life and to identify the weights of its dimensions and items. Indeed, the quality of life is linked with other constructs (environment, tourism, quality of services, networks and social relations, safety, subjective and economic well-being, education and training) representing the different dimensions, that are not directly observable but are connected to the single MVs by a reflective relationship. The choice of using the PLS-PM as the methodological framework was made for several reasons. Specifically, it provides:

- the possibility of obtaining, simultaneously and coherently with the estimation method, a ranking of individuals for specific indicators;
- the possibility of comparing systemic indicators in space and in time;
- the possibility of estimating the hypothesized relationships without making assumptions about data distribution;
- the possibility of defining an optimal system of weightings;
- the possibility of working with a large number of variables and a few observations;
- the possibility of estimating complex models without any problems of identification of the model; and
- the possibility of working with missing data and in the presence of multicollinearity.

The PLS-PM approach to SEM consists of an iterative algorithm that computes the estimation of the LVs, measured by a set of MVs, and the relationships between them, by means of an interdependent system of equations based on multiple and simple regression. The idea is to determine the scores of the LVs through a process, that, iteratively, computes first an outer and then an inner estimation. PLS-PM is a suitable tool for the investigation of models with a high level of abstraction, in cases where the building of a system of CIs depends on different levels of construction. Higher-order constructs in PLS-PM are considered as explicit representations of multidimensional constructs that exist at a higher level of abstraction and are related to other constructs at a similar level of abstraction, completely mediating their influence from or to their underlying dimensions (Chin 1998). This theoretical model is used in order to estimate the higher-order CI, "perceived quality of life". In particular, the Mixed Two-Step Approach has been developed, proposed by Cataldo (Cataldo 2016), using the "plspm" package in the R statistical software (Sanchez and Trinchera 2012).

The Dimensions of the Quality of Life in Naples Historic Centre

During the survey, a total of 312 completed questionnaires were collected. The sample of respondents is therefore characterized by a deep knowledge of the problems of the historic centre: many of these individuals have grown up in the neighbourhood and have chosen to live there even after leaving the nuclear family, moving to live on their own or to create their own family but staying in the same area. From a first analysis of the data, the main issues that seem to

Table 1 The dimensions of the quality of life

Interventions to improve the environmental quality	
(1 not important; 5 very important)	
	Mean
Cleaning the public area	3.6
Securing the buildings	3.0
Improving the street furniture	3.0
Tourist flows contribute to:	
(1 not agree; 5 completely agree)	
	Mean
Improving the economy of the area	4.8
Increasing the prestige of the area	4.3
Making the area more "lively"	4.0
Factors of social insecurity	
(1 not important; 5 very important)	
	Mean
Micro-criminality	3.4
Racketeering, the "camorra"	3.3
Subjective well-being: particular conditions	
(1 not satisfied; 5 completely satisfied)	
	Mean
Relationships	3.8
Health	3.6
Free time	3.1
Economic status	2.7
Safety	2.5

impact on the quality of life of the respondents can be summarized as follows (Table 1): on the environmental quality, "cleaning the public area" represents, in the perception of the interviewees, the factor on which it is necessary to take action, followed by "securing the buildings" and "improving the street furniture (roads, manholes, benches, sidewalks, etc.)". Specifically, the use of public spaces plays an important role in the respondents perceptions. For those who live in the city historic centre public spaces acquire a special significance in the everyday practices of socialization. Among the most significant features of this area are its lively night life and its high tourist density. This continuous crowding, however, sometimes hinders the collection of garbage thus reducing the public spaces cleanliness.

The aspects mentioned above are those that, more than the others, the interviewees regarded as important for the improvement of the whole area, whose relevance is even higher if we consider the huge growth of tourism during the last five years.

The dimension of tourism is, in fact, an important driving factor for the economic development of the area. The respondents seemed to be aware of the socio-economic and cultural value that tourist flows can generate. Although the particular urban structure of the whole area, characterized by narrow streets and lanes which can become very crowded during periods of strong tourism, can create inconvenience in many periods of the year, the majority of the respondents considered tourism as a resource for the local economy that enhances the prestige of the area and makes it more attractive and lively. No negative implications seem to emerge with respect to the way citizens perceive the dimension of tourism and relate it to the perception of their quality of life. All the items included in the questionnaire which explore any forms of inconvenience that might be attributed to the increase of tourist flows show low scores, confirming the positive effect that tourism has on the citizens of the area. Therefore, which are the main factors of social insecurity? Micro-criminality, racketeering and the Camorra (the main Neapolitan crime syndicate) are the phenomena that achieve the highest average rating among the issues examined. The respondents generally agree in confirming the presence of criminal episodes in the area, but the results of the survey do not allow us to assign these phenomena an important role in determining a clearly negative impression of the quality of life in this neighbourhood. Criminality does not seem to erode the satisfaction of living within the historic centre and, in spite of criminal episodes, the respondents do not perceive the area as particularly dangerous. Even the literature on crime security and the quality of life in Naples is ambiguous on this aspect, and our research did not show a very significant association either. Based on this analysis, insecurity does not seem to have a strong impact on the perception of the quality of life (average 2.5 Table 1). Generally, the respondents have a positive perception of their own life and well-being, positively related (above all) by the relationship and health dimensions. As shown in Table 1, no dimensions appear to have a significant importance on the quality of life of the citizens of the historic centre. Based on the average ratings, we can assume that the dimensions listed in the table do not condition the subjective perception of well-being. Additionally, economic conditions do not constitute a determining factor: the majority of the sample (65%) declared that they had no economic difficulties. The interviewees income did not modify their perception of quality of life and their styles of consumption. The same result emerges in an analysis of the student cluster, where economic status enters only marginally in the self-evaluation of their own well-being. The most significant aspects concern health and personal relationships. More than 70% of respondents had no serious health problems. The factor which best reveals the perceived individual well-being is that relating to relationships. The respondents are very satisfied with their own networks of family and friends which serve to construct their social capital.

From the Concept of Quality of Life to a Synthesis Indicator: Towards the Construction of a Composite Indicator

The graphical representation of the higher-order perceived quality of life construct is reported in Fig. 1. It represents the structural model that has been developed in order to analyse the quality of life perceived by the citizens of the historic centre of

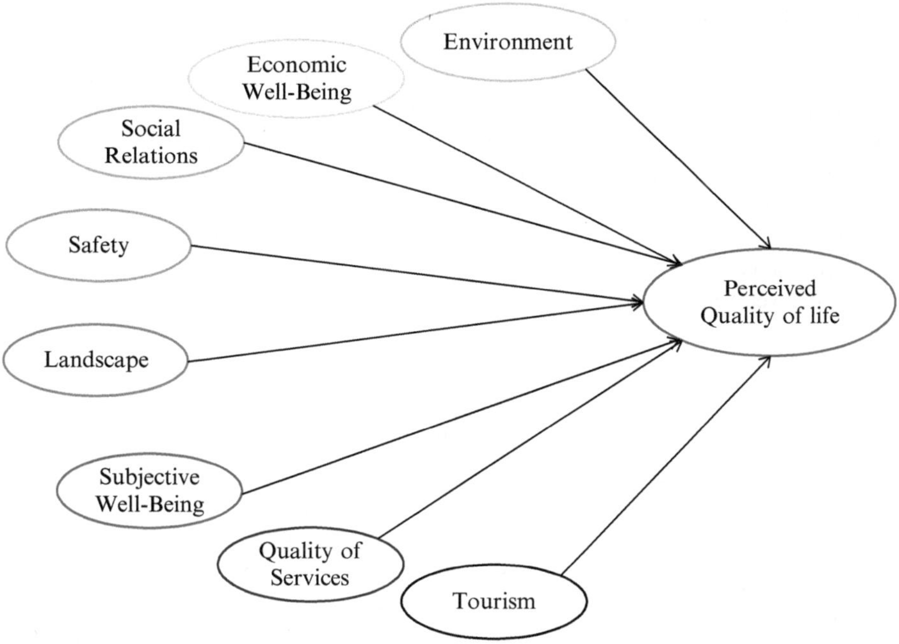

Fig. 1 PLS-PM structural model to analyse the perceived quality of life

Naples from different dimensions. This means that there is a formative relationship between the exogenous blocks and the endogenous block. It consists of 8 LVs, which represent the sections of the questionnaire, and 44 MVs, all measured on an ordinal Likert scale from 1 to 5. These LVs are linked to the higher-order LV "Perceived Quality of Life".

Before completing the PLS-PM analysis, a pre-treatment of the data was performed. First of all, the two scales were normalized with scores from 0 to 100 to make them homogeneous. Since the questionnaire was composed of items in a Likert Scale with a range from 1 to 5, the normalization made the data belonging to the different variables comparable. Next, the variables that had a low average and low correlation with the other variables in the block were removed from the analysis. The final database was composed of 44 variables on 312 individuals. The analysis was performed with a centroid scheme for the inner structural model, while the measurement model is reflective in each block. The reflective measurement model means that the LV is assumed to be a common factor that reflects itself in the MVs (Mode A). In the reflective case, the MVs should be highly correlated, due to fact that they are correlated with the LV of which they are an expression. In other words, the block should be homogeneous. There are several tools for checking the homogeneity and unidimensionality of a reflective block: Cronbachs Alpha; Dillon-Goldsteins Rho and Principal Component Analysis of a block. In this case all the blocks are unidimensional, as it is possible to verify from Table 2 in which the

Table 2 Block unidimensionality

LVs	Mode	MVs	Alpha Cronbach	Dillon Goldstein's Rho	First eigenvalue	Second eigenvalue
Environment	A	7	0.717	0.805	2.64	1.045
Safety	A	5	0.786	0.855	2.73	0.802
Economic well-being	A	5	0.705	0.758	2.17	1.011
Social relations	A	5	0.691	0.753	1.91	0.941
Landscape	A	7	0.805	0.858	3.26	0.982
Quality of services	A	5	0.767	0.742	1.57	0.707
Subjective well-being	A	5	0.724	0.820	2.40	0.904
Tourism	A	5	0.722	0.702	2.16	1.167

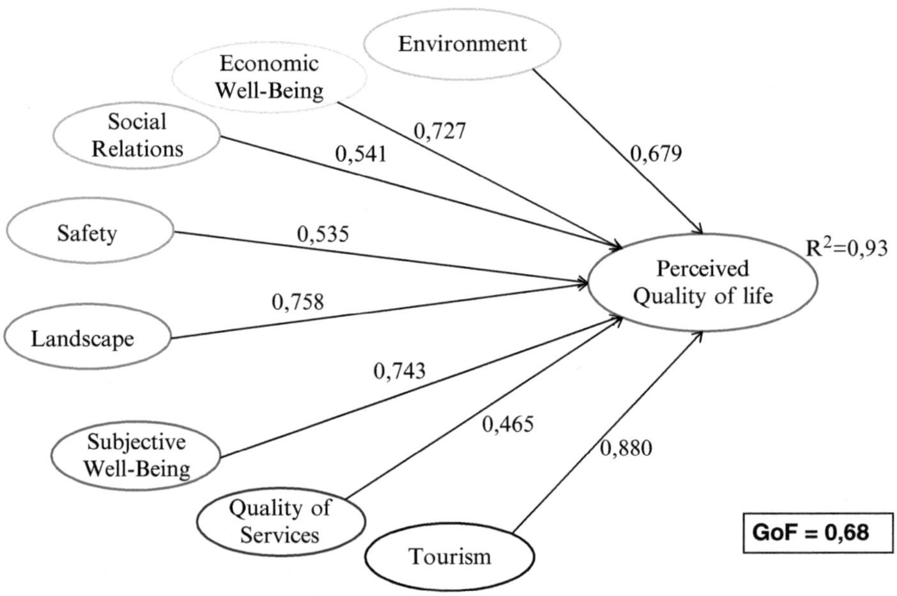

Fig. 2 Path coefficients and goodness of fit of a PLS-PM model to analyse the perceived quality of life

values of Cronbachs Alpha and Dillon-Goldsteins Rho are reported (the values of Dillon-Goldsteins Rho are greater than 0.7, and the first eigenvalues are greater than 1 for all LVs). This result shows that the outer model is well specified and that the LVs are well measured by the MVs, their synthesis being good.

The most interesting result of a SEM is the estimate of the values of the concepts of interest obtained through a weighting system assigned to both the indicators associated with each latent concept and the dependency network that links the different concepts to one another. A knowledge of these weights allows an evaluation of the influence of the different dimensions of the phenomenon on the final result. Figure 2 shows the value of the linear determination index $R2$ which reveals the goodness of the model in predicting LV scores, indicating how much of the information in the questionnaire is well synthesized by the model. The value on the arrows represents the impact of each LV on the final block. The coefficient indicates that an increase by one point in the LV level leads to an increase in value in the quality of life index.

As we can see from the graph, the high *R*2 indices show a good predictive power for all structural relations; the questionnaire information, thus, is well synthesized by the model. From an analysis of the path coefficients it emerges that each dimension has a significant impact on the final block: it is noteworthy that they all have a high impact, with the exception of the blocks of Quality of Services (0.465), Safety (0.535) and Social Relations (0.541). Tourism has the strongest impact among all the dimensions, this meaning that this dimension is an important lever to increase the perceived quality of life. Table 3 presents the loading for each MV, that is the ordinary least squares coefficient of a simple regression of the MV on its LV, which describes how the MV reflects the corresponding LV.

The loading measures the contribution that each single indicator separately makes to the relevance of the construct with which it is associated. As can be noted from Table 3, for all the dimensions of the model, almost all the variables have a loading greater than 0.60, with the exception of some variables, in particular "Noise" and the "Possibility of parking" for the Environment, "Home" and "Income" for the "Economic well-being", "Political parties" for the Social relations, "Kilometres travelled per day" and "Use of subways" for the Quality of services, and the "Possibility of creating employment" for Tourism. These considerations are very useful in identifying the most critical points and thus establishing a strategy that improves the scales of dimensions and individual factors with respect to the perceived quality of life.

In Table 4 the impacts and means of each dimensions are reported.

It is important to emphasize that, in addition to verifying which dimensions have a greater impact on the quality of life, we should also take into account the average scores calculated for these blocks. Only the combined reading of these two pieces of information (impacts and average scores) allows us to identify the so-called levers for improvement, as it suggests in which critical areas it is recommended to intervene and with what urgency. A key characteristic of the PLS-PM method is the construction of a decision matrix. This matrix is a simple and valid tool to support the diagnosis and detection of such levers. It consists of a dispersion graph that allows each variable to be positioned based on the average score (coordinated on the x-axis) and on the estimated impact on the target LV (coordinated on the y-axis). The matrix is divided into four areas: the first area is the most critical area, because the variables have a high impact but a low mean value; the second is the area of the monitoring, in which the variables have a low value both for the mean and the path coefficient; the third is the area to be improved because the variables have a high mean value and a low path coefficient; finally, the fourth is the area to be maintained, in which variables have a high value both for the mean and for the path coefficient. Figure 3 show a decision matrix of the perceived quality of life.

Table 3 Measurement model estimates

LV	MVs	Loadings
Environment	Street cleaning	0.652
	Possibility of parking	0.449
	Noise	0.390
	Public lighting	0.698
	Protected areas	0.624
	Street furniture	0.680
	Housing	0.601
	Selling drugs	0.759
	Selling smuggled goods	0.757
Safety	Micro-criminality	0.786
	Racketeering, camorra	0.734
	Vandalism against private property	0.598
	Home	0.393
	Home size	0.855
Economic well-being	Home aesthetics	0.845
	Home location	0.733
	Income	0.220
	Associations	0.871
	Union	0.410
Social relations	Political parties	0.229
	Religious initiatives	0.558
	Voluntary work	0.559
	Ecological days	0.696
	Electric bus	0.676
	Free transport	0.474
Landscape	Garbage disposal	0.738
	Cleaning common area	0.774
	Upgrading street furniture	0.715
	Police controls	0.662
	Kilometres travelled per day	0.351
	Use of trams/bus	0.598
Quality of services	Use of subways	0.322
	Use of cycle lanes	0.425
	Health service	0.689
	Happiness	0.750
	Economic conditions	0.710
Subjective well-being	Health	0.775
	Free time	0.602
	Relationships with family members	0.599
	Increase in economy	0.510
	Not creating inconvenience for residents	0.671
Tourism	Possibility of creating employment	0.396
	Not making the neighbourhood dirty	0.695
	Facilitating a multi-ethnic society	0.786

Table 4 Impacts and means of each dimension of the model

LVs	Path coefficients	Mean
Environment	0.679	4.44
Safety	0.727	5.92
Economic well-being	0.541	5.61
Social relations	0.535	5.46
Landscape	0.758	7.58
Quality of services	0.743	6.90
Subjective well-being	0.465	4.72
Tourism	0.880	5.54

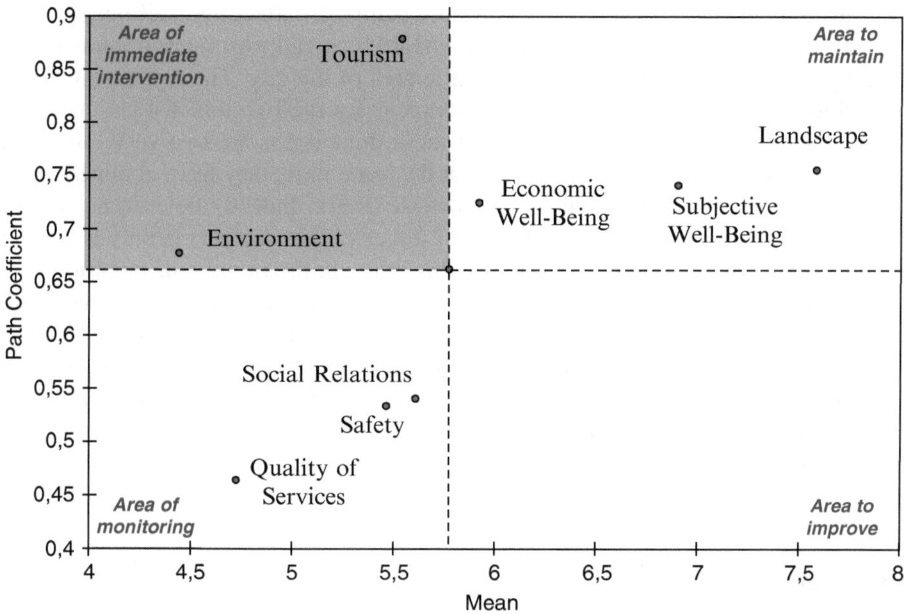

Fig. 3 The decision matrix of the quality of life

As you can immediately notice the dimensions of Tourism and Environment fall into the area of immediate intervention, as they have a very high impact but a low average. This means that these dimensions are two very important levers to increase the quality of life but, at the same time, they have obtained a low average rating from the citizens of the historic centre of Naples. They represent dimensions which need a great effort to be improved. It remains to be seen, however, if, in constructing this discourse, there can be a "voice" for all those Neapolitans whose quality of life is being affected by the future directions of the city.

Conclusions and Future Perspectives

The goal of this research has been to analyze the perceived quality of life in the historic centre of Naples by identifying the crucial aspects that influence and determine the level of well-being of individuals in this area of the city. The work is part of the project METRICS whose research area is the historic centres of cities. For this reason the statistical population forming the subject of this study has been the population of residents in this area of Naples, one of the most famous cities in the world. In this paper we have used Structural Equation Models, estimated using the Partial Least Squares-Path Modeling method, in order to understand how the various dimensions, considered in a questionnaire, can affect the well-being of the citizens and, above all, what dimensions should receive investment to improve the quality of life of the citizens of the historic area of the city. The results show that the dimensions of tourism and the environment are the two dimensions that need immediate intervention. This means that these dimensions are two very important levers to improve the quality of life but, at the same time, they have obtained a low average rating from the citizens of the historic centre. Indeed, the citizens declare little satisfaction with these two aspects of the city. This analysis is only a starting point, a first exploratory investigation of this issue. In the future, our intention is to extend the analysis to all citizens of the metropolis and above all to consider not only the perceptions of the citizens relating to these aspects but also to analyze objective indicators of each dimension. These are topics on which our research group is already working. Moreover, the idea is to propose this model with these dimensions to analyze the perceived quality of life in the historic centres of all the major Italian cities.

References

Baldwin, Sally and Godfrey, Christine and Propper, Carol: Quality of life: Perspectives and policies. Routledge (2002)

Campbell, Angus and Converse, Philip E and Rodgers, Willard L.: The quality of American life: Perceptions, evaluations, and satisfactions. Russell Sage Foundation (1976)

Cataldo, Rosanna: Developments in PLS-PM for the building of a System of Composite Indicators. Ph.D Thesis. Universita‘ degli Studi di Napoli Federico II (2016)

Chin, Wynne W: The partial least squares approach to structural equation modeling, Modern methods for business research, 295, 2, 295–336, (1998)

Cicerchia, Annalisa: Indicators for the measurement of the quality of urban life. Social indicators research, 39 (3), 321–358, Springer (1996)

Gadotti, G: Riflessioni sulla definizione e misurazione della qualit a‘ della vita.Sociologia ur- bana e rurale, 8 (21), 129–146, ITA (1986)

Gasparini, A.: La sociologia degli spazi. Carocci (2000)

Graziosi, M.: Problemi nella misurazione del benessere sociale: indicatori oggettivi e sogget- tivi. Quaderni di sociologia 28 (1), 71–101. (1979)

Hajiran, H.: Toward a quality of life theory: net domestic product of happiness. Social Indicators Research, 75 (1), 31–43, Springer (2006)

Inglehart, R: La rivoluzione silenziosa, ed. it. a cura di M, Rodriguez, Rizzoli, Milano (1983)
Lauro, Natale Carlo and Grassia, Maria Gabriella and Cataldo, Rosanna: Model Based Composite Indicators: New Developments in Partial Least Squares-Path Modeling for the Building of Different Types of Composite Indicators, Social Indicators Research, 1–35. (2017)
Martinotti, G.: Problemi di metodo per una analisi della qualit a' della vita urbana nelle grandi citta' italiane, Schmidt Di Friedberg P.(a cura di), Gli indicatori ambientali, valori, metri e strumenti nello studio dellimpatto ambientale, Angeli, Milano, 575–615 (1988)
Mazziotta, M and Pareto, A.: Nuove misure del benessere: dal quadro teorico alla sintesi degli indicatori, SISmagazine, rivista on-line della Societa´ Italiana di Statistica (2011)
Noll, Heinz-Herbert: Social indicators and Quality of Life research: Background, achievements and current trends, Advances in sociological knowledge 151–181, Springer (2004)
Nuvolati, G.: Quality of life in cities: A question of mobility and accessibility, Quality of life and the millennium challenge, 177–191, Springer (2009)
Nuvolati, G.: La qualit della vita, Quaderni di Sociologia, 52, 97–111 (2010)
Salzman, J.: Methodological choices encountered in the construction of composite indices of economic and social well-being, Centre for the study of living standards (2003)
Sanchez, G and Trinchera, L: plspm: Partial Least Squares data analysis methods, R package version 0.2–2, URL http://CRAN.R-project.org/package=plspm (2012)
Schifini, D'Andrea S.: Livello e qualit a' della vita, Dipartimento Statistico, Universita' degli Studi di Firenze, Firenze (1988)
Szalai, Alexander and Andrews, Frank M.: The quality of life: Comparative studies. Beverly Hills, CA: Sage (1980)
Spanò, A.: Benessere e felicita' nella prospettiva della teoria della qualita' della vita, La critica sociologica, (90) (91), 69–120 (1989)
Stiglitz, Joseph E and Sen, Amartya and Fitoussi, Jean-Paul: Report by the commission on the measurement of economic performance and social progress, Paris: Commission on the Measurement of Economic Performance and Social Progress (2010)
Stull, Donald E.: Conceptualization and measurement of well-being: Implications for policy evaluation, Critical issues in aging policy: linking research and values/edited by Edgar F. Borgatta, Rhonda JV Montgomery. Newbury Park, Calif.: Sage Publications (1987)
Tenenhaus, Michel and Vinzi, Vincenzo Esposito and Chatelin, Yves-Marie and Lauro, Carlo: PLS path modeling, Computational statistics & data analysis, 48, 1, 159–205 (2005)
Vergati, S.:Dimensioni sociali e territoriali della qualita'della vita, Euroma (1989) 26.Wold, Herman: Partial least squares, Encyclopedia of statistical sciences, (1985)
Wold, Herman: Partial least squares, Encyclopedia of statistical sciences, (1985)

The Incidence of Sin Taxes: Evidence from Italy

Enrico di Bella, Luca Gandullia, Lucia Leporatti, and Marcello Montefiori

Abstract The term "sin goods" is used to identify goods or services whose consumption can be considered self-destructive for individuals and source of negative externalities for the entire society. The potentially harmful nature of sin goods makes these categories of products subject to special fiscal rules. The regulation of sin goods markets in Italy deeply changed over the last 15 years, and it has now reached a particularly complex and potential unfair taxation system. In this paper, we analyse the fairness of the Italian taxation system applied to sin goods in order to measure their economic incidence. After investigating the Italian taxation on sin goods, we analyze and compare their degree of regressivity using data of the Italian Household Budget Survey (HBS). Results show that, among "sin taxes", gambling taxes can be considered the most regressive form of taxation, followed by cigarettes and beer.

Introduction

The term "sin taxes" is used to identify taxes charged on a class of products and services considered sources of risky behaviours, such as cigarettes, alcoholic beverages and gambling, generally called "sin goods". The peculiar nature of sin goods makes them subject to special rules both from the regulatory and taxation perspective. First, sin goods are not basic goods, and therefore a high taxation is generally accepted. Second, they themselves have an inelastic demand curve, and consequently they represent an efficient tax base. However, the intrinsic nature of sin goods opens a series of ethical and moral issues that make the identification of an optimal taxation scheme a particularly tricky task. Taxation of sin goods requires several decisions able to cope with the efficiency/equity trade off (Clotfelter 2005).

E. di Bella · L. Gandullia
Department of Political Science, University of Genoa, Genoa, Italy
e-mail: edibella@unige.it; luca.gandullia@unige.it

L. Leporatti (✉) · M. Montefiori
Department of Economics and Business Studies, University of Genoa, Genoa, Italy
e-mail: lucia.leporatti@unige.it; montefiori@unige.it

A. Bianco et al. (eds.), *Italian Studies on Quality of Life*, Social Indicators Research Series 77, https://doi.org/10.1007/978-3-030-06022-0_9

Several studies have been developed to guide policy makers and appropriate tax schemes have been identified to balance efficiency and equity (O'Donoghue and Rabin 2006). However, most of the countries still adopt particularly complex tax designs, difficult to be evaluated and in conflict with the economic theory (Bird 2015).

During the last decade, the regulation applied to sin goods in Italy have been widely reformed.

The tobacco industry has been recently involved in significant changes in terms of taxation rules (Liberati and Paradiso 2014), and available products (e.g. electronic cigarettes). In the alcoholic beverages' sector, most of the European countries have adopted new policy actions, such as the strict drinking and driving limits, addressed to the protection of adolescents and vulnerable individuals from the negative outcomes derived from an excessive alcohol consumption (Allamani et al. 2014).

Gambling has been by far the most broadly reformed sector. Several new forms of gambling have been legalized and the number of authorized retailers exploded, leading Italy to be by far the largest market in Europe, representing more than 20% of total EU27 (H2 Gambling Capital 2013). More in detail, the Italian gambling market received a great boost after 2003 when new forms of entertainment machines (i.e. New Slots) have been legalized outside casinos; since 2003 entertainment machines in Italy can indeed be placed in several economic activities (e.g. cafes, tobacconist, supermarkets, restaurants), and, consequently, gambling opportunities during routine life exploded. The liberalization of the Italian gambling market has been completed in the period 2003–2009 through the introduction of several instant lotteries tickets and through the legalization of remote gambling in 2008. The expansion of gambling opportunities led gambling turnover to increase by 483% from 2003 to 2015 with an average yearly per capita gross turnover equal to 1455 € and an effective expenditure, after subtracting winnings, of 282 € (AAMS 2015). Despite its relevance, the Italian gambling market and its taxation have not been deeply explored by the literature.

The present study is organized in two parts. The first part compares the different taxation schemes of sin goods in use in Italy. The investigation of national fiscal policies is the first step towards fiscal harmonization and towards the analysis of equity issues. The second part focuses on the evaluation of the regressivity of the current systems applied to such a category of products. More in detail, we make use of the Italian Household Budget Survey (HBS, ISTAT) data to evaluate the relationship between households' consumption of the four most relevant sin goods (i.e. cigarettes, beer, wine and gambling) and their socio-economic status. Additional comparisons will be provided with other five categories of consumption goods that have been found to be particularly relevant in households' budget (i.e. bread and cereals, meat and fish, vegetables, clothing, recreational and cultural products).

The Taxes on Sin

Sin Goods and Taxes

According to Galizzi (2012), decision makers, to control sin goods consumption, generally adopt three policy actions: releasing of information on health risks due to sin goods use or abuse; introducing financial disincentives; changing the taxation mechanism. This latter option to control risky behaviors is relatively new but it may be effective given that sin goods are subject to widely different tax regimes (i.e. excises) with respect to ordinary consumption goods[1]. Although one of the main goals of government's fiscal policy is income redistribution, suitable taxation schemes also should be intended to control and curb the consumption of "harmful products". Traditional economic theories argue that taxes on sin goods should be imposed to meet three objectives (Clotfelter 2005): (i) to maximize tax revenues; (ii) to devolve tax revenues to the treatment of the social costs arising from their consumption; (iii) to partially discourage the consumption of such goods. However, the identification of the correct level of sin taxes able to meet the aforesaid objectives represents a particularly challenging task and a high-pitched debate on the designing and implementation of appropriate taxation schemes is still open and supported by the World Health Organization. Several issues should indeed be taken into account. The consumption of sin goods causes an immediate or medium-long term negative impact on consumers' health also referred to as "negative internality" (Herrnstein et al. 1993) (i.e., "costs that consumers impose on themselves but that they do not sufficiently take into account in their decisions", Galizzi 2012). The government's intervention can be therefore justified as a way to make consumers of sin goods aware of the risks of smoking, drinking and gambling. A first controversy concerns the precarious balance between public policies addressed towards curbing consumption of sin goods and the freedom of choice of consumers (Lorenzi 2004; Haile 2009). Second, the consumption of sin goods generates negative externalities also for the entire society (e.g., additional healthcare costs due to smoking or heavy drinking) (Pigou 1920; Baumol 1972). As a result, it is common sense to consider sin taxes as an instrument of social compensation for the additional external costs borne by the society. Henceforth, setting sufficiently high tax rates to sin goods is generally considered a good instrument to yield social benefits (Pogue and Sgontz 1989). Moreover, collecting revenues from sin taxes represent a relatively easy task for the government due to the inelasticity of sin goods' demand curve: the addictive/habitual nature of this category of goods makes consumers' demand little responsive to a price increase (Lorenzi 2004).

In order to achieve the aforesaid goals, sin taxes systems should be properly designed and decision makers should take several decisions, particularly on the

[1]Excises are also applied to the consumption of petroleum products; we decided on purpose not to consider these products since excise taxation applied to oils has the main aim of contrasting traffic and pollution and not to reach healthier lifestyles.

composition between specific and *ad valorem* taxes as well as the adoption of uniform or differentiated rates. The internalization of externalities seems to favour the adoption of specific taxes, whereas *ad valorem* schemes tend to amplify price differences across products leading consumers to buy cheaper products rather than reducing their consumption (Clotfelter 2005).

In addition to these issues, previous studies have shown that the consumption of sin goods significantly varies over different demographic, social and racial groups leading to a problem of horizontal equity. People in the same economic condition but different for age, ethnicity or social background (just to quote some), can indeed contribute differently to sin tax revenues (Borg et al. 1990; Hansen 1995; Mikesell 1989). It has been showed (Kitchen and Powells 1991) that socioeconomic variables have a role in determining gambling expenditure, in particular the level of education, occupational status, family structure, geographical residence. In addition, the impact of the socio-economic variables turn out to be differentiated across different games (Layton and Worthington 1999). For what it concerns strictly economic determinants of sin goods expenditure, the results of most of the previous studies are concordant is stating that people belonging to the weaker social classes are those most attracted by the consumption of sin goods (Sammartino 1990; Clotfelter and Cook 1991; Hansen 1995). Even if expenditure increases as income rises, the increase is less than proportional. This means that lower income individuals contribute relatively more than higher income individuals to generate tax revenues and, consequently to pay the public services, making sin taxes regressive forms of taxation (Lyon and Schwab 1997; Price and Novak 1999; Remler 2004; Beckert and Lutter 2009). A vast debate exists on the selection of an appropriate measure of household's economic wellbeing on which regressivity should be assessed. Most of previous literature proposed an income-based approach; however, independently of income, the level of consumption can be smoothed by adjusting savings or borrowing money. As a consequence, IFS (2011) recommends the use of an expenditure approach since it allows to take into account borrowing and saving decisions. Differently from IFS, OECD (2014) suggests the use of an income-based approach when the interest is in the immediate distributional effects, whereas an expenditure-based approach would be more suitable to analyse the lifetime distributional effect.

In Italy, some studies have been proposed on the optimal taxation scheme for sin goods (Jones and Mazzi 1996; Liberati and Paradiso 2014). The research on potential regressivity of gambling tax is a rarity: this is partially due to the great difficulty in finding suitable data on gambling expenditure by a sufficiently disaggregated area (e.g. by ZIP code) or derived by surveys. The first attempt to fill this research gap has been proposed by Sarti and Triventi (2012) who used survey data deriving from the HBS to study the impact of income on households' gambling expenditure finding evidence of gambling tax regressivity. No previous Italian research has focused on the comparison among sin taxes.

The Italian Framework of Sin Goods

During 2014, sin tax revenues in Italy contributed to generate 22.8 billion €, roughly 5.5% of total tax revenues. Gambling represented the most relevant source of revenues (11.2 billion €), followed by tobacco (10.5 billion €) while alcoholic beverages contributed to a significantly lower share (1.1 billion €).

The taxation schemes applied to sin goods are particularly complex and they differ substantially in terms of tax base, tax rate and composition of specific and *ad valorem* taxes, not only among the three most important categories of products but also within each category of goods. Both specific and ad valorem mechanisms are applied and tax rates diverge, leading to different incidences of taxation on price for different sin goods. Therefore, the evaluation of the equity of the current system cannot leave out of consideration the current structure of the Italian system.

The taxation schemes applied to alcoholic beverages and tobacco products are partially ruled by the European Union, that is responsible for setting the minimum level of excise to be applied.

Alcoholic beverages in Italy are mainly taxed through a specific scheme, based on the alcoholic content of beverages. Beer is subject to an excise duty accounting to € 3.04 per hectolitre/degree Plato, whilst spirits are taxed with an excise duty equal to € 1035.52 per hectolitre of pure alcohol. Wine is exempt from excise duty; this fact can be attributed to cultural reason and to the importance of wine national productions[2]. All alcoholic products are also subject to VAT (22%).

Taxation of cigarettes is instead based on a mixed system, composed by a specific tax (i.e. fixed amount per 1000 cigarettes produced) that represents roughly 5% of retail price and by an ad valorem tax that is proportional to price and accounts for roughly 52% of retail price. 22% VAT is also applied on a tax base that includes the amount owed by excise ("tax on tax").

The Italian taxation of gambling differs substantially form that applied to other sin goods. If, on the one hand, taxation to the latter is partially ruled out at European level, on the other, no tax harmonization is currently present, across EU for the former. In the Italian framework, three main taxation schemes exist and the tax system is particularly complex (Giuricin 2013). The residual tax margin system is applied to lotto and lotteries; for these games, the fiscal withdrawal is equal to the difference between the winning in a fair game and the effective winning. In some situations, an additional 6% withdrawal is applied on winnings. The gross turnover system is applied to sport and horse related games and to entertainment machines:

---

[2]The fact that wine is not subject to an excise duty but only to 22% VAT obliges to be cautious when defining wine taxes as sin taxes. Indeed, from a taxation point of view, wine represents a luxury good. However, we decided to include wine in the analysis since it represents a particularly relevant share of alcoholic beverage consumption in Italy. Another issue that should be mentioned concerns the inability, of our analysis, to take into account quantity and price simultaneously. Indeed, the HBS survey only contains data on values consumed. This issue obliges us to consider equal a person who consumed only one expensive bottle of wine and a person who consumed several bottles of cheaper wine.

the tax base is the gross turnover (i.e. the total amount bet) but different tax rates are applied to different games varying between 6% and 26.8%. Entertainment machines, which in 2015 represented approximately the 55% of total gambling turnover are subject to a tax rate equal to roughly 13%. Lastly, in the gross expenditure mechanism, the tax base is the difference between gross turnover and winnings. This system is applied to poker games (20%) and casinos. Generally, recently introduced games (i.e. entertainment machines, remote gambling) are subject to lower tax rates than traditional games (e.g. lotto) and, consequently, the average tax rate applied on turnover decreased drastically over the years: from 23% in 2003 to 10% in 2015.

These complex taxation schemas led to different incidences of taxation on retail prices of sin goods. If we consider the four goods of interest in our analysis, for each euro spent in cigarettes, beer, wine, or gambling, taxes are equal to 0.77 €, 0.42 €, 0.22 €, and 0.47[3] € respectively. This information is relevant when looking at consumption data; as we are interested in comparing the regressivity level of different sin taxes, we need to convert consumption data into tax paid data. The overall level of regressivity of sin taxes is indeed dependent on two factors: the level of consumption of different socio-economic strata of the population and the incidence of taxation on price. In this context we assume that indirect taxes are fully passed through to the consumers and we do not take into account the potential changes in households' behaviour due changes in tax schemas.

Data and Methods

In order to measure the regressivity level of sin taxes in Italy, we use the 2014 data on consumption of cigarettes, beer, wine, and gambling[4] derived of the HBS (16,804 households); our aim is to detect the impact of socio-economic status on the demand for sin goods in order to compare the regressivity of sin taxes. The survey contains data on monthly expenditure in all the main consumption goods for a sample of Italian households. Sampled households are requested to fill in a daily diary on the amount spent for a 14-days period on a detailed list of consumption goods. An initial and a final Computer Assisted Personal Interview completed the collection of information for each household.

The dataset used has some limitations. First, information on risky behaviours collected through surveys tend to suffer for under-reporting. In addition, household income is not present in the dataset; typically, income surveys do not provide data on households' income and vice versa. However, a proper analysis of household living condition should jointly consider the level of consumption and the available

[3]This represents an average incidence on effective expenditure on gambling, globally considered.

[4]While specific questions on the consumption of cigarettes, beer, and wine are available, the question on gambling aggregates all gambling products, and therefore it does not allow an analysis of intra-market differences across different games.

Table 1 Number of observations, average individual income (EU-SILC) and average estimated income (HBS) for each working category of individuals

	HBS		EU SILC	
Category	Number of observations	Estimated individual average income	Number of observations	Average individual income
Not employed	15,769	€ 3984	13,186	€ 4987
Employed full time	9043	€ 24,340	10,862	€ 23,531
Employed part time	1879	€ 13,083	2162	€ 13,245
Self-employed	4199	€ 20,404	4307	€ 23,425
Pensioners	7554	€ 17,154	9712	€ 18,028

economic resources. Consequently, a common approach consists in the use of matching techniques to exploit the information derivable from different sets of micro data (Donatiello et al. 2014). In this context, we use the propensity score matching technique as an instrument to attribute to each household member an estimated income exploiting the information contained in the 2014 Statistics on Income and Living Conditions (EU-SILC, 40,280 records) survey. The propensity score matching has been obtained through different steps:

1. process of re-coding of the variables to make comparable HBS and EU-SILC data;
2. selection of the variables to be included after evaluating the balancing hypothesis;
3. matching has been estimated through the STATA function psmatch2 (Nearest neighbours matching approach).

Matching has been run on 5 datasets divided by 5 categories of individuals (not employed; employed full time; employed part time; self-employed; pensioners) using as matching variables: age, marital status, gender, educational level, region of residence, occupational position, home ownership.

Table 1 reports some synthetic results of the propensity score matching and the number of observations used in HBS and EU –SILC surveys for the five groups on which propensity score matching has been computed. The final yearly average household income on HBS data accounts to 31,110 €.

We assess the regressivity of sin taxes using three different indices: the Suits (1977) index, the Reynolds-Smolensky (1977) index and the Kakwani (1977) index.

The Suits Index (Suits 1977), similarly to the Gini Index, represents a measure of concentration and it expresses the degree of regressivity or progressivity of a tax looking at the area between the Lorenz curve and the diagonal, which represents the condition of tax proportionality. The Lorenz curve is a two-dimensional representation that reports, on the x-axis the cumulative proportion of income, and on the y-axis the cumulative proportion of tax paid. Thus, Suits Index can be computed as:

$$S = 1 - \frac{L}{K} \tag{1}$$

where L indicates the area below the Lorenz curve and K the area below the diagonal representing proportional taxes. The index varies between $+1$ and -1 such that positive values indicate a progressive tax, negative values a regressive tax whilst zero identifies a proportional tax.

The Kakwani (1977) index looks at the disproportionality of tax payments relative to pre-tax incomes; it measures the progressivity as the difference between the concentration coefficient of taxes (C_T) and the Gini of pre-tax income (G_Y)

$$K_T = C_T - G_T \tag{2}$$

A positive number indicates progressivity, while a negative number identifies a regressive tax. With a proportional tax, the two components, C_T and G_Y are the equal and $K_T = 0$.

The Reynolds-Smolensky (1977) index, allows to obtain an overall measure of the redistributive effect of taxation. It is computed as the difference between the Gini coefficient of pre-tax income (G_Y) and the concentration coefficient of post-tax income (G_{YN}):

$$RS = G_Y - G_{YN} \tag{3}$$

If the Reynolds-Smolensky index assumes a negative value this means that the introduction of the tax increases the concentration coefficient and, consequently, the tax can be considered regressive.

In this paper, we compute the three indices for the four previously mentioned categories of sin goods and for some other consumption goods used as a benchmark (bread and cereals, meat and fish, vegetables, clothing, cultural goods)[5]. We use as alternative measures of the households' economic wellbeing income and total expenditure; this allows us to take into account savings and borrowing decision and to obtain an immediate and a lifetime measure of tax redistributive effects. To assess their statistical significance, we also estimate confidence intervals for Suits indices using the bootstrap approach suggested by Anderson et al. (2003) and already used in similar contexts (Combs et al. 2008).

[5]When different tax rates are applied to goods belonging to the previously mentioned macro-category of products, we computed the total amount of tax paid as a weighted average.

Results

Table 2 shows that Italian households spend, on average 2488 € per month that, taking into account family composition, corresponds to an average equivalised[6] monthly expenditure of 1709 €. Most of the total expenditure is devoted to "House, water, electricity" (36.7%), "Food and non-alcoholic beverages" (17.5%), "Transportation" (10.3%), "Recreational and cultural products" (4.9%), and "Clothing" (4.6%). The households' expenditure in tobacco products, alcoholic beverages and gambling correspond to 0.9%, 0.8% and 0.2% of their total expenditure. Cigarettes are the 93% of tobacco products' expenditure whereas beer and wine account for 84% of alcoholic beverage expenditure.

Table 3 shows that, overall, the average monthly amount of money spent in gambling, by those households who spent at least 1 €, accounted to 31 € in 2014.

Table 2 Consumption pattern and taxation scheme applied

Macrocategory	% total	Tax scheme	Tax incidence
Food and an-alcoholic beverages	17.5		
Meat and fish	30.4	VAT	10%
Bread and cereals	16.8	VAT	4%–10%
Vegetables	13.5	VAT	4%
Alcoholic beverages	0.8		
Beer	26.40	Excise + VAT	42%[a]
Wine	57.90	VAT	22%
Tobacco	0.9		
Cigarettes	92.9	Excise + VAT	77%[b]
Gambling	0.2	Excise	47%[c]
Clothing	4.6	VAT	22%
House, water, electricity, gas	36.7	VAT	10%
Transportation	10.3	VAT	0%–10%–22%
Cultural products	4.9	VAT	0%–4%–10%–22%
Other goods	24.2	VAT	0%–4%–10%–22%
Total	100.00		

Source: Our elaboration on HBS, year 2014
[a]Average incidence (Excise + VAT) computed considering a beer with 12 degree Plato (4.8%)
[b]Average incidence on cigarettes, considering both specific, ad valorem excises and VAT
[c]This represents an average incidence on gambling

[6]Different equivalent scales have been proposed in the literature (Atkinson et al. 1995). The two most common approaches for equivalising income and expenditure include: divide by the square root of the number of the household members; divide by the number of "equivalent adults" (1.0 to the first adult; 0.5 to the second and each subsequent person aged 14 and over; 0.3 to each child aged under 14). Since our dataset only contains information on people aged under 18 years old, in this study, we employed the first approach (i.e. divide by the square root of the number of the household members).

Table 3 Descriptive statistics

	Quartile		Sin goods				Other consumption goods				
			Cigarettes	Beer	Wine	Gambling	Bread and cereals	Meat and fish	Vegetables	Clothing	Cultural goods
Average amount (in €) spent by those who spent at least 1 €		Total	90.0	16.4	28.5	31.3	74.4	137.5	61.1	174.0	140.6
	Expenditure	1st	76.2	13.8	16.1	21.0	50.4	89.6	39.2	82.3	39.9
		2nd	86.1	14.9	21.4	27.2	68.4	129.1	55.6	122.7	77.7
		3rd	94.6	16.0	27.9	33.2	81.9	149.2	66.8	158.1	129.2
		4th	98.4	19.5	41.6	36.7	96.9	181.4	82.0	281.2	275.7
	Income	1st	86.6	15.4	22.8	30.9	60.7	112.9	52.8	122.2	91.5
		2nd	88.0	17.2	25.8	30.4	72.1	136.0	59.9	160.5	120.8
		3rd	91.5	15.6	29.7	33.9	77.1	142.6	62.1	180.7	151.0
		4th	93.1	17.1	34.0	29.9	87.6	158.3	69.6	221.5	191.8
% households spending at least 1 €		Total	23.5	33.1	41.8	17.7	98.7	96.7	96.1	65.2	85.9
	Expenditure	1st	16.4	23.9	29.5	9.6	98.0	94.9	93.5	46.9	66.6
		2nd	23.3	32.9	40.3	17.2	99.1	97.5	96.8	63.9	87.0
		3rd	26.4	35.3	45.9	21.0	98.8	96.7	96.5	70.9	94.0
		4th	27.9	40.5	51.2	23.2	98.7	96.8	97.3	81.3	97.9
	Income	1st	19.2	26.4	36.3	17.1	98.5	95.9	95.4	57.3	89.3
		2nd	24.4	32.1	40.8	17.8	98.4	96.0	95.5	65.5	91.2
		3rd	23.8	35.5	42.9	17.4	38.6	96.5	96.1	68.7	91.8
		4th	26.7	38.5	47.0	17.7	99.1	97.3	97.2	71.6	93.4

% of total expenditure		Total	3.96	0.72	1.12	1.30	3.33	6.05	2.72	6.04	4.92
	Expenditure	1st	6.08	1.16	1.37	1.78	4.29	7.44	3.33	6.26	3.04
		2nd	4.50	0.81	1.16	1.44	3.60	6.78	2.98	6.07	3.89
		3rd	3.70	0.61	1.10	1.35	3.15	5.70	2.60	5.86	4.83
		4th	2.50	0.47	0.97	0.96	2.30	4.31	1.99	6.04	6.15
	Income	1st	4.84	0.87	1.19	1.63	3.65	6.61	3.12	5.89	4.11
		2nd	4.16	0.83	1.11	1.32	3.44	6.31	2.85	6.20	4.41
		3rd	3.79	0.65	1.13	1.30	3.17	5.76	2.51	5.91	4.74
		4th	3.28	0.57	1.07	1.00	3.08	5.53	2.40	6.12	5.16

Source: Our elaboration on HBS, 2014

This value is close to the monthly average expenditure in alcoholic beverage (34 €, 16 € in beer and 29 € in wine) but significantly lower than the average expenditure for cigarettes (90 €). However, only 17% of households bought gambling products in the period analysed; one household over four (25%) consumed tobacco products (23% cigarettes), and slightly less than 60% consumed alcoholic beverages (33% and 43% consumed beer and wine, respectively). If we split households by their total expenditure/income quartiles we can see that the amount of money spent in sin goods increases with total expenditure. If we consider gambling, households belonging to the first expenditure quartile spend significantly less than those belonging to the forth expenditure quartile (21 € and 37 €); the pattern is similar to that recorded for cigarettes (76 € vs 98 €), beer (14 € vs 19 €) and wine (16 € vs 41 €). Also other consumptions goods (e.g. meat and fish, clothing, vegetables, clothing and recreational goods) show a similar behaviour. However, when splitting the households by income quartiles the differences in gambling and beer consumption across different income quartiles is not evident anymore. It is interesting to notice that the share of total expenditure in most of consumption goods decreases with total expenditure, meaning that lower income/expenditure households spend disproportionally more on most of the consumption goods. Two exceptions in this pattern are recorded for recreational and cultural products and clothing.

Figure 1 shows the results of the Suits indices (year 2014) based on households' income. The coefficients turn out to be lower than zero for all the goods considered, recording a minimum of −0.41 for gambling and a maximum of −0.28 for wine. The first 20% and 60% of cumulative income correspond, respectively, to more than 40% and 80% of cumulative gambling tax paid, highlighting the regressivity pattern in gambling taxation.

As confirmed by looking at the confidence intervals (Table 4), gambling is the most regressive form of taxation, followed by cigarettes, and beer. Among sin goods, wine is instead the least regressive. A comparison with the regressivity level of other consumption goods taxes reveals that, with the exception of wine, sin taxes are substantially more regressive. When measured in terms of households' expenditure, the regressivity level is generally lower suggesting that the degree of regressivity is stronger in the short term rather than under a lifetime point of view. Consistently with existing literature (e.g. OECD 2014) when regressivity is measured in terms of income we got lower values of the coefficients; this result can be explained by the fact that saving rates tend to increase with income. As a consequence, higher income individuals would have a lower proportion of their income subject to VAT or excise. Under a lifetime approach (i.e. expenditure approach) the most regressive taxes turn out to be cigarettes, followed by vegetables, bread and cereals, beer and gambling.

Table 5 shows the results of the Reynolds-Smolensky and Kakwani indices. When measured in terms of income all the Reynolds-Smolensky and Kakwani indices turn out to be negative, suggesting the regressivity nature of the consumption goods analysed. However, when measured in terms of expenditure, taxes connected to cultural goods and clothing turn out to have a small redistributive effect.

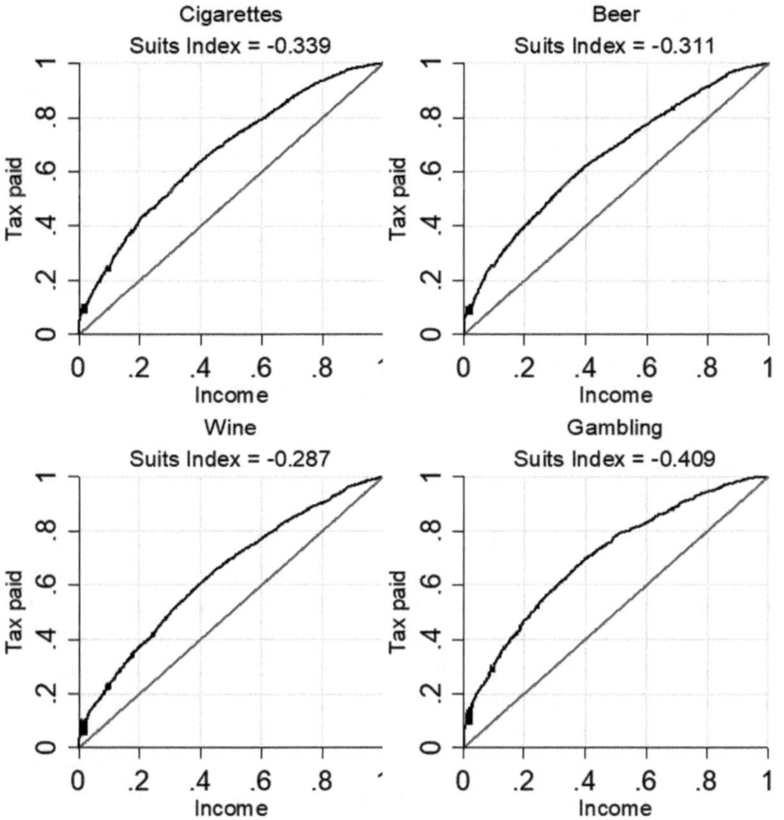

Fig. 1 Suits indices (year 2014)

Table 4 Bootstrapped confidence intervals for the Suits indices

	Income			Expenditure		
Good	Suits index	IC1	IC2	Suits index	IC1	IC2
Gambling	−0.41	−0.41	−0.41	−0.09	−0.09	−0.09
Cigarettes	−0.34	−0.34	−0.34	−0.13	−0.13	−0.13
Total sin taxes	−0.34	−0.34	−0.34	−0.11	−0.11	−0.11
Beer	−0.31	−0.31	−0.31	−0.10	−0.10	−0.10
Vegetables	−0.36	−0.37	−0.36	−0.12	−0.12	−0.12
Meat and fish	−0.32	−0.32	−0.31	−0.11	−0.11	−0.11
Bread and cereals	−0.30	−0.30	−0.30	−0.10	−0.10	−0.10
Wine	−0.29	−0.29	−0.29	0.01	0.01	0.01
Cultural goods	−0.30	−0.30	−0.30	0.06	0.06	0.06
Clothing	−0.26	−0.26	−0.26	0.13	0.13	0.13

Table 5 Kakwani and Reynolds-Smolensky indices computed on income and expenditure

	Income		Expenditure	
Good	Reynolds-Smolensky	Kakwani	Reynolds-Smolensky	Kakwani
Gambling	−0.0004	−0.3974	−0.0001	−0.0570
Cigarettes	−0.0022	−0.3209	−0.0008	−0.1022
Beer	−0.0003	−0.3006	−0.0001	−0.0809
Vegetables	−0.0003	−0.3228	−0.0001	−0.1018
Meat and fish	−0.0016	−0.3002	−0.0005	−0.0934
Bread and cereals	−0.0005	−0.2847	−0.0002	−0.0810
Wine	−0.0003	−0.2715	0.0000	0.0115
Cultural goods	−0.0021	−0.2628	0.0005	0.0652
Clothing	−0.0022	−0.2021	0.0012	0.1200

Discussion and Conclusions

Results show that sin goods are highly regressive and that lower income households spend larger proportion of their income on risky behaviours than higher income ones. Differences persist among different sin taxes; when measured in terms of income, gambling taxation turns out to be the most regressive recording a Suits Index, almost twice those of other sales taxes. This fact raises doubts on the fairness of public policies adopted towards gambling during the last 15 years. The results obtained are in line with previous international studies: Beckert and Lutter (2009) comparing the results of several previous researches on gambling show that Suits indices are almost unanimously negative ranging from −0.10 (Livernois 1987) to −0.44 (Brinner and Clotfelter 1975). Focusing on the Italian context we can conclude that the tax regressivity of gambling seems to have increased in the last 6 years, from −0.21 in 2008 (Sarti and Triventi 2012) to −0.41 in 2014. When measured in terms of expenditure (i.e. lifetime approach), cigarettes taxes are the most regressive among the ones herein discussed.

The fact that low income individuals tend to contribute to a larger share of sin tax revenues highlights the need for designing policies aimed at protecting vulnerable consumers. Selecting the best way to organize sin markets minimizing the social problems and the inequality without allowing for the widespread of illegal gambling represents a challenging task. The majority of studies support, as an alternative way to partially correct inequality, the imposition of constraints on the destination of state revenues collected though sin taxes according to the model of earmarked taxes. This means that sin taxes revenues should be spent mostly in the interest of consumers, satisfying the benefit principle or giving revenues to good causes (Scudiero 2014). It cannot be ignored that sin goods consumption is characterized by the presence of social costs. In the Italian context, healthcare problems connected to heavy smoking and drinking, are indeed universally and freely guaranteed to all Italian citizens and from 2012 services addressed towards the prevention and care of pathological gamblers have also been included in services guaranteed by the National Healthcare System (Decree Law 158/2012). However, at the moment, in the Italian framework, there is a spatial mismatch between gains raised through tax revenues (that are collected at central level) and costs of dealing with negative externalities and social costs (which are organized and financed by regional governments). As a consequence, more attention should be paid in the redistribution of tax revenues collected through sin taxes. Gambling tax revenues are also affected by a strong marketing effect (Smith 2000); however, advertisement through sponsorship or school and sporting events may be responsible to attract vulnerable individuals, particularly young people. Therefore, the potentially harmful nature of gambling consumption makes necessary the definition of responsible and not misleading promotion and advertising campaign.

References

AAMS - Agenzia delle Dogane e dei Monopoli (2015). Organizzazione, attività e statistica. Available at: www.agenziadoganemonopoli.gov.it. Accessed: 10 February 2018.

Allamani, A., Pepe, P., Baccini, M., Massini, G., Voller, F. (2014). Europe. An analysis of changes in the consumption of alcoholic beverages: the interaction among consumption, related harms, contextual factors and alcoholic beverage control policies. *Substance use & misuse*, 49(12), 1692–1715.

Anderson J.E., Roy A.G., Shoemaker P.A. (2003). Confidence intervals for the Suits Index. *National Tax Journal*, 56(1), 81–90.

Atkinson A.B., L. Rainwater, T.M. Smeeding, (1995). Income Distribution in the OECD Countries: The Evidence from the Luxembourg Income Study, *Social Policy Studies*, 18, OECD, Paris, France.

Baumol W.J. (1972). On taxation and the control of externalities. *The American Economic Review*, 62(3), 307–322.

Beckert J., & Lutter M. (2009). The inequality of fair play: Lottery gambling and social stratification in Germany. *European Sociological Review*, 25(4), 475–488.

Bird R.M. (2015). Tobacco and alcohol excise taxes for improving public health and revenue outcomes: marrying sin and virtue? *World Bank Policy Research Working Paper* No. 7500. http://documents.worldbank.org/curated/en/577831467986372982/. Accessed: 20 February 2018.

Borg, M.O., Mason, P.M., & Shapiro, S.L. (1990). An economic comparison of gambling behavior in Atlantic City and Las Vegas. *Public Finance Review*, 18(3), 291–312.

Brinner R.E., & Clotfelter C.T. (1975). An economic appraisal of state lotteries. *National Tax Journal*, 28(4), 395–404.

Chaloupka F.J., Yurekli A., & Fong, G.T. (2012). Tobacco taxes as a tobacco control strategy. *Tobacco control*, 21(2), 172–180.

Clotfelter C.T. (1979). On the regressivity of state-operated “numbers” games. *National Tax Journal*, 32(4), 543–548.

Clotfelter C.T., & Cook P.J. (1991). Selling hope: State lotteries in America. Harvard University Press.

Clotfelter, C.T. (2005). Gambling taxes. In: S. Cnossen (Ed.), *Theory and practice of excise Taxation: Smoking, drinking, gambling, polluting, and driving*, (pp. 84–119). Oxford University Press.

Combs K.L., Kim, J., Spry, J.A. (2008). The relative regressivity of seven lottery games. *Applied Economics*, 40(1), 35–39.

Donatiello G., D'Orazio M., Frattarola D., Rizzi A., Scanu M., & Spaziani M. (2014). Statistical matching of income and consumption expenditures. *International Journal of Economic Sciences*, 3(3), 50.

Fink S.C., Marco A.C., & Rork J.C. (2004). Lotto nothing? The budgetary impact of state lotteries. *Applied Economics*, 36(21), 2357–2367.

Galizzi M.M. (2012). Label, nudge or tax? A review of health policies for risky behaviours. *Journal of Public Health Research*, 1(1), 14–21.

Giuricin A. (2013). La tassazione del settore dei giochi, Special Report, Istituto Bruno Leoni. http://www.brunoleoni.it/special-report-la-tassazione-del-settore-dei-giochi Accessed: 20 February 2018.

Gambling Capital (2013). Benchmark of gambling taxation and license fees in eight European member states. https://www.tweedekamer.nl/downloads/document?id=b53d39ec-957b-4c51-8760-31554671a428&title=Advies%20Gambling%20Capital.pdf. Accessed: 20 October 2017.

Haile A.J. (2009). Sin taxes: When the state becomes the sinner. *Temple Law Review*., Elon University Law Legal Studies Research Paper No. 2009–05. https://ssrn.com/abstract=1425621. Accessed: 20 October 2017.

Hansen A. (1995). The tax incidence of the Colorado state lottery instant game. *Public Finance Quarterly*, 23(3), 385–398.

Herrnstein R.J., Loewenstein G.F., Prelec, D., & Vaughan, W. (1993) Utility maximization and melioration: Internalities in individual choice. *Journal Of Behavioral Decision Making*, 6(3), 149–185.

IFS (2011). Quantitative analysis of VAT rate structures, in IFS et al., A retrospective evaluation of elements in the EU VAT system, Institute for Fiscal Studies, Report prepared for the European Commission. https://www.ifs.org.uk/publications/5947. Accessed: 15 November 2017.

Jones A., & Mazzi M.G. (1996). Tobacco consumption and taxation in Italy: an application of the QUAIDS model. *Applied Economics*, 28(5), 595–603.

Kakwani, N. (1977). Measurement of tax progressivity: an international comparison. *Economic Journal*, 87 (345), 71–80.

Kitchen, H., & Powells, S. (1991). Lottery expenditures in Canada: A regional analysis of determinants and incidence. *Applied Economics*, 23(12), 1845–1852.

Layton, A., & Worthington, A. (1999). The impact of socio-economic factors on gambling expenditure. *International Journal of Social Economics*, 26(1/2/3), 430–440.

Liberati P., & Paradiso M. (2014). Sulla composizione dell'accisa sui tabacchi: un'ipotesi di modifica del sistema di tassazione in Italia. No. 55906, University Library of Munich, Germany. https://ideas.repec.org/p/pra/mprapa/55906.html. Accessed: 15 November 2017.

Livernois J.R. (1987). The redistributive effects of lotteries: Evidence from Canada. *Public Finance Quarterly*, 15(3), 339–351.

Lorenzi P. (2004). Sin taxes. *Society*, 41(3), 59–65.

Lyon A.B., & Schwab R.M. (1997). The Regressivity of Sin Taxes: The Lifetime Tax Burden of Taxes on Alcohol and Cigarettes. Tax Foundation. https://taxfoundation.org/regressivity-sin-taxes-lifetime-tax-burden-taxes-alcohol-and-cigarettes/. Accessed: 15 November 2017.

Mikesell, J. L. (1989). A note on the changing incidence of state lottery finance. *Social Science Quarterly*, 70(2), 513.

O'Donoghue T., & Rabin, M. (2006). Optimal sin taxes. *Journal of Public Economics*, 90(10), 1825–1849.

OECD (2014). The Distributional Effects of Consumption Taxes in OECD Countries, *OECD Publishing, Paris*. https://doi.org/10.1787/9789264224520-en. Accessed: 15 November 2017.

Pigou A.C. (1920). The economics of welfare. McMillan&Co., London.

Pogue T.F., & Sgontz L.G. (1989). Taxing to control social costs: the case of alcohol. *The American Economic Review*, 79(1), 235–243.

Price D.I., & Novak E.S. (1999). The tax incidence of three Texas lottery games: Regressivity, race, and education. *National Tax Journal*, 52(4), 741–751.

Remler D.K. (2004). Poor smokers, poor quitters, and cigarette tax regressivity. *American Journal of Public Health*, 94(2), 225–229.

Reynolds, M. & Smolensky, E. (1977). *Public Expenditures, Taxes, and the Distribution of Income: The United States, 1950, 1961, 1970*, New York, Academic Press.

Sammartino F. (1990). Federal taxation of tobacco, alcoholic beverages, and motor fuels. Congress of the United States, Congressional Budget Office, Washington DC.

Sarti S., & Triventi M. (2012). Il gioco d'azzardo: l'iniquità di una tassa volontaria. La relazione tra posizione socio-economica e propensione al gioco. *Stato e mercato*, (3), 503–534.

Scudiero L. (2014). Quando il fisco "dipende" dal gioco. Special Report, Istituto Bruno Leoni.

Smith, J. (2000). Gambling taxation: Public equity in the gambling business. *Australian Economic Review*, 33(2), 120–144.

Suits D.B. (1977). Gambling taxes: Regressivity and revenue potential. *National Tax Journal* 30(1), 19–35.

With Whom Do We Compare Our Income? The Effect of Gendered Income Comparisons on Subjective Well-Being

Laura Ravazzini and Marcin Piekałkiewicz

Abstract Income comparisons are often performed through the construction of reference groups based on sociodemographic characteristics. Gender is usually included in these characteristics only when the number of cases is large. However, it has not been demonstrated empirically that people compare their income within or between genders. This study analyses these comparisons using questions collected in three waves of the pretest of the German Socio-Economic Panel. Results suggest that income comparisons are mainly within groups of the same gender. On average, women compare more than men, and this is the case regardless of the gender composition in their sector of employment. Despite the predominance of within-gender comparisons, between-gender comparisons also exist. Indeed regressions that test the impact of income comparisons and reference groups on subjective well-being explain the data better when gender is not included as a dimension of reference.

Introduction

The analysis of the impact of relative income on subjective well-being (SWB) is often limited by the correct construction of reference groups. Previous studies show that income comparisons among colleagues and friends affect people's SWB (Clark and Oswald 1996; Senik 2009; Clark and Senik 2010; Friehe et al. 2014; Goerke and Pannenberg 2015). While people's close networks would be the most appropriate group for income comparisons, normal survey data do not provide such detailed

L. Ravazzini (✉)
Université de Neuchâtel, Neuchâtel, Switzerland

Université de Lausanne, Lausanne, Switzerland
e-mail: laura.ravazzini@unine.ch

M. Piekałkiewicz
Department of Economics and Statistics, University of Siena, Siena, Italy

Happonomy, Leuven, Belgium

A. Bianco et al. (eds.), *Italian Studies on Quality of Life*, Social Indicators Research Series 77, https://doi.org/10.1007/978-3-030-06022-0_10

information due to data anonymisation. For this reason, reference groups are often used to identify a feasible set of comparison possibilities. Indeed the construction of reference groups with survey data is fundamental for many empirical applications, among which the estimation of the impact of income comparisons on SWB. The most frequent characteristics used in survey data for the construction of reference groups include the region where people live, their level of education and their age. Gender is often omitted or included only if the number of observations is large enough for this additional test. This study addresses this issue and tests references groups depending on gender to obtain the correct construction. In particular, the analysis investigates whether income comparisons occur mainly between or within genders and how they affect SWB. The analysis uses data from three pretests of the German Socio-Economic Panel (pretest SOEP 2008–2010). Germany is a country with high female and male labour force participation rates (respectively around 70% and 82% in the reference period) and a traditional division of labour (i.e. the labour market follows a modified male-breadwinner model according to which men usually work full-time and women work part-time (Trappe et al. 2015)).[1] Previous studies based on Germany and the SOEP have investigated the importance of income comparisons between specific groups, such as neighbours (Knies 2012), co-workers, friends, family members and people of the same age (Friehe et al. 2014; Goerke and Pannenberg 2015), but have omitted gendered effects. This study investigates the importance of gender for the construction of reference groups and for the effect of relative income on SWB.

The study is structured as follows. We start by presenting hypotheses based on findings from the relevant literature about the intensity of within and between gender comparisons and their impact on SWB. We continue with the description of the data and the empirical specifications. Next, we explain the descriptive and analytical evidence provided by our findings and in the last section, we conclude with recommendations on how to best construct reference groups with survey data.

Hypotheses

Previous studies have shown that not all people compare their income with others, but those who do tend to compare upwards (Ferrer-i-Carbonell 2005; Boyce et al. 2010). This means that people generally compare with individuals with higher, not lower, income. However, whether women compare more than men and whether the relevant factors differ are still open questions due to the lack of data about specific gender comparisons. Our first hypothesis is that women, given their lower position in the income distribution and thus higher probabilities of finding individuals with higher income, compare their incomes with both men and other women and

[1] 92% of active men worked full-time and 62% of active women worked part-time in the reference period.

therefore more than men in general (H1). Confirming this hypothesis would support results from Clark and Senik (2010), who find that comparison intensity is higher for those with lower income.

We also formulate hypotheses about several possible mediators of income comparisons that depend on gender. All else being equal, we expect that the macroeconomic context and the sector of employment influence gendered comparisons. With respect to the sector of employment, we expect that those who work in sectors dominated by one gender ("gendered sectors") compare more with the opposite gender (H2). This hypothesis assumes that individuals who work in gendered sectors conform less to gender norms and compare more between genders. We define a sector as gendered if at least 70% of its workers are of the same sex. Given the unbalanced sex ratio of these sectors, the gender minorities who work in gendered sectors may have more opportunities to compare with the opposite gender.

With respect to the macroeconomic context, we advance the hypothesis that a greater gender pay gap[2] increases women's comparisons with men but decreases men's comparisons with women (H3). It could also be the case that a sufficiently high gender-pay gap creates a barrier between genders and discourages all forms of comparisons. For these reasons, women and men might behave as separate groups with different potential outcomes in the labour market.

With this in mind, we build further expectations for the analysis on SWB. The relationship between the importance of comparisons (IC) and SWB is expected to be negative (Clark and Senik 2010; Goerke and Pannenberg 2015). In other words, this means that people that place more importance on the income differentials are expected to be less happy. Combining our expectations for H1 and knowing that those who have a higher IC are less satisfied, we expect, ceteris paribus, women to be significantly less satisfied than men (H4). We base this hypothesis on the envy effect, which states that people's SWB decreases when the reference group does better than the individual (Clark and Senik 2010; Fiske 2011). An alternative effect of reference income is the tunnel effect (also known as the 'ambition' or 'signal' effect (Hirschman and Rothschild 1973; Clark and Senik 2010)). According to this effect, individuals should be happier when the income of the reference group increases because this change contains information about their future prospects. Supporting evidence for the tunnel effect is typically found in countries with high mobility such as Russia or Eastern Europe (Senik 2008). Given that our study is based on a Western country, namely Germany, we believe the envy effect will dominate, but we acknowledge that the tunnel effect might be more important in the Eastern part of the country.

Previous works have implicitly assumed within-gender comparisons are plausible when calculating the income of reference groups (Bartolini et al. 2013; Piekalkiewicz 2016). Ferrer-i-Carbonell (2005) constructed reference groups with and without gender using the SOEP 1992–1997 and found that the inclusion of gender did not change the importance of reference income for an individual's

[2]In 2008, the gender pay gap was 23% in Germany.

wellbeing.[3] In those years, however, the SOEP did not allow for an evaluation of the importance of income comparisons. This study contributes to the literature by assessing the intensity and the direction of gender comparisons. According to H1 and H3, we expect to find men to compare mainly with men, but women to compare with both women and men. According to H4, we also expect to see a negative impact of these comparisons on SWB. Combining these hypotheses, we expect to find an impact of income comparisons between genders on SWB (H5). Therefore, we expect gender to be an important determinant of reference groups. We test this hypothesis in the last part of the study where the inclusion of gender in the reference income assesses whether gender should or should not be included in the definition of the reference group.

Data, Empirical Specifications and Descriptive Evidence

Data

The analysis is based on three pretests (2008, 2009 and 2010) of the SOEP. Each SOEP pretest consists of an independent set of questions asked to a representative random sample of the resident population in Germany (around 1000 individuals per year). Even though the pretest samples are limited, this is the only existing data source that allows to test the hypotheses about between- and within-gender income comparisons. Other surveys (for instance the European Social Survey, Round 3) that contain information on the declared importance of comparing income within particular groups do not consider gender among the definitions of these reference groups.

In the years 2008–2010 the SOEP pretest included the following question: *If you evaluate your earned income, the comparison of the gross-income of other people matters. If you compare your current gross-income with others: How important is the comparison of your gross-income with: (a) your neighbours, (b) your friends, (c) your colleagues, (d) people who exercise your profession, (e) people of your age, (f) your parents when they were your age, (g) your partner, (h) (other) women, (i) (other) men?*[4] Respondents were asked to evaluate the importance they give to income comparisons on a seven-point scale, ranging from "(1) completely unimportant" to "(7) extremely important", for every reference group. Scores

[3]In a footnote, the author mentions that she added gender only because "The two referees of this paper asked to include gender in the reference group definition". Therefore, the inclusion of gender was not originally planned in the article.

[4]The question wording comes from https://paneldata.org/questions/12781 (accessed 18 May 2017). The term (other) refers to people of the same sex. This term is excluded when the question is asked to people of the opposite sex. For more information about SOEP pretests see https://paneldata.org/studies/5 (accessed 18 May 2017).

reported for the two last reference groups (h and i) measure the importance given to gendered income comparisons.

It is crucial to note that the income comparison question was asked only to working respondents in the years 2009 and 2010; we therefore impose the same restriction for the year 2008 to construct the sample. We also pool each of the cross-sectional samples resulting in an overall sample that includes 1119 workers who reported the importance of income comparisons and life satisfaction between 2008 and 2010.

In order to test the last hypotheses related to SWB (H4 and H5) and to assess whether gender should be included in reference groups, we use responses to a standard life satisfaction question: *In conclusion, we would like to ask you about your satisfaction with your life in general. Please answer according to the following scale: 0 means "completely dissatisfied", 10 means "completely satisfied". All things considered, how satisfied are you with your life?.*

Empirical Specifications

In the analysis of gendered income comparisons, our three key explanatory variables are *Gender* (male/female), *Sector*, and the *Gender Pay Gap (GPG)*. To construct the *Sector* variable, we adhere to the statistical classification of economic activities in the European Community (two-digit NACE). The NACE sectors are grouped into three categories corresponding to the prevailing gender in a given sector: male dominated sector, female dominated sector, and gender-neutral sector. *GPG* is the unadjusted gender pay gap calculated at the regional level (German Länder), defined as the "difference between the average gross hourly earnings of men and women expressed as a percentage of the average gross hourly earnings of men".[5]

We introduce several control variables based on our hypotheses and the existing literature related to the determinants of income comparisons (Clark and Senik 2010; Friehe et al. 2014). We include regional Gini indices because general income inequality may increase the motivation for individuals at the bottom of the income ladder to reach the top or discourage competition when the position on the income ladder is judged unfair. The Gini is also relevant for life satisfaction because income inequality has been found to be negatively correlated with SWB in Europe (Schneider 2016; Ravazzini and Chávez-Juárez 2018). We also include the logarithm of equivalised disposable income (deflated with the consumer price index for each year).[6] This income variable is derived from household income

[5]See http://ec.europa.eu/eurostat/statistics-explained/index.php/Gender_pay_gap_statistics

[6]To calculate the equivalised disposable income, we follow the so-called modified OECD equivalence scale, which gives a weight to all members of the household: 1.0 to the first adult; 0.5 to the second and each subsequent person aged 14 and over; 0.3 to each child aged under 14. Due to the dataset construction, we define adults as individuals aged 16 and over.

due to the high number of missing values of alternative earnings measures, i.e. individual income from work. This control is crucial because the IC declines with disposable income (Boyce et al. 2010; Ferrer-i-Carbonell 2005). A further set of controls is work-related and includes variables related to working full-time, being self-employed, having a university degree, status as a "white collar" employee (i.e. an employee with extensive managerial duties), and working in the public sector. This set of controls captures the importance that individuals attribute to work and consequently the IC (Friehe et al. 2014). The last set of controls is composed of common socio-demographic variables (age, age squared (divided by 100), a dummy for being married, a dummy for having dependent children in the household, a dummy for living in a town with more than 100,000 inhabitants, and a dummy for East Germany (Knies 2012)), and year dummies.

The model for the importance of income comparison *IC* of individual *i* is specified as follows:

$$IC_i = \alpha + \beta_1 * Gender_i + \beta_2 * Sector_i + \beta_3 * GPG_i + \boldsymbol{X_i \delta} + \epsilon_i \tag{1}$$

where ε is the standard error clustered by region and **X** is the vector of control variables listed above. The estimation is run first for the whole sample and then separately for women and men to obtain gender-specific income comparisons. We employ an OLS regression assuming that the declared importance of income comparison can be treated as a cardinal variable. An ordered probit is performed as a robustness check.

In the second part of the analysis, we investigate the relationship between gendered income comparisons and SWB. Individual's *i* life satisfaction *LS* is estimated as:

$$LS_i = \alpha + \beta * IC_i + \boldsymbol{X_i \delta} + \epsilon_i \tag{2}$$

where ε is defined as in eq. (1) and **X** includes the already mentioned control variables as well as *Gender*. To simplify the interpretation of coefficients we use an OLS model, which yields similar results to those coming from a probit regression (Ferrer-i-Carbonell and Frijters 2004). The second *LS* specification includes reference income, defined as the average income of the reference group:

$$LS_i = \alpha + \beta * RefInc_i + \boldsymbol{X_i \delta} + \epsilon_i \tag{3}$$

with ε and **X** defined as in Eq. (2). To check which type of income comparisons (within- or between-gender) has a greater explanatory power, we introduce two definitions of the reference group: the first one includes individuals of the same sex, and age group, living in the same region, while the second one excludes gender. Therefore, the average income of the reference group differs according to the definition of the reference group. Both *LS* regressions are first estimated for the whole sample and then separately for women and men.

Table 1 IC for different reference groups (weighted averages)

IC with:	Neighb.	Friends	Colleag.	Profess.	Age	Parents	Partner	Women	Men	N
Male	1.76	2.17	3.15	3.49	2.67	1.95	2.50	1.94	2.34	540
Female	1.71	2.11	3.21	3.62	2.67	1.93	2.55	2.71	2.52	579
Difference	0.08	0.06	−0.06	−0.13	0.00	0.02	−0.05	−0.77*	−0.18	
Total	1.74	2.14	3.18	3.55	2.67	1.94	2.52	2.28	2.42	1119

Note: *Indicates a significant difference between males and females at the 1% level

Descriptive Evidence

Table 1 shows the average declared IC (on a 1–7 scale) with neighbours, friends, colleagues, people of the same profession, people of the same age, parents, partners, women, and men. Consistent with the literature, respondents are mostly concerned about work-related comparisons (i.e. with colleagues and within a profession), whereas they are not highly interested in comparing with neighbours or parents. The average IC calculated for various reference groups are similar among males and females; however, they differ when it comes to gendered comparisons. Comparing with women is substantially more important for women than for men: the difference amounts to 0.77 and is statistically significant at the 1% level. The gender difference in mean IC is smaller for male comparisons with men: it is equal to 0.18 and is not statistically significant. All other reported differences in mean IC are also statistically insignificant.

Figure 1 presents the distributions of the importance to compare with people of the same and of the opposite sex. Consistent with Table 1, the distributions differ considerably between genders in the importance of comparisons with women. The percentage of responses indicating an elevated importance to compare with women (5–7) is equal to 8.2% for males and 20.4% for females. The distributions of answers regarding comparisons with men are quite similar for both genders. Comparing with men is highly relevant (5–7) for 15.1% of males and for 15.9% of females. About 64% of men versus 47% of women declare that between-gender comparisons are completely unimportant. From the descriptive results, H1 seems to be supported because women compare more than men.

Concerning the analysis related to SWB, we also compute average life satisfaction, measured on a 0–10 scale, for women and men. We remark that life satisfaction is slightly higher for women (7.51) than for men (7.42). There is also a considerable gap in life satisfaction between individuals who report that comparing their income is “extremely important” (7.30 and 7.40, respectively for individuals who compare with women and men) and those who state that it is “completely unimportant” (7.55 and 7.60).

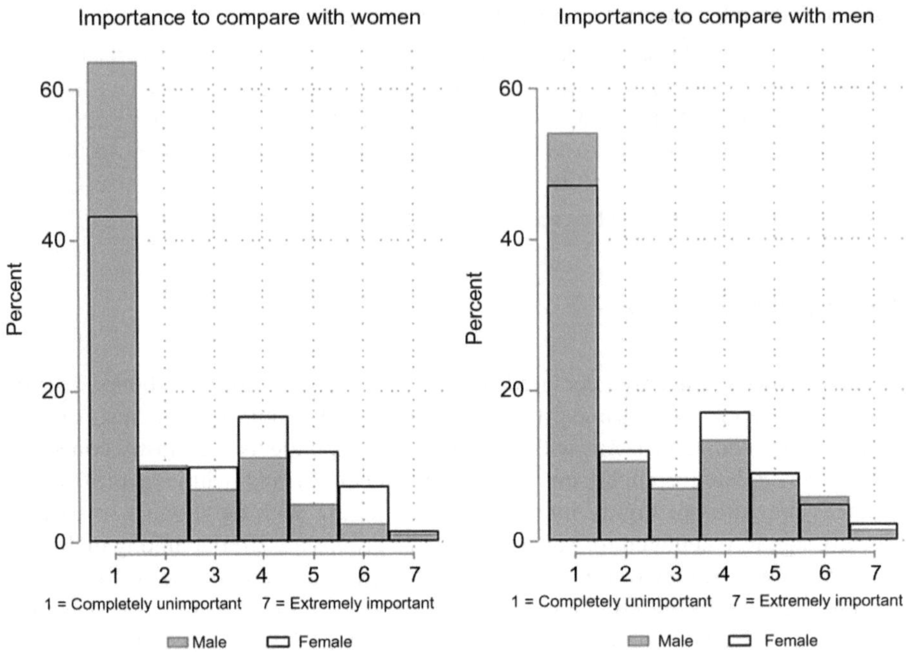

Fig. 1 IC with women and men: distributions by gender (weighted statistics)

Regression Results

Determinants of Gendered Income Comparisons

Table 2 reports the estimated coefficients for various OLS specifications of Eq. (1).[7] We first estimate the coefficients for the whole sample, then separately for women and men in order to investigate within and between gender comparisons.

Consistent with the descriptive analysis, we observe that women compare more to individuals of both sexes. Women do compare their incomes more with other women, but they also compare with men. We can therefore confirm that H1 is supported by empirical evidence.

Results about the sector of employment do not support our expectations (H2). In male dominated sectors, men report significant IC with both women and men, whereas in female dominated sectors, men compare significantly only with other men. We can therefore conclude that men compare more intensively when they are the predominant gender of the sector, whereas they compare only with the same sex when they are the minority of the sector. Women are overall not sensitive to the sector of employment. This means that the sector does not influence ICs for women.

[7]Similar results have been found using ordered probit models (omitted for brevity and available upon request).

Table 2 Determinants of gendered income comparisons

	(1)	(2)	(3)	(4)	(5)	(6)
	All: IC to w.	All: IC to m.	Men: IC to w.	Women: IC to w.	Men: IC to m.	Women: IC to m.
Female	0.865***	0.296**				
	(6.28)	(2.16)				
Gender neutral sector (ref.)						
Male dominated sector	0.331**	0.474***	0.452***	0.304	0.548***	0.391
	(2.54)	(3.07)	(3.61)	(1.29)	(3.92)	(1.64)
Female dominated sector	0.089	0.242*	0.260	0.027	0.362*	0.148
	(0.56)	(1.79)	(1.27)	(0.16)	(1.86)	(1.04)
Gender pay gap	−0.015	−0.031*	−0.035	0.004	−0.064**	−0.002
	(−0.84)	(−1.86)	(−1.42)	(0.14)	(−2.26)	(−0.09)
Gini index	−2.724	−3.770	−3.375	−2.139	−5.491*	−1.424
	(−1.02)	(−1.66)	(−1.27)	(−0.51)	(−1.83)	(−0.43)
Log of equivalised income	−0.127	−0.159	−0.310	0.021	−0.271	−0.067
	(−0.73)	(−1.00)	(−1.38)	(0.12)	(−1.64)	(−0.31)
Full time	0.312**	0.448***	0.067	0.522***	0.513**	0.461***
	(2.36)	(3.86)	(0.32)	(3.97)	(2.88)	(4.02)
Self-employed	−0.260	−0.250	0.043	−0.590**	−0.090	−0.454
	(−1.08)	(−1.17)	(0.10)	(−2.74)	(−0.23)	(−1.56)
University degree	0.063	−0.063	0.230	−0.081	0.105	−0.119
	(0.32)	(−0.26)	(0.93)	(−0.25)	(0.34)	(−0.39)
White collar	0.030	0.057	0.020	0.008	−0.250	0.250
	(0.23)	(0.40)	(0.14)	(0.04)	(−1.01)	(1.67)
Public sector	−0.079	−0.063	0.081	−0.130	−0.100	−0.036
	(−0.39)	(−0.39)	(0.27)	(−0.67)	(−0.45)	(−0.20)

(continued)

Table 2 (continued)

	(1)	(2)	(3)	(4)	(5)	(6)
	All: IC to w.	All: IC to m.	Men: IC to w.	Women: IC to w.	Men: IC to m.	Women: IC to m.
Age	0.005	−0.012	0.064*	−0.045	0.021	−0.049
	(0.17)	(−0.41)	(1.92)	(−0.83)	(0.57)	(−1.28)
Age squared/100	−0.010	0.010	−0.067*	0.043	−0.019	0.047
	(−0.29)	(0.29)	(−1.86)	(0.65)	(−0.42)	(1.00)
Married	−0.005	−0.012	−0.178	0.148	−0.136	0.059
	(−0.06)	(−0.09)	(−1.11)	(1.09)	(−0.71)	(0.33)
Children	−0.096	0.089	−0.311	0.151	0.017	0.151
	(−0.78)	(0.51)	(−1.34)	(0.89)	(0.05)	(0.99)
Town size 100,000+	−0.095	0.209	−0.229	0.002	0.191	0.237
	(−0.49)	(1.31)	(−0.99)	(0.01)	(0.66)	(1.38)
East Germany	−0.215	−0.380	−0.426	0.031	−0.652**	−0.110
	(−0.75)	(−1.73)	(−1.40)	(0.08)	(−2.88)	(−0.26)
2008 (ref.)						
2009	0.070	0.022	−0.169	0.229	−0.281	0.203
	(0.36)	(0.09)	(−0.87)	(1.00)	(−1.29)	(0.67)
2010	0.173	0.194	0.118	0.204	−0.031	0.337
	(0.78)	(0.81)	(0.58)	(0.70)	(−0.14)	(1.06)
Constant	3.306*	5.222***	5.210**	4.040*	7.251***	4.062*
	(2.08)	(3.27)	(2.64)	(1.82)	(3.34)	(2.13)
Observations	979	979	458	521	458	521
R^2	0.065	0.040	0.057	0.040	0.065	0.050
Adjusted R^2	0.046	0.021	0.018	0.005	0.027	0.016

Note: OLS estimates with standard errors clustered by region. Dependent variable: IC to w. indicates the importance of income comparisons with women and IC to m. with men (measured on a 1–7 scale)

*$p < 0.1$, **$p < 0.05$, ***$p < 0.01$, t statistics in parentheses

Concerning macroeconomic context (H3), we observe that the gender pay gap predominantly reduces the IC. There is thus an effect of the macroeconomic conditions on gendered income comparisons, but in most cases, it is not strong enough to be statistically significant. Moreover, the relationship is significant only for the importance of comparisons among men. H3 is therefore not supported by empirical evidence. The other IC-regression results confirm standard findings from the literature related to income comparisons. Although we do not discuss all of the coefficients in detail for purposes of brevity, we find it important to mention that women compare less to other women if they are self-employed and that men-to-men comparisons are also significantly less important in the Eastern part of Germany.

Gendered Income Comparisons and SWB

To analyse the relation between SWB and gendered income comparisons, we first regress individual life satisfaction on declared IC (Table 3), and then on the average income of the reference group (Table 4).

Table 3 Gendered income comparisons and SWB

	(1)	(2)	(3)	(4)	(5)	(6)
	LS: all	LS: all	LS: men	LS: men	LS: women	LS: women
IC with women	−0.094***		−0.086**		−0.100***	
	(−4.24)		(−2.24)		(−3.40)	
IC with men		−0.094***		−0.083***		−0.108***
		(−5.13)		(−4.57)		(−3.26)
Gender neutral sector (ref.)						
Male dom sector	−0.077	−0.065	−0.264**	−0.259**	0.069	0.081
	(−0.69)	(−0.60)	(−2.26)	(−2.19)	(0.48)	(0.59)
Female dom sector	−0.108	−0.094	−0.250*	−0.244*	−0.039	−0.026
	(−1.20)	(−1.03)	(−1.94)	(−1.96)	(−0.33)	(−0.22)
Gender pay gap	0.005	0.004	0.011	0.009	−0.002	−0.002
	(0.28)	(0.20)	(0.59)	(0.47)	(−0.06)	(−0.09)
Controls	Yes	Yes	Yes	Yes	Yes	Yes
Observations	979	979	458	458	521	521
R^2	0.127	0.128	0.159	0.160	0.134	0.135
Adjusted R^2	0.112	0.112	0.122	0.124	0.106	0.107

Note: OLS estimates with standard errors clustered by region. Dependent variable: LS indicates life satisfaction (measured on a 0–10 scale). Controls include: sector of employment, gender pay gap, female (in columns 1 and 2 only), Gini index, log of equivalised income, full time worker, self-employed, university degree, white collar, public sector, age, age squared, married, having children, town size, East Germany, year dummies

$*p < 0.1$, $**p < 0.05$, $***p < 0.01$, t statistics in parentheses

Table 4 Gendered income comparisons and SWB: testing reference groups

	(1)	(2)	(3)	(4)	(5)	(6)
	LS: all	LS: all	LS: men	LS: men	LS: women	LS: women
Log of equivalised	0.715***	0.705***	0.808***	0.813***	0.733***	0.730***
Income	(6.46)	(6.42)	(7.15)	(7.81)	(3.53)	(3.54)
Log of ref. inc.:	−0.121		−0.547*		0.355	
With gender	(−0.49)		(−1.97)		(0.95)	
Log of ref. inc.:		−0.040		−1.130**		0.921
Without gender		(−0.10)		(−2.52)		(1.65)
Gender neutral sector (ref.)						
Male dom sector	−0.110	−0.108	−0.315**	−0.301**	0.029	0.019
	(−0.96)	(−0.95)	(−2.78)	(−2.55)	(0.21)	(0.15)
Female dom sector	−0.116	−0.115	−0.288**	−0.282**	−0.051	−0.067
	(−1.22)	(−1.22)	(−2.25)	(−2.37)	(−0.45)	(−0.59)
Gender pay gap	0.008	0.008	0.020	0.024	−0.005	−0.014
	(0.45)	(0.45)	(1.21)	(1.72)	(−0.20)	(−0.56)
Controls	Yes	Yes	Yes	Yes	Yes	Yes
Observations	979	979	458	458	521	521
R^2	0.116	0.116	0.158	0.164	0.121	0.125
Adjusted R^2	0.101	0.100	0.118	0.124	0.093	0.097

Note: OLS estimates with standard errors clustered by region. Dependent variable: LS indicates life satisfaction (measured on a 0–10 scale). Controls include: sector of employment, gender pay gap, female (in columns 1 and 2 only), Gini index, full time worker, self-employed, university degree, white collar, public sector, age, age squared, married, having children, town size, East Germany, year dummies

*p < 0.1, **p < 0.05, ***p < 0.01, t statistics in parentheses

The IC with women and with men is negatively and significantly related to SWB in the whole sample and in gender-specific regressions.[8] A unit increase on the 1–7 scale of the IC is associated with a decrease of between 0.08 and 0.11 points in life satisfaction (measured on a 0–10 scale). Even though the coefficients appear larger for women, an additional test reported in Table A1 shows that the effect of IC on SWB is not different depending on gender. Hypothesis (H4) about women being more affected than men by income comparisons is therefore not supported. In Table 3 (columns 3–6), it is however interesting to note that men who work in gendered sectors have a lower SWB than those who work in gender neutral sectors, and this effect is not significant for women. This result differs from studies in the UK, which found working in gender neutral sectors is associated with higher job satisfaction for

[8]We always regress the two IC measures in separate equations because they are highly collinear (Spearman's rho = 0.83).

both men (Peccei and Lee 2005) and women (Haile 2012). This discrepancy may be because the relations depend on context (e.g., macroeconomic) or the measure of satisfaction (life in contrast to job). Estimated mean relationship directions for the control variables are consistent with the existing happiness literature (MacKerron 2012) and are not displayed for purposes of brevity.[9]

In the last analysis on SWB, we estimate a negative relationship between reported life satisfaction and the average income of the reference group (Table 4). The relationship is statistically significant only in the regressions for men. This means that when men have a lower income than their reference group, their satisfaction is negatively affected. In contrast, the relationship is positive and insignificant for women. It is rather surprising that for women, the group that compares the most, reference income shows no significant effect on life satisfaction. This might be explained by the fact that women do not place the same emphasis on economic and job-related factors as men when evaluating their life satisfaction (Della Giusta et al. 2011). This is also displayed by the lower R-squareds in the regressions for women as compared to men. Contrary to what is observed for men, the evidence for women suggests that an increase in the income of peers creates offsetting effects. For some women, an increase in the average income of the reference group might generate positive expectations about their own future income (tunnel effect) thereby increasing life satisfaction. While for other women, probably those who compare the most as in Table 3, this same increase might produce unfavourable comparisons (envy effect) thus reducing life satisfaction. Finding no significant effect on life satisfaction suggests that the envy effect does not predominate among women, in contrast to men, for which the evidence supports the envy effect. Finally, consistent with H5, we observe that the coefficients of the reference income constructed without gender are larger than the coefficients that include gender. Most importantly, the adjusted R-squared measures are greater when excluding gender, implying SWB is better explained when allowing for between gender comparisons.

Conclusions

Reference groups are used for many applications in social sciences, but their construction is often tailor-made and dependent on the sample size. The present paper addresses the question of whether gender should be included as a characteristic for the definition of reference groups. The analysis uses three pretests of

[9]Results produced without controls are reported in the Appendix (Table A2 and Table A3).

the German Socio-Economic Panel with specific questions on gender comparisons. Results show that income comparisons happen mainly within people of the same sex. Women compare more than men regardless of the gender composition in their sector of employment. This result is probably because women have on average more possibilities of upward comparisons. Men, in contrast, compare less, but for those that do, the gender composition of the sector matters. Men compare with both women and men in male-dominated sectors, whereas they compare with only other men in female-dominated sectors. This study also confirms that more intense income comparisons decrease the SWB of all individuals. In spite of this evidence, we find that women's SWB is not affected by increasing income of their reference group. There may be two explanations for this finding. On the one hand, women's SWB could benefit from a possible tunnel effect, which occurs when an increase in reference income has the effect of increasing an individual's belief in future upward mobility. On the other hand, even though they found income comparisons to be important, women may not place much weight on economic and job-related factors in evaluating their overall life satisfaction. In contrast, men find income comparisons to be less important, but they suffer when the average income of their reference group increases. Therefore, the envy effect is the dominating effect compared to the tunnel effect for men. In the regressions estimating the effects of reference income on SWB, the reference groups constructed without gender better explain the overall variation. The coefficient magnitude of reference income is also larger when gender is not included in the creation of reference groups. This implies that reference groups for income comparisons should not include gender as a determinant even when the number of observations allows for its inclusion. As a cautionary note, it must be mentioned that the external validity of these results is limited to Western European countries characterised by a predominantly male breadwinner model. The relations may change in countries where women are more strongly selected into the labour market (e.g. Southern European countries) or where traditional gender norms are less common (e.g. Northern European countries). Moreover, the order in which questions were asked may have masked the effect of gendered comparisons; particularly because questions about colleagues and people who work in the same profession are asked before questions on men and women. New questionnaires with separate or distanced questions about gender comparisons might help with respect to this response bias. Future research might also investigate more closely why men, and not women, report a lower SWB when they work in gendered sectors.

Appendix

Table A.1 Gendered income comparisons and SWB: interactions between IC and gender

	(1)	(2)
	LS	LS
IC with women	−0.085**	
	(−2.49)	
Female * IC with women	−0.016	
	(−0.33)	
IC with men		−0.080***
		(−5.24)
Female * IC with men		−0.026
		(−0.70)
Controls	Yes	Yes
Observations	979	979
R^2	0.127	0.128
Adjusted R^2	0.111	0.112

Note: OLS estimates with standard errors clustered by region. Dependent variable: LS indicates life satisfaction (measured on a 0–10 scale). Controls include: female (main effect), Gini index, log of equivalised income, full time worker, self-employed, university degree, white collar, public sector, age, age squared, married, having children, town size, East Germany, year dummies

*p < 0.1, ** p < 0.05, *** p < 0.01, t statistics in parentheses

Table A.2 Gendered income comparisons and SWB

	(1)	(2)	(3)	(4)	(5)	(6)
	LS: all	LS: all	LS: men	LS: men	LS: women	LS: women
IC with women	−0.091***		−0.120**		−0.088**	
	(−5.13)		(−3.04)		(−3.12)	
IC with men		−0.099***		−0.110***		−0.092**
		(−5.99)		(−4.83)		(−3.16)
Controls	No	No	No	No	No	No
Observations	979	979	458	458	521	521
R^2	0.011	0.013	0.015	0.017	0.011	0.011

Note: OLS estimates with standard errors clustered by region. Dependent variable: LS indicates life satisfaction (measured on a 0–10 scale)

*p < 0.1, **p < 0.05, ***p < 0.01, t statistics in parentheses

Table A.3 Gendered income comparisons and SWB: testing reference groups

	(1)	(2)	(3)	(4)	(5)	(6)
	LS: all	LS: all	LS: men	LS: men	LS: women	LS: women
Log of equivalised	0.856***	0.841***	0.898***	0.903***	0.875***	0.862***
Income	(8.30)	(8.13)	(7.93)	(7.81)	(6.03)	(5.97)
Log of ref. inc.:	−0.322		−0.675**		0.110	
With gender	(−1.43)		(−2.77)		(0.37)	
Log of ref. inc.:		−0.323		−1.076***		0.295
Without gender		(−1.27)		(−4.62)		(0.96)
Controls	No	No	No	No	No	No
Observations	979	979	458	458	521	521
R2	0.070	0.070	0.078	0.084	0.073	0.074

Note: OLS estimates with standard errors clustered by region. Dependent variable: LS indicates life satisfaction (measured on a 0–10 scale)
*$p < 0.1$, **$p < 0.05$, ***$p < 0.01$, t statistics in parentheses

References

Bartolini, S., Bilancini, E., Sarracino F. (2013). Predicting the trend of well-being in Germany: How much do comparisons, adaptation and sociability matter? *Social Indicators Research,* 114(2), 169–191.

Boyce, C.J., Brown, G.D., Moore, S.C. (2010). Money and happiness: rank of income, not income, affects life satisfaction. *Psychological Science,* 21(4), 471–475.

Clark, A.E., & Oswald, A.J. (1996). Satisfaction and comparison income. *Journal of Public Economics*, 61(3), 359–381.

Clark, A.E., & Senik, C. (2010). Who compares to whom? The anatomy of income comparisons in Europe. *The Economic Journal,* 120(544), 573–594.

Della Giusta, M., Jewell S.L., Kambhampati, U.S. (2011). Gender and life satisfaction in the UK. *Feminist Economics,* 17(3), 1–34.

Ferrer-i-Carbonell, A. (2005). Income and well-being: An empirical analysis of the comparison income effect. *Journal of Public Economics,* 89(5), 997–1019.

Ferrer-i-Carbonell, A., & Frijters, P. (2004). How important is methodology for the estimates of the determinants of happiness? *The Economic Journal,* 114(497), 641–659.

Fiske, S. T. (2011). *Envy up, scorn down: How status divides us.* New York: Russell Sage Foundation.

Friehe, T., Mechtel, M., Pannenberg, M. (2014). Positional income concerns: Prevalence and relationship with personality and economic preferences. SOEPpapers on Multidisciplinary Panel Data Research 712. http://www.diw.de/documents/publikationen/73/diw_01.c.492426.de/diw_sp0712.pdf. Accessed 13 May 2018.

Goerke, L., & Pannenberg, M. (2015). Direct evidence for income comparisons and subjective well-being across reference groups. *Economics Letters,* 137, 95–101.

Haile, G. A. (2012). Unhappy working with men? Workplace gender diversity and job-related well-being in Britain. *Labour Economics,* 19(3), 329–350.

Hirschman, A.O., & Rothschild, M. (1973). The changing tolerance for income inequality in the course of economic development with a mathematical appendix. *The Quarterly Journal of Economics,* 87(4), 544–566.

Knies, G. (2012). Income comparisons among neighbours and satisfaction in East and West Ger *Social Indicators Research*, 106(3), 471–489.

MacKerron, G. (2012). Happiness economics from 35 000 feet. *Journal of Economic Surveys,* 26(4), 705–735.
Peccei, R., & Lee, H. J. (2005). The Impact of Gender Similarity on Employee Satisfaction at Work: A Review and Re-Evaluation. *Journal of Management Studies,* 42(8), 1571–1592.
Piekalkiewicz, M. (2016). Money, social capital and materialism. Evidence from happiness data. MPRA Paper No 70522. https://mpra.ub.uni-muenchen.de/70522/1/MPRA_paper_70522.pdf. Accessed 13 May 2018.
Ravazzini, L., & Chávez-Juárez, F. (2018). Which inequality makes people dissatisfied with their lives? Evidence of the link between life satisfaction and inequalities. *Social Indicators Research*, 137(3), 1119–1143.
Schneider, S. M. (2016). Income inequality and subjective wellbeing: Trends, challenges, and research directions. *Journal of Happiness Studies*, 17(4), 1719–1739.
Senik, C. (2008). Ambition and jealousy: Income interactions in the 'old' Europe versus the 'new' Europe and the United States. *Economica*, 75(299), 495–513.
Senik, C. (2009). Direct evidence on income comparisons and their welfare effects. *Journal of Economic Behavior & Organization,* 72(1), 408–424.
Trappe, H., Pollmann-Schult, M., Schmitt, C. (2015). The rise and decline of the male breadwinner model: institutional underpinnings and future expectations. *European Sociological Review,* 31(2), 230–242.

Part II
Social Sustainability, Lifestyle, Cultural Aspects and Local Applications

Sustainability of Wellbeing: An Analysis of Resilience and Vulnerability Through Subjective Indicators

Maria Bachelet, Fabiola Riccardini, and Filomena Maggino

Abstract Many scholars have focused on how the concepts of vulnerability and resilience may be employed in the analysis of sustainability. Different approaches have been proposed, concerning different fields of application (from environmental to financial settings). While much of the existing literature on vulnerability and resilience is sector-specific, we propose a more holistic approach that allows the sustainability of human well-being to be analyzed as a whole. In particular we apply those concepts to BES (*Benessere, Equo e Sostenibile*) framework, where 12 domains are included. Moreover, while the majority of studies consider the vulnerability and resilience as aspects of the sustainability of a "system" (a society, a country, or even the whole planet), we focus on an individual dimension of well-being, considering the exposure to risk and the ability to recover of the single persons. We show how the proposed scheme lends itself to the use of both objective and subjective indicators of well-being. Finally, using Italian data provided by the National Institute of Statistics (ISTAT), we propose an example of how to analyses the subjective aspects of wellbeing in terms of sustainability.

Introduction

In recent years, the concept of sustainability has received much attention both from the political and the academic world. Born in the realm of environmental economics, it has been gradually extended to many other domains. The fact that

M. Bachelet (✉)
Università degli Studi di Roma "Tor Vergata", Rome, Italy

F. Riccardini
Italian National Institute of Statistics (ISTAT), Rome, Italy
e-mail: fabiola.riccardini@istat.it

F. Maggino
Università degli Studi di Roma "La Sapienza", Rome, Italy
e-mail: filomena.maggino@uniroma1.it

A. Bianco et al. (eds.), *Italian Studies on Quality of Life*, Social Indicators Research Series 77, https://doi.org/10.1007/978-3-030-06022-0_11

sustainability is at the heart of the current international debate about the post-2015 agenda (the UN General Assembly met in September to deliver the final set of "Sustainable Development Goals") is still another proof of the relevance of such topic and an encouragement to provide rigorous research. Nonetheless, a shared universal definition of the concept of sustainability is still to be found and, more importantly, how the concept can be formalized to allow practical applications is a highly debated question. With the present study we hope to contribute to this debate by proposing a conceptual scheme to analyze sustainability of wellbeing. While most studies concentrate on specific fields, we propose a very general framework to analyze human well-being, which can be adapted to different situations according to the available data and needs. To do so, we exploit the concepts of "vulnerability" and "resilience" borrowed from the environmental and psychological disciplines. We reckon that the aim of analyzing human wellbeing as a whole is an ambitious goal, and that further research is certainly needed to complete and improve our framework. However, we feel that this preliminary discussion may actually provide very useful insights and ideas for future studies.

Secondly, we provide an application of such scheme with Italian data on subjective variables provided by the National Institute of Statistics (ISTAT) and included in the BES set of indicators. Indeed, the wide-range of information included in the BES project offers a unique opportunity to explore objective and subjective dimensions of individual wellbeing and jointly consider indicators related to different life domains. In this application we will focus on the cognitive aspect of subjective wellbeing, using "life satisfaction" as the outcome indicator and other subjective evaluations (linked to specific life domains) as instruments to check its sustainability.

Previous works exist which have studied the relationship between life-satisfaction and other aspects of life but they have done it for specific fields (mainly health, job, and social relations). Instead, we want to build a dynamic framework with interactions between all the different life domains and cognitive subjective wellbeing.

Besides while results in empirical studies are often weakened by the difficulty of identifying the correct causality nexus in the observed correlation, results on our specific research question yield straightforward implications even without finding a decisive answer to the causality problem. This is because the simple correlation we observe is already exploitable for the analysis of sustainability: if vulnerability and resilience factors significantly correlate with future overall life-satisfaction this implies that the subjective indicators under scrutiny must be taken into account to analyze sustainability of subjective wellbeing and forecast future trends. Preliminary results provide support to our hypotheses.

The chapter proceeds as follow. In section "Literature review on subjective wellbeing" we review the literature on subjective wellbeing, while in section "The BES framework for sustainability" we outline the theoretical framework setup by the BES scientific commission based on the concepts of vulnerability and resilience to analyze sustainability of wellbeing. In the third section we show how the proposed scheme lends itself to the use of subjective indicators of wellbeing. In section

"Application to subjective indicators", we use subjective indicators coming from the BES framework to test our hypothesis and present preliminary results of our analysis. In the final section, we draw conclusions and outline future steps that needs to be accomplished in order to complete our research.

Literature Review on Subjective Wellbeing

Traditionally, wellbeing has been identified with a single objective dimension: material progress measured by GDP per capita. However, it is now widely accepted that the concept of wellbeing is multidimensional, encompassing all aspects of human life that are not included in the GDP (housing, working conditions, health, social relations etc.). In latest years, and particularly after the recommendations included in the Sen, Stiglitz and Fitoussi commission's report (2009), many national statistical institutes and international institutions have recognized the need to measure quality of life with set of indicators covering different aspects of individual and community life.[1] It is worth noting that the identification of the domains to be included in the definition of wellbeing and the choice of indicators to measure them of such a complex concept inevitably reflects values and norms and priorities of those who are involved in the selection process.

There is particular disagreement on whether the subjective dimension, which can indicate how a condition is perceived by people as distinct from an objective observable assessment of conditions, should be included in the measurement of wellbeing. In the wellbeing literature, despite some attempts to reconcile them, two opposite approaches still exist: Objective Well-being theories (such as the basic need approach) are usually supported by a list of requirements that people should have satisfied in order to lead a good life, those requirements are universal and do not vary among societies. On the other hand, Subjective Well-being theories base their notion of well-being on the fact that people are reckoned to be the best judges of the overall quality of their lives, and it is a straightforward strategy to ask them about their well-being (Frey and Stutzer 2002).

It has in fact been observed in many studies how objective or external indicators do not always track with self-reported measures, so that people may be highly satisfied with a life way that seems poor by standard measures. Thus, information on subjective wellbeing can usefully complete other objective information by allowing divergences between what persons perceive and what is objectively observed (Diener and Seligman 2004). Since perceptions and evaluations influence the way persons face life and benefit from opportunities, it is crucial to consider subjective

[1]Following the recommendation of the SSF commission ISTAT has incorporated in the BES framework both objective and subjective assessments of wellbeing "Measures of both objective and subjective well-being provide key information about people's quality of life. Statistical offices [worldwide] should incorporate questions to capture people's life evaluations, hedonic experiences and priorities in their own survey." [Executive Summary of Commission Report (32), pp. 12 and 16].

dimensions within the concept of general wellbeing, thus allowing attention to be oriented towards individuals' evaluation of living conditions, opportunities, preferences, expectations and adaptations (Eurofound 2005). This fact has been recognized also by the OECD, which has recently clarified that "measuring subjective well-being is an essential part of measuring quality of life alongside other social and economic dimensions" (OECD 2013). However, reconciling subjective accounts of well-being and objective measures such as availability of housing, school or health facilities has proven to be a challenging task (Gasper 2004).

Among the many theoretical framework that have been set out, we will refer to the one proposed by Wolfgang Zapf (1984) which divides wellbeing into two macro dimensions: (i) living conditions, (ii) subjective wellbeing (SWB). It is important to note that the subjective component is relevant in both dimensions. Living conditions can mainly be distinguished in objective living conditions and subjective evaluation of living conditions, observed, respectively, through objective and subjective measures and indicators (e.g. the concept of "security" can be seen in objective terms but also in its dynamics related to subjective perceptions). Objective living conditions relate to the different (personal and social) domains which each individual is involved in. In other words, objective living conditions refer mainly to material resources, standards of living, working conditions and status, state of health, social relationships. Objective indicators allow each aspect of living conditions to be evaluated. Their specificity is in the possibility to define and recognize external objective references, so that they are verifiable. The same living conditions can be subjectively evaluated by individuals by asking questions about their level of satisfaction with specific matter (e.g. "how satisfied are you with your job?" "would you say your health is very good, good, bad, very bad?").

Concerning the second component, SWB, the most accepted and adopted definition envisages two distinct dimensions, cognitive and affective (Diener 1984).The cognitive component is related to the process through which each individual retrospectively evaluate (in terms of "satisfaction") her/his life, as a whole. In other words, satisfaction with life is the result of a cognitive process, allowing the individual to evaluate her/his present situation with reference to standards individually defined (Nuvolati 2002). The affective component, on the other hand, refers to the emotions experienced by individuals during their daily lives and relates to the individuals' present situation. The emotions can be positive (pleasant affects) or negative (unpleasant affects), which are considered conceptually distinct and influenced by different variables (Bradburn 1969; Diener and Emmons 1984; Argyle 1987). A third component of SWB is actually recognized, the so-called eudaimonia, mainly has been proposed by Ryff (1989). This third dimension encompasses concepts such as authenticity, self-actualization, engagement, and purpose in life, which are crucial elements of people's subjective perceptions about their own wellbeing, and are not captured by either the cognitive or the affective measures. However, this latter dimension is not usually recorded in national and international surveys, like life satisfaction. Besides, unlike the affective component of SWB, life satisfaction ensures a higher level of reliability and comparability (Diener 2006). This is why in this study we focus our attention only on the cognitive dimension of SWB.

The interpretative models allow determinants of subjective wellbeing to be identified. The different ways through which the relationship between living conditions and subjective wellbeing is defined relate to different conceptualization of quality of life. In an attempt to define the quality of happiness and, in general, subjective wellbeing, two structural elements have to be considered, the community and the future. With reference to the former element, the relationship between the individual wellbeing and the community's wellbeing should be considered by exploring two issues. On one hand, even though the concept of "community wellbeing" could be covered by referring to aggregation of individual outcomes, the simple sum of all individuals' wellbeing composing that community cannot represent in itself the community wellbeing, which should include also other different characteristics. On the other hand, the discussion concerns if a compromise is needed between pursuing community's and pursuing individuals' wellbeing. In other words, it should be verified whether any individual wellbeing is pursued at the expense of other individuals' wellbeing. Concerning the latter element, the future perspective directly refers to the individual future as well as the community one. The discussion involves the costs of maintaining, improving, or declining of the present situation. While the former element involves the concept of equity, the latter refers to the concept of sustainability.

The concept of sustainability can be considered with reference to different perspectives (present and future; objective and subjective) and different levels (community and individual). The concept of sustainability can be referred to the capitals which should be preserved for present and future generations and at individual and community levels. By focusing on subjective perspective, two approaches should be identified, subjective aspects of sustainability and the sustainability of subjective wellbeing. Assessing sustainability of subjective wellbeing generally does not necessarily require ad-hoc measures and the identification of particular aspects (and indicators) but different analytical approaches of those already monitored (Stiglitz et al. 2009; Giovannini et al. 2012). In the next section we will discuss how the BES scientific commission has adopted and elaborated on this latter approach.

The BES Framework for Sustainability

The theoretical framework produced by the sub-group of the Scientific Commission of the Scientific Committee of BES project has focused its attention on a concept of sustainability that, means the concept of sustainability not as a "noun" in its own right, but rather as an "adjective" of well-being; therefore avoids facing the question of systemic sustainability as such, and rather focuses on checking whether the levels of wellbeing being achieved are sustainable - in the sense of "maintainable" - over time. The subgroup on the sustainability of the Scientific Committee of BES then traced the path for the identification of appropriate measures for sustainable wellbeing. In this process, the conceptual aspects of measuring sustainability have been treated in line the current debate on overcoming of GDP and with the United Nations

Declaration of 2013 for which there is sustainable development when the well-being of individuals is sought.

In the discussion on the indicators for sustainable well-being the committee also considered the framework on the measurement of sustainable development provided by the CES (Conference of European Statisticians) and the UNECE (United Nations Economic Commission for Europe), as well as suggestions included in the EU Development Strategy and the program Europe2020.

In deciding how to measure sustainability, the subgroup of the Scientific Committee of the BES project has made the basic choice of connecting the concept of sustainability to that of wellbeing of people, considering the interconnection of the three dimensions: economic, social and environmental. The commission acknowledged that wellbeing is a multidimensional concept that changes with time, places and cultures, and identified some key features in the measurement of sustainability such as insecurity, complexity, dynamism, global scope and, above all, interconnection between different BES domains (trade-offs between the components of the different domains have been considered like the tensions that can exist between policies on energy, environmental protection, social welfare and economic development).

The final outcome of the work of the BES committee is a theoretical model that considers whether it is possible to improve or maintain the level of wellbeing achieved without compromising the conditions, opportunities and resources of the present and future generations. Sustainability is understood as a balance between elements of vulnerability and elements of resilience referred to a country, a group of people, or an individual.

Vulnerability and resilience are reflected, respectively, in the risk factors that can undermine the level of wellbeing, and the factors of risk mitigation and/or ability to react that allow to recover after a negative shock. This theoretical framework based on resilience and vulnerability factors is in fact applicable to all aspects of wellbeing, both at the individual and at the collective level. It also permits to highlight the interconnections between indicators of different domains and to identify existing trade- off. The scheme of the theoretical framework developed by the Scientific Committee is summarized in Fig. 1.

The sustainability of the wellbeing (and not sustainable ecosystem *tout court*) is understood as a state of balance/equilibrium (of conditions, factors, resources ...) with respect to the level of well-being achieved in a given time. In this equilibrium there is a simultaneous presence of vulnerabilities and resilience, which can be existing or potential.

These aspects, present in the different domains of the BES framework, may refer to individuals, specific social groups or the whole country, thus justifying the use of both micro- and macro-level indicators (e.g. individual policies put in place to ensure good governance of the resources, condition of specific social groups, state of the environment etc.). Therefore by considering these individual and collective dimensions, the concepts of vulnerability and resilience can be divided into indicators that pick at the individual and collective exposure to adverse shocks, with reference to the first concept, or the ability to restore the lost equilibrium, with regard to the second concept.

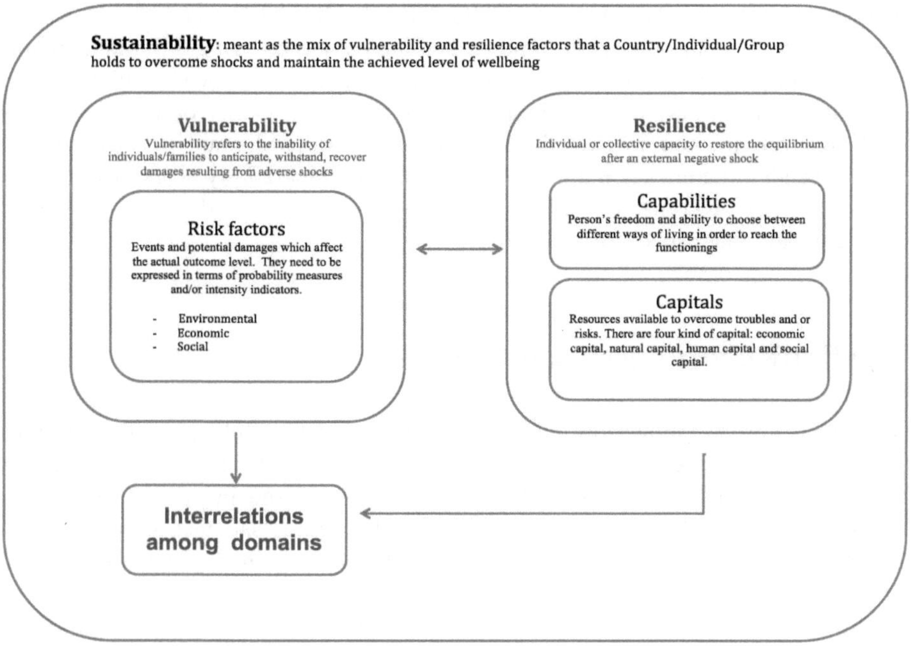

Fig. 1 Scheme for sustainability

Indicators of vulnerability should measure the main risk factors that threaten the current levels of well-being, considering the economic, social and environmental context, and all those structural aspects that can alter the equilibrium achieved in terms of well-being (including excessive levels of socio-economic inequality). Conversely the indicators of resilience must consider those elements that, as a result of adverse shocks, allow to restore the level of wellbeing previously reached, including individual capacities and collective capitals (economic, social and environmental) available. In this case, recourse is made to the concepts of capital and capacity indicators. For capacity means states and activities of people that reflect the freedom and the ability of the same to choose between different ways of living, in order to achieve personal well-being, where are those for capital resources (wealth) that can be used to meet the needs and/or to face individual and collective future risks, net of liabilities (considering measures of capital stocks and flows that determine the variation over time of the stock through investment and depreciation). The measures developed by the National Accounts, such as physical capital, human capital and trials of some satellite accounts (such as the estimation of non-market household), natural capital and its environmental accounts are then placed in this conceptual framework.

The most critical aspect of the BES theoretical framework, is that the functional division that has allowed us to consider the well-being divided into separate domains cannot be maintained when discussing sustainability, as the interrelations between phenomena and their trade-offs that exist in real life necessarily lead to simultaneously consider aspects (and related indicators) covering different domains of wellbeing. For this reason vulnerabilities and resilience elements, which in their mutual dynamics may affect the equilibrium, must necessarily be conceptualized and analyzed in their interrelations among the various domains (an element of resilience identified in a domain can be an aspect of vulnerability in another domain, as well as an outcome indicators of a domain can be considered as factors of resilience to other aspects of wellbeing).

Application to Subjective Indicators

In this section we show how the theoretical framework outlined in the previous section can be applied to subjective indicators of wellbeing. The outcome indicator is considered to be "life-satisfaction", which is analyzed in order to check its vulnerability or resilience. As highlighted in the literature, 'satisfaction with life as a whole" reflects the cognitive dimension of SWB and arises naturally as an outcome indicator.

Vulnerability and resilience factors in this case are represented by subjective evaluations of different aspects of life (such as health, social relations, job etc.). As will be clarified later on, these indicators come from the BES framework and are grouped into ten life-domains. However, the scheme is very general and could be easily enlarged and adapted to other sets of subjective indicators referring to different domains (Fig. 2).

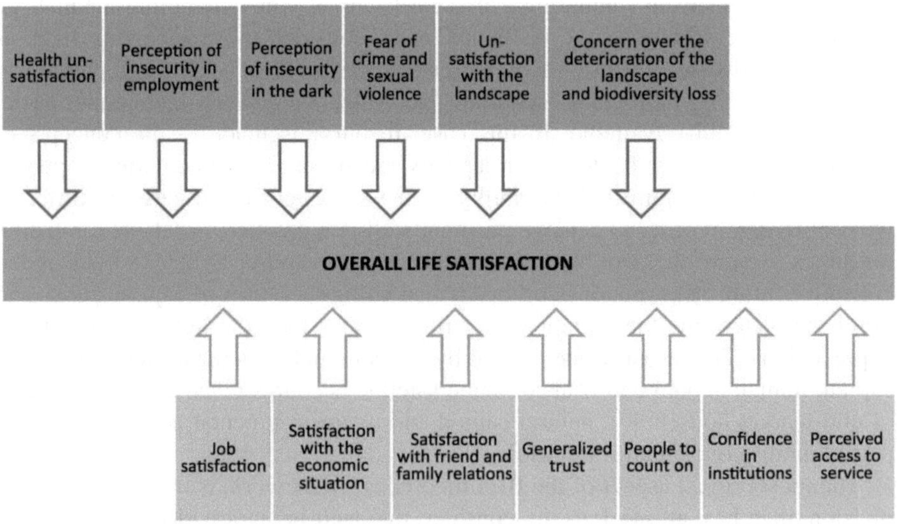

Fig. 2 Vulnerability/resilience scheme applied to subjective indicators

We start by dividing the available variables based on what we think could affect the outcome indicator in a positive or negative way (see Fig. 1). As clarified in the previous section, we define as vulnerability factors those elements that increase the probability of experiencing a negative shock on the outcome variable. In this setting, the definition translates into the following hypothesis: if the vulnerability indicator is high at time t−1, we should observe on average a lower level of the outcome indicator (life- satisfaction) at time t. On the other hand, resilience factors are those factors that increase the ability of recovering after a negative shock. In this case, if the resilience indicator is high at time t−1, we should observe a stable or higher level of the outcome indicator at time t. Given these definitions, we will test our hypothesis by analyzing the trends and the correlation coefficients of the outcome variable (life satisfaction) with each indicator lagged one period. If our model is correct, we should observe negative coefficients for all vulnerability indicators and positive coefficients for resilience indicators.

Data Description

We created the "BES subjective database" by assembling data about the subjective indicators of the BES framework. Since, with the exception of education, each domain contains at least one subjective indicator, the BES framework offers the perfect environment to jointly analyze aspects of subjective wellbeing linked to different life- domains (see Fig. 1). With respect to the original framework, two indicators were substituted for practical reasons so as to obtain a cleaner database, namely the indicators on the health and the economic situation.

The original indicator on subjective health was the PCS.[2] Since it consists in a complex mixture of subjective and objective assessments of the health status, it was difficult to interpret and not exploitable as a pure subjective indicator. It was therefore substituted with an indicator based on the widely used and universally accepted question: "How is your health in general? Very good, Good, Fair, Bad, Very bad" (in particular the indicator consists in the percentage of people responding "Bad" or "Very Bad"). The initial subjective indicator on economic wellbeing was the so-called "Index of subjective evaluation of economic distress" which combines different pieces of information about the economic situation of the household.[3] For

[2]The "Physical Component Summary, PCS" computed as the summary of the scores of each individual answering the 12 questions on the questionnaire SF12 on physical state.

[3]The Index of subjective evaluation of economic distress combines three indicators: (a) share of individuals living in households answering "with great difficulty" to the question "Considering all the available income, how does your household manage to get to the end of the month?"; (b) proportion of individuals living in households with insufficient resources to face an unexpected expense of a given amount, fixed as a fraction of the median of the distribution of previous year equivalent income; (c) share of individuals who expect to be unable to make savings in the next 12 months.

the same reasons as before, this indicator was substituted with the more standard and simple indicator based on the question: "How satisfied are you with your economic situation? Very Satisfied, Somewhat Satisfied, Not very satisfied, Not at all satisfied" (in particular the indicator is the percentage of people responding "Very satisfied" or "Somewhat satisfied').

After these two substitutions, all indicators come from multiple-item questions (a complete description of indicators is presented in Table 1 in the Appendix). Most of the questions entails a ladder were the respondent has to place himself (the following indicators belong to this category: "Health un-satisfaction", "Satisfaction with economic situation", "Friend relations", "Family relations", "Confidence in all kind of institutions", "Fear of sexual violence", "Insecurity in the dark", "Life satisfaction", "Landscape un-satisfaction", "Access to service"). All these indicators are expressed as the percentage of people who chooses either the "most positive" or the "most negative" items, with the important exception of confidence in all kind of institutions which is expressed as the average score (the scale goes from 0 to 10).

The remaining indicators come from questions that have only two options (i.e. "Generalized trust", "People to count on", "Insecurity of employment", "Fear of crime", "Landscape deterioration", "Biodiversity loss"). These indicators are expressed as the percentage of people who answered one of the two items (actually most of the questions also involves the extra option "I don't know"). Finally, the indicator on job satisfaction is different from all the others and more complicated. It consists in the average satisfaction with the following aspects of the work done (scale of 0 to 10): wage, number of hours worked, type of schedule, labor relations, stable place, distance from home to job, interest of the job. We could not substitute it because we could not find data from surveys where a simpler question was asked (such as "How satisfied are you with your job overall?").

Concerning the level of aggregation, all indicators refer to data aggregated at regional level. Each indicator refers to a given year and to a region. Since Italian regions are 23,[4] this means we have 23 observations on each indicator for each year. Moreover, we also consider in our analysis the macro-areas of Northern, Centre and Southern Italy. The resulting dataset is a panel database where $i =$ Italian regions, and $t =$ year, containing 2470 observations. The time-ranges from 1998 to 2013, but unfortunately the availability of years varies greatly depending on the indicator, and some indicators are available for very few years (see Table 2 in the Appendix).

The main drawback of this database is that it contains information coming from different ISTAT surveys (and thus from different samples). This means that we must rely on regional averages in order to compare the indicators, while it would be more appropriate to compare them at the individual level. Nonetheless, the analysis of regional data may provide interesting insights and a first empirical support to our hypothesis. Finally, it is important to note that the indicator on life satisfaction (the

[4]Piemonte, Valle d'Aosta, Liguria, Lombardia, Trentino-Alto Adige, Bolzano, Trento, Veneto, Friuli-Venezia Giulia, Emilia-Romagna, Toscana, Umbria, Marche, Lazio, Abruzzo, Molise, Campania, Puglia, Basilicata, Calabria, Sicilia, Sardegna.

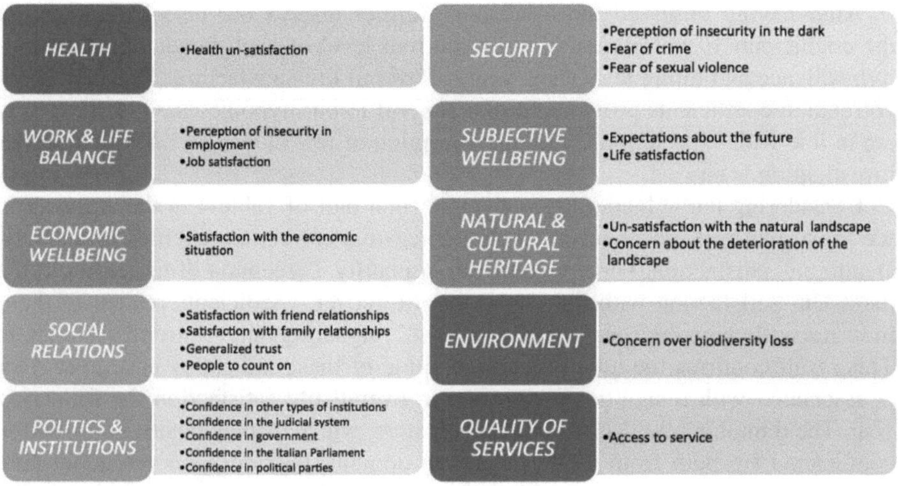

Fig. 3 Subjective indicators in the BES framework

outcome variable) is available only for the last 4 years (i.e. from 2010 to 2013). Beyond the general consideration that it would be better to have longer time series, this means that for the purpose of our analysis we must rely on data that refers to the post-crisis period. This fact potentially biases the results, or at least make them less robust and externally valid (Fig. 3).

Descriptive Findings

To test the hypotheses described in section "Application to subjective indicators", we first examine data through the analysis of trends and then through the computation of correlation coefficients (Table 3).

Actually, by considering jointly the trends of subjective indicators, it is already possible to draw preliminary conclusions in support of our hypothesis (see Figs. 4, 5, 6 and 7 in the Appendix). The figures show clearly that while vulnerability indicators have generally experienced an increase over the considered years, all subjective indicators of resilience displayed a negative trend. Even though for some indicators the series is short, these tendencies are clearly visible. These two realities are matched with a significant decrease of the outcome indicator, i.e. life satisfaction. This same pattern is replicated in all macro-areas of the country (North, Center and South), with very little variations. This fining demonstrates that the overall trend observed at the country level is not the result of compensations between subsets of the sample (the pattern is actually the same also for each Italian region, but we do not show all the graphs here for the sake of brevity).

After having observed the trends, we further inspect our data by computing the coefficients of correlation between current level of each factor of vulnerability/resilience and future level (next year) of overall life-satisfaction. The analysis of correlation coefficients provides further support to our hypotheses. Overall, results are in line with expectations, with the exception of few indicators on which deeper investigation is needed.

Considering the vulnerability indicators (first half of Table 4 in the Appendix), we found that five out of seven display a negative correlation coefficient; namely, Health un- satisfaction, Perception of job insecurity, Perception of insecurity in the dark, Un- satisfaction with the landscape. Moreover, coefficients related to these indicators all range between −0.65 and −0.82, signaling quite a strong correlation. This result confirms the idea that a high value of these indicators in a given year is associated with a significant decrease in overall life satisfaction the following year. The remaining two vulnerability indicators, which display positive correlation coefficients are both from the environment domain (they are Concern about land deterioration, and Concern over biodiversity loss). Despite the positive sign of the coefficient, we cannot infer that these two would be better classified as resilience factors, since there are probably other reasons for this result. First of all for these indicators we have data about just 1 year, which is not sufficient to draw robust conclusions. Secondly, it could be that the link between problems of the environment and evaluation of quality of life is not strong and direct enough (compared for instance to job or social relations). As a matter of fact, consequences of biodiversity loss and land deterioration do not directly affect everyday life, or at least not in the short-run. Besides, the two indicators actually come from the same question, which has and the wording of the questions from which the indicators come is actually ambiguous: "Which are the top 5 environmental problems among the following?" and then there are 15 items among which we find: "Biodiversity loss", and "Decay of landscape due to overbuilding". It is thus probable that the unexpected signs of the coefficients are related to a measurement problem linked to this atypical question.

About the analysis on resilience indicators, we found positive and relevant correlation coefficients (see second half of Table 4 in the Appendix) for the following factors: Job satisfaction, Economic satisfaction, Satisfaction with friend relations, Satisfaction with family relations, Generalized trust, People to count on, Perceived access to services. These positive coefficients confirm the idea that a high value of these indicators in a given year is associated with a significant increase in overall life satisfaction the following year. On the other hand, no clear pattern is observed in the subset of indicators referring to confidence in institutions (i.e., Confidence in the judicial system, Confidence in the government, Confidence in the government, Confidence in the Italian Parliament, Confidence in political parties, Confidence in other types of institutions).

Some of these indicators display negative coefficients while the others are positive but very small. To interpret this outcome we must recall that these are the only indicators computed as average score (scale 0–10) instead of percentage. This difference in measurement may be responsible for the unexpected results. Besides, also in this case very few years are available (just one or 2 years). Finally, another possible explanation is that, as in the case of environmental problems, these factors do not directly affect everyday life (even though the government and the parliament clearly have the possibility to change people's life, many people still perceive them as distant and not very relevant in their everyday matters). Moreover, in this case we must also consider that not everybody have direct contact with institutions such as the judicial system. For all these reasons we believe that future investigation is needed on this subset and that we cannot conclude weather these indicators should or should not be included among vulnerability factors (Tables 5, 6, 7 and 8).

Conclusions and Next Steps

The paper has highlighted how the sustainability of wellbeing could be analyzed through the lenses of vulnerability and resilience. The scheme proposed is an original contribution and a very general framework that could be fruitfully adapted to other contexts and fields. Also, we have shown an example of how to apply the scheme to subjective indicators of wellbeing, using the framework of the BES project. With the available data we delivered preliminary results that provide support to our hypothesis. We found that almost all vulnerability factors correlate strongly and negatively with future life- satisfaction, while resilience factors correlate positively. Policy implications of our theoretical framework and results are that through the analysis of vulnerability and resilience factors it is possible to say something about the sustainability of the current level of wellbeing and predict future changes in overall life satisfaction.

Although the analysis provided interesting insights and a first empirical support to our theoretical model, further research is needed to complete our work. Indeed, as highlighted earlier, some limitations on data availability prevented us from completing the study. We are thus planning to continue and improve he research through the following steps.

First of all, we plan to recover micro-level data from the ISTAT database. Since information come from different surveys and samples, we are planning to apply a "record linkage", a statistical methodology that permits to link data from different surveys (already used in Italy to connect surveys on enterprises). Once we have a complete database with data at the individual level, it will be possible to perform an econometric analysis. Using a regression model will allow us to include control variables and thus disentangle the specific effect of each vulnerability and resilience factor on the outcome variable. Moreover, we wish to find extra data to obtain longer time series on life-satisfaction and extend the analysis to include the years before the financial crisis. Finally, we would like to deepen the research on the role of "future expectations" and "satisfaction with leisure time", two subjective indicators belonging to the BES framework, which we could not exploit yet.

Appendix

Table 1 Variable legend (BES)

Variable	Label	Description
health_insat	Health un-satisfaction	Percentage of people aged 14 and over who respond "very bad" or "bad" to the question "How is your health in general?"
insec_job	Perception of insecurity in employment	Percentage of employees who believe that in the next 6 months they are likely to lose current job and that they have little probability of finding another job on the total employed.
job_sat	Job satisfaction	Media satisfaction with the following aspects of the work done (scale of 0 to 10): wage, number of hours worked, type of schedule, labor relations, stable place, distance from home to job, interest of the job.
eco_sat	Satisfaction with the economic situation	Percentage of people aged 14 and over who are very satisfied with their economic situation
rel_friend	Satisfaction with friend relationships	Percentage of people aged 14 and over who are very satisfied with their relationships with friends
rel_family	Satisfaction with family relationships	Percentage of people aged 14 and over who are very satisfied with family relationships
gen_trust	Generalized trust	Percentage of people aged 14 and over who believes that most of the people are trustworthy
rel_count	People to count on	Percentage of people aged 14 and over who have relatives, friends or neighbors they can count on
conf_inst	Confidence in other types of institutions	Average score of confidence in the police and fire department (on a scale from 0 to 10) expressed by persons aged 14 and over.
conf_jud	Confidence in the judicial system	Average score of trust in the judicial system (on a scale from 0 to 10) expressed by persons aged 14 and over.
conf_gov	Confidence in government	Average score of confidence in the regional government, the provincial and municipal level (on a scale from 0 to 10) expressed by persons aged 14 and over.
conf_parl	Confidence in the Italian Parliament	Average rating of confidence in the Italian Parliament (on a scale from 0 to 10) expressed by persons aged 14 and over.
conf_party	Confidence in political parties	Average score of trust in political parties (on a scale from 0 to 10) expressed by persons aged 14 and over.
insec_dark	Perception of insecurity in the dark	Percentage of people aged 14 and over who does not feel safe walking alone in the dark in the area where they live
fear_crime	Fear of crime	Percentage of people aged 14 and over who have been afraid of being about to suffer a crime in the last 12 months
fear_viol	Fear of sexual violence	Percentage of people aged 14 and over who are worried (very or somewhat) to undergo a sexual assault
future_exp	Expectations about the future	Percentage of people aged 14 and over who feel that their personal situation will improve over the next 5 years

(continued)

Table 1 (continued)

Variable	Label	Description
life_sat	Life satisfaction	Percentage of people aged 14 and over who have expressed a life satisfaction score between 8 and 10
land_insat	Un-satisfaction with the landscape	Percentage of people aged 14 and over stating that the landscape near their place of living is affected by evident degradation
land_det	Concern about the deterioration of the landscape	Percentage of people aged 14 and over who place among the top 5 environmental problems landscape deterioration caused by excessive construction of buildings
bio_loss	Concern over biodiversity loss	Percentage of people aged 14 and over who place biodiversity loss among the top 5 environmental concerns
serv_acc	Access to service	Percentage of households who do not have difficulties in reaching three or more essential services (pharmacy, emergency room, Post office, police, police, municipal offices, kindergarten, maternal, elementary school, middle school lower, grocery stores, markets, supermarkets)

Table 2 Availability of years

	Variable	1998	2003	2004	2005	2006	2007	2008	2009	2010	2011	2012	2013
V	*health_insat*	.	.	.	.	.	.	.	X	X	X	X	X
V	*insec_job*	.	.	.	.	.	.	.	.	.	.	.	X
R	*job_sat*	.	X	.	.	.	.	.	X	.	.	.	X
R	*eco_sat*	X	X	X	X	X	X	X	X	X	X	X	X
R	*rel_friend*	.	.	.	X	X	X	X	X	X	X	X	X
R	*rel_family*	.	.	.	X	X	X	X	X	X	X	X	X
R	*gen_trust*	.	.	.	.	.	.	.	.	X	X	X	X
R	*rel_count*	X	X	.	.	.	.	.	X	.	.	.	X
R	*conf_inst*	.	.	.	.	.	.	.	.	.	.	X	X
R	*conf_jud*	.	.	.	.	.	.	.	.	.	X	X	X
R	*conf_gov*	.	.	.	.	.	.	.	.	.	.	X	X
R	*conf_parl*	.	.	.	.	.	.	.	.	.	X	X	X
R	*conf_party*	.	.	.	.	.	.	.	.	.	X	X	X
V	*insec_dark*	.	.	.	.	.	.	.	.	X	X	X	X
V	*fear_crime*	.	.	.	.	.	.	.	X	.	.	.	.
V	*fear_viol*	.	X	.	.	.	.	.	X	.	.	.	.
V	*land_insat*	.	.	.	.	.	.	.	.	.	.	X	.
V	*land_det*	X	.	.	.	.	.	.	.	.	.	X	.
V	*bio_loss*	X	.	.	.	.	.	.	.	.	.	X	X
R	*serv_acc*	.	.	.	.	X	X	X	X	X	X	X	.
O	*future_exp*	.	.	.	.	.	.	.	.	.	.	X	X
O	*life_sat*	.	.	.	.	.	.	.	.	X	X	X	X

Table 3 Correlation coefficients with life satisfaction in the same year (table on the left) and Correlation coefficients with life satisfaction in the next year (table on the right)

	2010	2011	2012	2013		2009	2010	2011	2012
Vulnerability					**Vulnerability**				
health_insat	−0.7573	−0.7165	−0.6691	−0.7835	*health_insat*	−0.6940	−0.6859	−0.7586	−0.7020
insec_job	.	.	.	−0.8306	*insec_job*	.	.	.	.
insec_dark	−0.6896	−0.7676	−0.7995	−0.7090	*insec_dark*	.	−0.7499	−0.6480	−0.8238
fear_crime	.	.	.	.	*fear_crime*	−0.6934	.	.	.
fear_viol	.	.	.	.	*fear_viol*	−0.8110	.	.	.
land_insat	.	.	−0.7786	.	*land_insat*	.	.	.	−0.7439
land_det	.	.	0.7100	.	*land_det*	.	.	.	0.7225
bio_loss	.	.	0.8926	0.8471	*bio_loss*	.	.	.	0.8919
Resilience					**Resilience**				
job_sat	.	.	.	0.9362	*job_sat*	0.8782	.	.	.
eco_sat	0.9127	0.9113	0.9310	0.8846	*eco_sat*	0.8610	0.8373	0.9071	0.9312
rel_friend	0.7732	0.7429	0.8967	0.8819	*rel_friend*	0.7242	0.7487	0.8242	0.8840
rel_family	0.7276	0.7277	0.8402	0.8268	*rel_family*	0.7035	0.6611	0.8145	0.7959
gen_trust	0.8738	0.7728	0.7534	0.8540	*gen_trust*	.	0.8047	0.8166	0.7882
rel_count	.	.	.	0.7375	*rel_count*	0.7134	.	.	.
conf_inst	.	−0.1037	0.6864	0.5592	*conf_inst*	.	.	.	0.6293
conf_jud	.	.	−0.2624	−0.2335	*conf_jud*	.	.	−0.2985	−0.2201
conf_gov	.	−0.4252	0.8418	0.8287	*conf_gov*	.	.	.	0.8532
conf_parl	.	0.4431	−0.4835	−0.7473	*conf_parl*	.	.	−0.6313	−0.4525
conf_party	.		0.5594	0.4148	*conf_party*	.	.	0.2644	0.6212
serv_acc	0.6228	0.4556	0.6526	.	*serv_acc*	0.6406	0.4929	0.6830	0.6425

Table 4 Correlation coefficients between resilience indicators

	job_sat	*eco_sat*	*rel_friend*	*rel_family*	*gen_trust*	*rel_count*	*conf_inst*	*conf_jud*	*conf_gov*	*conf_parl*	*conf_party*	*serv_acc*
job_sat	1											
eco_sat	0,7939	1										
rel_friend	0,8019	0,7693	1									
rel_family	0,7666	0,7288	0,9467	1								
gen_trust	0,8572	0,8217	0,7199	0,7162	1							
rel_count	0,5172	0,3403	0,5172	0,5557	0,771	1						
conf_inst	0,6607	0,5404	0,7219	0,7521	0,5258	0,5209	1					
conf_jud	−0,2138	−0,0632	−0,2276	−0,2515	−0,1051	−0,1697	−0,2242	1				
conf_gov	0,9183	0,8398	0,8272	0,8021	0,7723	0,6549	0,7602	−0,2579	1			
conf_parl	−0,7199	−0,3382	−0,3152	−0,3743	−0,4223	−0,5909	−0,1971	0,421	−0,2552	1		
conf_party	0,3134	0,5183	0,295	0,2038	0,3342	0,192	0,1357	0,49	0,4382	0,2989	1	
serv_acc	0,7608	0,6222	0,7434	0,7424	0,658	0,7121	0,6917	−0,4846	0,7066	−0,3278	0,1706	1

Table 5 Correlation coefficients between vulnerability indicators

	health_ insat	*insec_job*	*insec_ dark*	*fear_ crime*	*fear_viol*	*land_ insat*	*land_det*	*bio_ loss*
health_insat	1							
insec_job	0,7231	1						
insec_dark	0,3637	0,5361	1					
fear_crime	0,3215	.	.	1				
fear_viol	0,431	.	.	0,8459	1			
land_insat	0,4593	.	0,6946	.	.	1		
land_det	−0,5921	.	−0,4102	.	.	−0,5769	1	
bio_loss	−0,6919	−0,7747	−0,5426	.	.	−0,7465	0,6979	1

Table 6 Correlation coefficients with future expectations in the same year

		2012	2013
Vulnerability	*health_insat*	0.2185	−0.1228
	insec_job	.	−0.3189
	insec_dark	0.0181	−0.2087
	fear_crime	.	.
	fear_viol	.	.
	land_insat	−0.3565	.
	land_det	0.3179	.
	bio_loss	0.2548	0.4286
Resilience	*job_sat*	.	0.3254
	eco_sat	0.1531	0.3147
	rel_friend	0.4009	0.3161
	rel_family	0.3662	0.2966
	gen_trust	0.0697	0.2713
	rel_count	.	0.4436
	conf_inst	0.1444	0.0105
	conf_jud	−0.6275	−0.5467
	conf_gov	0.1401	0.1758
	conf_parl	−0.2656	−0.3413
	conf_party	−0.1152	−0.0174
	serv_acc	0.4317	.

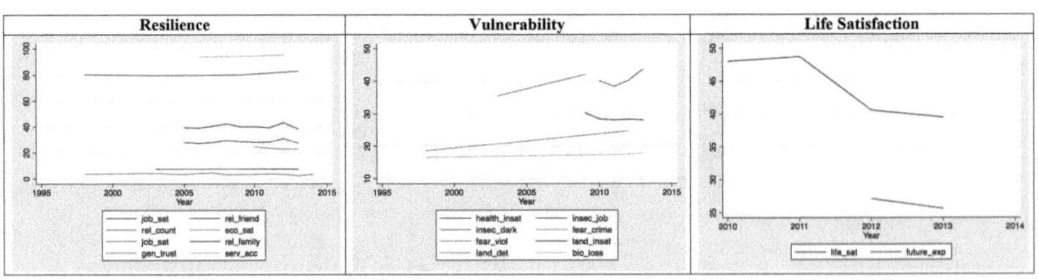

Fig. 4 Resilience and vulnerability in the North

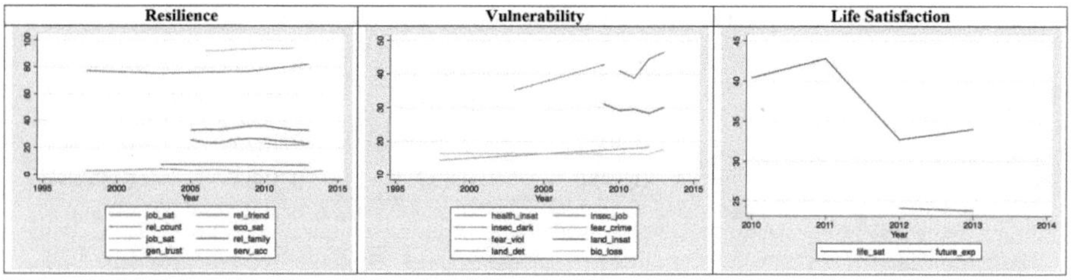

Fig. 5 Resilience and vulnerability in the Center

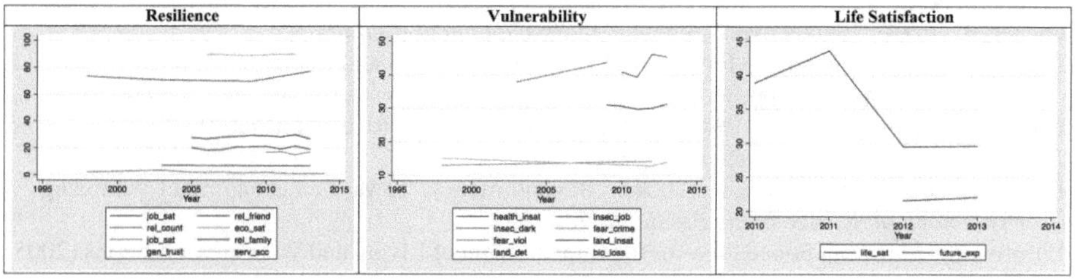

Fig. 6 Resilience and vulnerability in the South

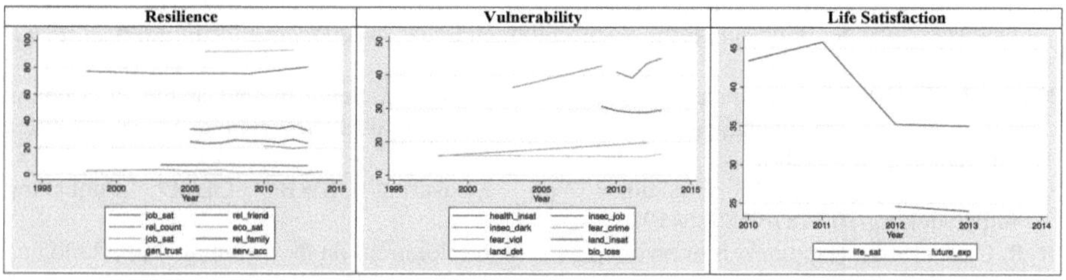

Fig. 7 Resilience and vulnerability in Italy

Table 7 Variables legend (SHARE)

Name	Variable	Description
health_sat	Perception of health status	"Would you say your health is... 1. Excellent 2. Very good 3. Good 4. Fair 5.Poor"
life_insat	Life satisfaction	"On a scale from 0 to 10 where 0 means completely dissatisfied and 10 means completelysatisfied,how satisfied are you with yourlife?"
job_insat	Job insatisfaction	"All things considered I am satisfied with my job. Would you say you strongly agree, *agree, disagree or stronglydisagree?*"
eco_sat	Satisfaction about economic conditions	"Thinking of your household's total monthly income, would you say that your household is able to make ends meet... 1. With great difficulty 2. With some difficulty 3. Fairly easily 4. Easily"

Table 8 Correlation coefficients with life satisfaction by year (SHARE)

	2006	2007	2010	2011	2012
health_insat	−0,3969	−0,406	−0,3352	−0,3957	−0,3111
job_insat	−0,2787	−0,3007	−0,3486	−0,2675	−0,3394
eco_sat	0,3396	0,3758	0,377	0,3681	0,3198

References

Argyle, M. (1987). *The Psychology of Happiness,* Methuen, London.

Bradburn, N.M. (1969). *The Structure of Psychological Wellbeing.* Aldine, Chicago.

Diener, E. (1984). "Subjective Wellbeing" in *Psychological Bullettin,* 95.

Diener, E. (2006). Guidelines for National Indicators of SWB and Ill-Being, Applied Research in Quality of Life, No. 1, pp. 151–157.

Diener E. & Emmons R.A. (1984). "The independence of positive and negative affect" in *Journal of Personality and Social Psychology,* 47 (5).

Diener, E. & Seligman, M. E. P. (2004). "Beyond money: Toward an economy of wellbeing" in *Psychological Science in the Public Interest,* 5.

Eurofound – European Foundation for the Improvement of Living and Working Conditions (2005). *First European Quality of Life Survey: Life satisfaction, happiness and sense of belonging.*

Frey and Stutzer (2002). *The Economics of Happiness World Economics*, Vol. 3, No. 1

Gasper, D.R. (2004). *Subjective And Objective Well-Being In Relation To Economic Inputs: Puzzles And Responses,* WeD Working Paper 09.

Giovannini, E., A. Morrone, T. Rondinella, L.L. Sabbadini (2012). "L'iniziativa CNEL- ISTAT per la misurazione del Benessere Equo e Sostenibile in Italia" in *Autonomie locali e servizi sociali,* n. 1, Il Mulino, Bologna.

Nuvolati, G. (2002). *Qualità della vita e indicatori sociali.* Seminar held at the PhD degree programme "Scienza tecnologia e società", Dipartimento di Sociologia e di Scienza Politica, Università della Calabria.

OECD (2013), OECD Guidelines on Measuring SWB, OECD Publishing. https://doi.org/10.1787/9789264191655-en

Ryff, C. D. (1989). Happiness is everything, or is it? Explorations on the meaning of psychological well-being. *Journal of personality and social psychology,* 57(6), 1069.

Stiglitz, J. E., A. Sen & J.-P. Fitoussi (Eds.) (2009). *Report by the Commission on the Measurement of Economic Performance and Social Progress*, Paris.

Zapf, W. (1984), "Individuelle Wohlfahrt: Lebensbedingungen und Wahrgenommene Lebensqualität", in W. Glatzer & W. Zapf (Eds.) *Lebensqualität in der Bundesrepublik*, Frankfurt a. M. – New York, Campus.

A Multi-stakeholder Framework to Facilitate Policy Making in the Use of BES Data: A Focus on Health in South Tyrol

Andrea Salustri and Federica Viganò

Abstract We present a statistical analysis aimed at investigating the quality of the health domain of BES in South Tyrol. After having summarized the academic debate on the distinction between objective and subjective indicators and on the use of subjective measures in policy making, we illustrate the rationale behind the approach adopted to interpret the available data. We observe how the heterogeneity of the stakeholders influences the way in which information is turned into policy action and the conflicts of interests that might arise must be resolved. Therefore we merge the information collected in a harmonized policy framework and we use it to identify the most critical issues regarding the improvement of health conditions in South Tyrol. Due to the high level of standardization, the exercise can be replicated for other BES domains and territories, promoting a more effective use of well-being data within policy making in Italy.

Introduction

In recent decades, the international debate on the inadequacy of the gross domestic product (GDP) as the dominant measure of prosperity has highlighted the necessity of integrating economic evaluations with an assessment of citizens' well-being (Stiglitz et al. 2009; Layard 2011; OECD 2013). At an academic level, the debate has focused on the use of both objective and subjective indicators, but the "extended" statistical background re-evoked the unexplained issue of their latent conflicting nature. The achievement of a clear understanding of citizens' subjective perspective is crucial also in the policy-making process; however, the debate is still open, and two groups of arguments are to be found in literature: one in favor and one against the use of subjective indicators (Veenhoven 2001; Noll 2013; Kroll and Delhey 2013).

A. Salustri (✉) · F. Viganò
Free University of Bozen, Bolzano, Italy
e-mail: federica.vigano@unibz.it

A. Bianco et al. (eds.), *Italian Studies on Quality of Life*, Social Indicators Research Series 77, https://doi.org/10.1007/978-3-030-06022-0_12

On the basis of these general premises, we present a statistical analysis aimed at investigating the health domain of BES (Equitable and Sustainable Well-being) in South Tyrol. Specifically, after summarizing the state of research on the distinction between objective and subjective indicators and the debated question of the use of subjective measures in policy making (section "Literature overview"), we illustrate the rationale behind the statistical approach adopted to interpret the available data on health in South Tyrol (section "A statistical analysis based on a multi-stakeholder approach"), and we discuss the statistical evidence gathered (section "The analysis of the health domain of BES in South Tyrol"). Finally, on the basis of the results of a multi-stakeholder analysis we draw up a set of recommendation policies that in our view integrate the major issues collected (section "Concluding remarks").

Literature Overview

The distinction between objective and subjective measures of well-being can be traced back to the Sixties (Abrams 1973; Campbell et al. 1976), when Quality-of-Life (QoL) indicators and key national indicators were initially published. The Seventies gave birth to data collection programs resulting in several QoL Surveys ("American Quality of Life Survey", "Quality of Life in Britain Survey", "Comparative Scandinavian Welfare Survey" and "German Welfare Survey"), while during the Eighties the issue of comparing several measures of subjective and objective well-being to show convergences and divergences among observed and perceived "state of the art" became a major field of investigation. In the late Eighties, QoL studies achieved political relevance and became strictly related to human development studies. Since the beginning of the new Millennium, the frontier of well-being measurement has been extended by combining objective and subjective approaches (Veenhoven 2001; Helliwell 2006; Kahneman et al. 2004).

Nowadays, surveys concerning self-reported measures of well-being are growing in number (from the general data on well-being worldwide, collected by the Gallup World Poll, World Database of Happiness and World Values Survey to more specific topics like health, household conditions, youth problems, employee and employer relations like in Gallup's surveys), and sampling methods are improving to avoid bias in self-reporting data (Kahneman et al. 2004). Two questions that are still debated, however, are firstly those concerning the use of subjective indicators in the policy-making process (Dolan and White 2007; Dolan and Peasgood 2008; Diener et al. 2009; Dolan et al. 2011; Forgeard et al. 2011; Adler and Seligman 2016), and secondly the role of public policies in boosting the average level of well-being in society (Helliwell et al. 2012). At a methodological level, there is a vast amount of literature on the construction of well-being subjective indicators and on the pros and cons of their use in policy making (Noll 2013; Kroll and Delhey 2013). Finally, we have recognized an old controversy and a rather philosophical question regarding the approach (top-down versus bottom-up) that policy makers should adopt (Duncan 2010; Frey and Stutzer 2002, 2010).

With these historical and methodological premises, we notice how, even if QoL studies were already implemented during Seventies in US, research on QoL flourished but with a consistent delay in Europe, and also with less ambitious purposes, often confined to the sphere of objective approaches to well-being. France, Germany, the Netherlands, Italy, Slovenia and Spain were the first European countries to organize surveys and publish well-being data collections (Noll 2008). Specifically, Italy started the BES project in 2013, producing the first Report on Equitable and Sustainable Well-being (ISTAT 2015). The Italian initiative follows the purpose of the Stiglitz-Sen-Fitoussi Report, i.e. going beyond the economic measure of well-being to understand welfare deficiencies and set effective policy measures.

The BES project has been implemented at a metropolitan level in several URBES[1] projects, which were devised to analyze the state of well-being of Italian cities, in order to highlight inequalities and trends that may affect future development models. At this spatial level, data indicates differences among the metropolitan areas involved, and in particular among central Municipalities and Regions (or Provinces). Therefore, the integration of the URBES approach with the activities of policy making might be an effective starting point in making a correct use of the statistical data and might represent a way of fostering territorial cohesion and people's empowerment and participation at all levels of the political and economic process of development (ISTAT 2015).

A Statistical Analysis Based on a Multi-stakeholder Approach

Having recognized the major issues concerning well-being analysis and its use in policy making, we will now present a statistical analysis aimed at identifying the latent conflicts within the plurality of goals that characterize South Tyrol's political process in the health domain. Specifically, we have adopted a multi-stakeholder approach based on four levels of analysis, i.e. people's subjective well-being, people's objective well-being, the relative efficiency of South Tyrol's local administrations compared to other similar Italian administrations, the level of South Tyrolean's economic well-being measured in terms of per capita GDP and other macroeconomic measures.[2]

Against this theoretical background, we initially performed a simple exercise consisting in representing the available data through appropriate graphs in order

[1]"URBES" stands for equitable and sustainable development of cities.

[2]The economic variables included in the analysis are: GDP measured at market prices, per capita GDP measured at current prices, GDP growth, per capita GDP growth, households' health care expenditure and the public sector's healthcare expenditure.

Table 1 Order used to sort the available data for each indicator (our elaboration)

Variable	Indicator	Order
Life expectancy at birth	Life expectancy at birth	Descending
Infant mortality	Infant mortality rate	Ascending
Mortality for traffic accidents (Y15–34)	Traffic accidents (15–34 years old)	Ascending
Mortality for dementia and related illnesses (Y > 65)	Age-standardised mortality rate for dementia and related illnesses (people aged 65 and over)	Ascending
Cancer mortality (Y19–64)	Age-standardised cancer mortality rate (19–64 years old)	Ascending

to highlight the observed levels and changes in the available time series.[3] We associated this interpretation of descriptive statistics with the widely-observed stakeholders' approach: having provided an initial scenario, when observing an increasing (decreasing) indicator, positive (negative) changes imply an upgrading, while negative (positive) changes imply a downgrading in the average level of well-being.

Secondly, we used URBES data (ISTAT, CNEL, Città di Bolzano 2015) on health to obtain a comparative measure of well-being by observing the relative position of South Tyrol in the ranking of Italian Provinces. Specifically, we sorted data according to a descending order if the indicator monitored a "good item", and according to an ascending order if it monitored a "bad item" (see Table 1). We then assigned a score reflecting the position achieved in the overall ranking to each observation.

In general, URBES data refers to all 110 Provinces that participated in the project, but the number of observations varies across time due to missing values and changes in the overall number of Provinces. To obtain a more precise measure of South Tyrol's position in the final rank, we used the following normalization criterion:

$$\text{dis.\%} = 100 - (\text{pos.\%}) = 100 - \left(\frac{\mathrm{n} - 1}{\mathrm{N} - 1 - \mathrm{m.v.}} \times 100\right)$$

where, "dis. %" indicates how far (in percentage points) South Tyrol is from the bottom of the ranking (therefore, 0% means the bottom, while 100% means the top of the ranking), while "pos.%" is a real number included in the interval [0, 100], and indicates at which position from the top of the overall ranking lies South Tyrol (0 means on top, 100 means at the bottom). The value "*n*" indicates the position of

[3]The full URBES Database is available at the following URL: http://www.istat.it/it/archivio/153995 (retrieved the 22nd of October 2017). For this initial step we only used data regarding the health domain in South Tyrol. For the descriptive statistics exercise, we have used the sub-sample of data referring to the health domain in South Tyrol.

South Tyrol in the ranking, "*N*" indicates the overall number of local administrations ranked and "m.v." indicates the number of missing values. We associated this comparative interpretation of rankings to widely-observed social planners' behavior (in this case, national policy makers): given the initial distribution of data, we assumed that the central administration is interested in fostering some sort of convergence toward an equitable level of well-being.

Thirdly, since URBES data only refers to objective measures of well-being, we integrated the initial dataset with the data surveyed by the local statistical office (ASTAT) on South Tyrolean's satisfaction over their health status and local health services, which we used as proxies of subjective well-being (ASTAT 2014, 2015). As widely debated in QoL and subjective well-being (SWB) literature, surveyed data on satisfaction might refer to several kinds of judgments (feelings, expectations, common sense...) so their interpretation might be biased. For the purpose of our exercise, however, we included the available data surveyed by ASTAT in order to provide at least a rough picture of citizens' habits and self-assessment on health.

Finally, we investigated the economic performance of South Tyrol using ASTAT economic data regarding GDP and other macroeconomic variables of interest. Specifically, we used economic data to identify the association between well-being and economic indicators in terms of linear correlation. The rationale is that in case of positive association among a positive (negative) well-being indicator and a positive (negative) economic indicator (i.e. life expectancy at birth and GDP growth) firms and other market players might be interested in financing initiatives aimed at achieving a higher level of well-being independently of the direct economic returns, as the indirect economic returns might, in the long run, overcome the initial costs.

The Analysis of the Health Domain of BES in South Tyrol

The descriptive analysis of URBES data show how the South Tyrolean level of health is high and increasing, even if some critical issues remain concerning the slight increment in female infant mortality rate, and the increase in cancer mortality rate for both sexes[4] (Fig. 1).

Moreover, the data highlights the existence of several gender gaps in favor of women, but in the period 2006–2011 most of them became either insignificant or turned in favor of men. The only persistent and significant gender gap is that in favor of women's life expectancy at birth (85 years for female, 80 years for male).

The comparative analysis of South Tyrolean's level of health with respect to the other Italian Provinces shows that while life expectancy at birth improved over time also in comparative terms (see Fig. 2), the other indicators often follow oscillating or decreasing trends for both sexes.

---

[4]Indeed, the interval 19–64 selected in the URBES database for this indicator is wide, therefore, even in a short period of 5 years, population ageing could affect results.

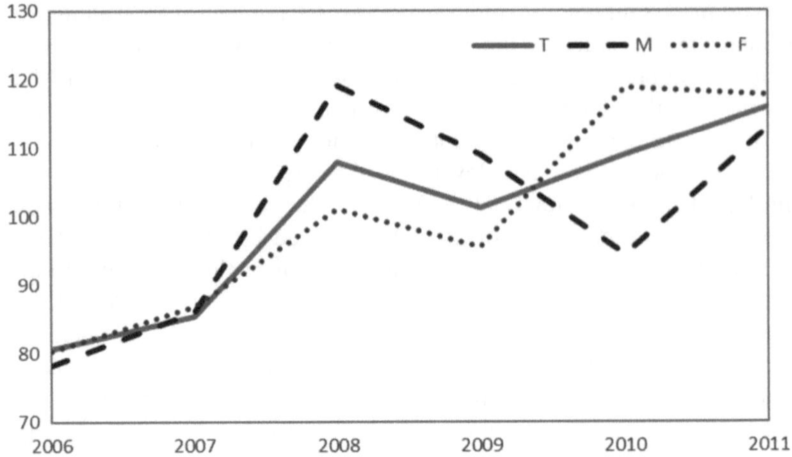

Fig. 1 Age-standardized cancer mortality rate (19–64 years old), deaths over 10,000 residents. Average 2006–2011 = 100 (our elaboration on URBES-ISTAT data, 2016). "M" = male, "F" = female, "T" = total

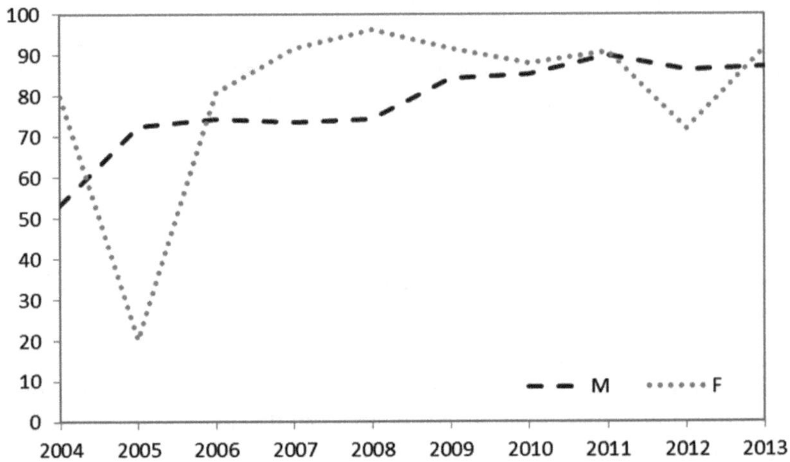

Fig. 2 Female and male life expectancy at birth, ranking 2004–2013. Average number of years, 100 means top, 0 means bottom (our elaboration of URBES-ISTAT data, 2016). "M" = male, "F" = female

While in absolute terms cancer among people aged 15–64 appeared the major issue that needed to be addressed among the target-specific causes of mortality, in relative terms the relevance of dementia and related illnesses for people aged 65 and over emerged (Fig. 3). In comparative terms, there is less evidence of an overall gender gap in favor of female (rather, in many rankings the gap is in favor of male).

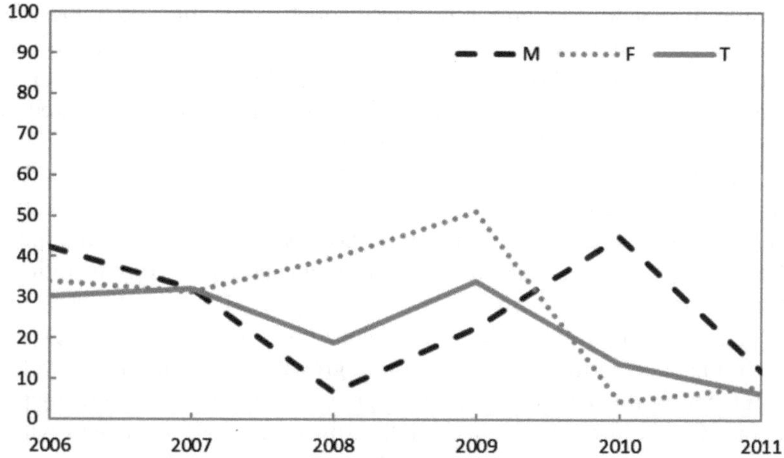

Fig. 3 Age-standardized mortality rate for dementia and related illnesses (people aged 65 and over), deaths over 10,000 residents (ranking 2004–2011), 100 means top, 0 means bottom (our elaboration of URBES-ISTAT data, 2016). "M" = male, "F" = female, "T" = total

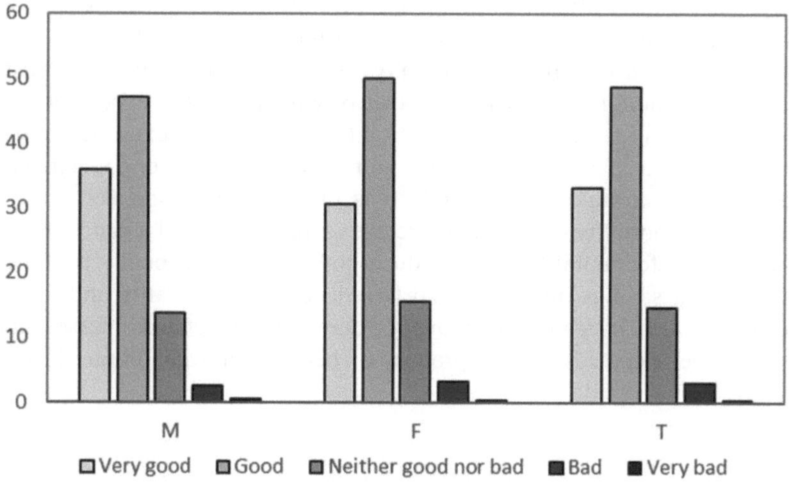

Fig. 4 South Tyrolean's self-reported health status, estimated relative frequency (our elaboration of ASTAT data, 2014). "M" = male, "F" = female, "T" = total

As regards subjective well-being and citizens' satisfaction, ASTAT data suggests that South Tyrolean's perceived health is good: more than 80% of people declared to have a good state of health, while only less than 3.5% of the total population self-assessed poor health (Fig. 4).

Furthermore, self-reported chronic diseases exhibited a negative change between 2005 and 2013, both for total population and for people aged over 65. On the supply side, it is worth noticing how physicians benefit from the highest level of trust among professionals in South Tyrol (88.2% of people trust them), and the health-care system as a whole generates a high level of citizen satisfaction (80.7% of citizens aged 18 or more are satisfied with its performance) but compared to other welfare services this result is less favorable (ASTAT 2015).

The statistical exercise ends with a correlation analysis (see Appendices). As regards the interdependence of economic and well-being health indicators, we noticed how life expectancy at birth of both sexes is strictly and positively correlated to the level of per capita GDP, household and public administration health expenditure, and negatively correlated to per capita GDP growth. Therefore, we suspect that there might be a trade-off between growth and longer life expectancy, at least in the short term, i.e. that economic growth might "dissipate" well-being, while high per capita income might ensure greater opportunities for raising personal well-being. On the other hand, high GDP growth rates are associated with lower life expectancy at birth for both sexes, a higher infant mortality rate (even if with a significant gender gap), a lower 15–34 male traffic-accident mortality rate, a lower 15–64 cancer mortality rate, and a higher over-65 male dementia and related illnesses mortality rate. Therefore, it seems that GDP growth has ambiguous effects, as it leads to negative effects on infant and over-65 well-being (i.e. people not at a working age), while it has positive effects on the well-being of people aged 15–65 (i.e. people at a working age). Finally, households and public administration health-care expenditure is closely and positively related to life expectancy at birth for both sexes, and to 15–64 cancer mortality rate for both sexes. Moreover, it is negatively associated with male infant mortality rate and over-65 dementia and related illnesses mortality rates, while it is only weakly associated with 15–34 traffic accident mortality rates. Therefore, we suspect that regular cancer preventive checkups and safer mobility might reduce both private and public health expenditure, and that savings might be used to reduce infant mortality and raising life expectancy at birth. Instead a higher over-65 dementia and related illnesses mortality rate should be accepted as a by-product of better health conditions in previous years.

A Multi-stakeholder Interpretation of the Evidence Collected

In this paragraph we provide a multi-stakeholder interpretation of the statistical evidence collected for South Tyrol for each indicator in the URBES health domain. The plurality of interests influences the way in which information is turned into policy action. Indeed, the interpretation of the same data might lead to different conclusions and therefore the conflicts of interests that might arise must be resolved.

Our research aims to develop and test a method for identifying a multi-stakeholder perspective that accounts for differences in viewpoints among stakeholders. Furthermore, the exercise proposed integrates the plurality of issues collected in a harmonized policy framework.

First of all, it is worth noting how South Tyrolean people have on average a perception of their level of health as being good. Their perception reveals itself to be correct, as it is consistent with high life expectancy at birth, both in absolute and relative levels. The correlation analysis shows how life expectancy at birth is positively correlated with the levels of per capita GDP and health-care expenditure, while it is negatively correlated with the GDP growth rate. If the latter correlation is not spurious (it might depend on some sort of saturation effect in GDP and in the health care expenditure growth pattern), there might be a trade-off between economic growth and longevity. This trade off might raise the issue of whether financial intermediaries (and other profit-oriented institutions) might be interested in financing projects aimed at increasing South Tyrolean's longevity, or if the latter should be rather achieved through the implementation of participated processes and commoning practices.

Secondly, even if we could not find any subjective assessment on this topic, we observed how the level of infant mortality is low both in absolute and in relative terms in South Tyrol. The correlation analysis shows how female infant mortality is negatively correlated to GDP growth, while male infant mortality is positively correlated to GDP growth and negatively correlated to GDP levels and public and private health care expenditure. In the light of the results of the correlation analysis, financial intermediaries and other market institutions might have an interest in financing projects aimed at reducing female infant mortality, but this issue requires an in-depth analysis of the causality nexus between the two indicators.

Thirdly, even if we could not find any subjective assessment on this topic, we observed how the mortality for traffic accidents among people aged 15–34 is low in absolute terms in South Tyrol, but high if compared to the data observed for other Italian territories. The correlation analysis shows how for males the related indicator is positively correlated to private healthcare expenditure and negatively correlated to GDP growth, while for female it is negatively correlated to both variables. Given the results of the correlation analysis, financial intermediaries and other market institutions might have an interest in financing projects aimed at reducing male mortality for traffic accidents among the young but this issue requires an in-depth analysis of the causality nexus between the two indicators.

Fourthly, notwithstanding South Tyrolean's good habits in terms of preventive healthcare (ASTAT 2014), we observed a high absolute level of cancer mortality among people aged 20–65, but compared to other Italian territories, the observed value is of low magnitude. The correlation analysis shows how for both sexes cancer mortality among people aged 20–65 is positively correlated to the levels of

GDP and public and private healthcare expenditure, but it is negatively correlated to GDP growth (the latter correlation might be spurious as it might reflect some sort of saturation effect in the GDP growth pattern). Therefore, we suggest how the interdependence of economic wealth and quality of life in South Tyrol might be an interesting topic for an in-depth analysis, as it might provide evidence of at least some non-linearity. Moreover, we suspect that policies aimed at reducing cancer mortality among people aged 20–65 might be supported at a local level but would hardly find the support of national policy makers, as South Tyrol does not appear to be a national priority in this sector.

Fifthly, the level of mortality for dementia and related illnesses among people aged 65 and over is low in absolute terms but is high if compared to other Italian territories. The correlation analysis reveals that for male this item is positively correlated to GDP growth, while for both sexes it is negatively correlated to private and public healthcare expenditure. Given also its negative correlation with cancer mortality among adults, we can consider this indicator as a proxy of healthcare expenditure sustainability and well-being, as it implicitly signals a good health status in previous ages. Finally, projects aimed at reducing mortality for dementia and related issues in people aged 65 and over might benefit from national policy makers' and profit-oriented institutions' support, but do not seem to be a priority at a local level.

Concluding Remarks

In this statistical exercise we identified several stylized facts regarding the health domain of well-being in South Tyrol, but also several issues concerning policy making and the role of social scientists.

First of all, at a local level South Tyrolean people have on average a perception of their state of health as good, and at a local level data paints a good picture of South Tyrolean health with the exception of the increase in cancer mortality for people aged 15–65. At a national level the picture is less clear, as there are indicators that show high relative levels of health (high life expectation at birth, low infant mortality, low cancer mortality rate for people aged 19–65), but there are also indicators on the basis of which South Tyrol is at the bottom of the national ranking (15–34-year-old male and female mortality for traffic accidents, mortality for dementia and related illnesses for people aged 65 and over). Finally, while the level of GDP positively affects all indicators except cancer mortality for people aged 15–65, only two out of four causes of death are negatively related to per capita

GDP growth (specifically, those related to people aged 15–65), suggesting that the interest of profit-oriented institutions in supporting projects aimed at increasing South Tyrolean's level of health might be limited to actions in favor of people of working age.

Secondly, we summarized the main methodological issues that emerged in the previous paragraphs. Firstly, reading data through a multi-criteria approach emphasizes the multi-stakeholder nature that intrinsically characterizes the interpretation of the results obtained. Specifically, when drawing up policy recommendations, the multi-agent perspective contributes to a more critical policy inquiry and sheds light on a range of different policy actions. A second consideration refers to the administrative and institutional availability of data: when collected, subjective data on well-being (often in the form of customer satisfaction) is not related to objective measures such as those included in the BES or URBES databases. If citizens' surveys were more correlated to the available objective data, especially at local government level, the comparison between subjective and objective well-being indicators would be more effective, and this might help authorities and municipalities to develop better local policies. A third consideration regards the well-publicized debate surrounding an integrated approach to policy making: both objective and subjective data should be used, and the statistical evidence collected should be discussed in a well-informed public debate on specific social objectives and on the trade-offs between them. Data and statistical analyses have their limits, but a multi-stakeholder perspective, including the subjective well-being indicators, has the advantage of disentangling problems emerging at different levels, and of focusing attention on important issues which might otherwise be ignored, perhaps because they refer to relatively powerless groups or because they were not previously identified as a problem (Seaford 2013; Kroll and Delhey 2013).

Finally, we highlighted how the exercise was limited to one single dimension and one single territory, but it could be easily replicated in other well-being domains and regions or municipalities. This approach helps to establish a dialogue among statisticians and policy makers and identifies a specific role for social scientists in policy-making processes. Indeed, the main purpose of social scientists is to mediate between quantitative and qualitative approaches, to collect all the information available and assess its quality, and to support policy makers in acquiring an integrated view of the phenomena under investigation, assessing policies' inner consistency and correspondence with the statistical evidence gathered.

Appendices

Appendix A: Legend

Label	Description	Territorial level	Time length	Unit of measure
gdp_	Gross domestic product at current prices	ST	2004–2013	Million euro
pcy_	Per capita gross domestic product at market prices	ST	2004–2013	Euro
gdpg	GDP growth at current prices	ST	2004–2013	%
pcyg	Per capita GDP growth at market prices	ST	2004–2013	%
heho	Resident and non resident household final consumption expenditure at economic territorial level (COICOP) - health expenditure	ST	2004–2013	Million euro
hepa	Public administration health expenditure (COFOG)	ST	2004–2013	Million euro
lebm	Life expectancy at birth for male	ST	2004–2013	Average number of years
lebf	Life expectancy at birth for female	ST	2004–2013	Average number of years
imrm	Infant mortality rate, male	ST	2004–2011	Deaths during the first year of life per 10.000 born alive
imrf	Infant mortality rate, female	ST	2004–2011	Deaths during the first year of life per 10.000 born alive
imrt	Infant mortality rate, total	ST	2004–2011	Deaths during the first year of life per 10.000 born alive
timm	Traffic accidents (15–34 years old), male	ST	2006–2011	Mortality rate for traffic accidents (initial cause) by 5 year age groups for people aged 15–34 years, standardized by the Italian 2001 Census population of the same age groups.
timf	Traffic accidents (15–34 years old), female	ST	2006–2011	Mortality rate for traffic accidents (initial cause) by 5 year age groups for people aged 15–34 years, standardized by the Italian 2001 Census population of the same age groups.

(continued)

(continued)

Label	Description	Territorial level	Time length	Unit of measure
timt	Traffic accidents (15–34 years old), total	ST	2006–2011	Mortality rate for traffic accidents (initial cause) by 5 year age groups for people aged 15–34 years, standardized by the Italian 2001 Census population of the same age groups.
drim	Age-standardised mortality rate for dementia and related illnesses (people aged 65 and over), male	ST	2006–2011	Mortality rate for nervous system diseases and psychical and behavioural disorders (initial cause) by 5 year age groups for people aged 65 years and over, standardized by the Italian 2001 Census population of the same age groups.
drif	Age-standardised mortality rate for dementia and related illnesses (people aged 65 and over), female	ST	2006–2011	Mortality rate for nervous system diseases and psychical and behavioural disorders (initial cause) by 5 year age groups for people aged 65 years and over, standardized by the Italian 2001 Census population of the same age groups.
drit	Age-standardised mortality rate for dementia and related illnesses (people aged 65 and over), total	ST	2006–2011	Mortality rate for nervous system diseases and psychical and behavioural disorders (initial cause) by 5 year age groups for people aged 65 years and over, standardized by the Italian 2001 Census population of the same age groups.
cmrm	Age-standardised cancer mortality rate (19–64 years old), male	ST	2006–2011	Mortality rate for cancer (initial cause) by 5 year age groups for people aged 19–64 years, standardized by the Italian 2001 Census population of the same age groups.
cmrf	Age-standardised cancer mortality rate (19–64 years old), female	ST	2006–2011	Mortality rate for cancer (initial cause) by 5 year age groups for people aged 19–64 years, standardized by the Italian 2001 Census population of the same age groups.
cmrt	Age-standardised cancer mortality rate (19–64 years old), total	ST	2006–2011	Mortality rate for cancer (initial cause) by 5 year age groups for people aged 19–64 years, standardized by the Italian 2001 Census population of the same age groups.

NW: "ST" = South Tyrol. The value of timf 2009 has been interpolated

Appendix B: Correlation Analysis

	gdp_	pcy_	gdpg	pcyg	heho	hepa	lebm	lebf	inmm	Inmf	inmt	timm	timf	timt	drim	drif	drit	cmrm	cmrf	cmrt
gdp_	1.0																			
pcy_	1.0	1.0																		
gdpg	−0.4	−0.4	1.0																	
pcyg	−0.4	−0.3	1.0	1.0																
heho	0.9	0.9	−0.3	−0.3	1.0															
hepa	0.9	0.9	−0.3	−0.3	0.9	1.0														
lebm	1.0	1.0	−0.5	−0.4	0.9	0.8	1.0													
lebf	0.9	0.9	−0.4	−0.3	0.9	0.8	0.9	1.0												
inmm	−0.7	−0.7	0.5	0.4	−0.8	−0.5	−0.8	−0.7	1.0											
inmf	0.1	0.0	−0.6	−0.6	−0.1	−0.1	0.3	0.1	−0.2	1.0										
inmt	−0.7	−0.6	0.2	0.1	−0.8	−0.6	−0.6	−0.6	0.9	0.2	1.0									
timm	0.2	0.1	−0.4	−0.3	0.4	0.1	0.4	0.2	−0.4	−0.1	−0.4	1.0								
timf	−0.5	−0.5	0.1	0.0	−0.4	0.1	−0.5	−0.5	0.5	−0.4	0.4	0.3	1.0							
timt	−0.1	−0.2	0.1	0.1	0.0	0.1	0.0	−0.2	0.1	−0.4	−0.1	0.7	0.8	1.0						
drim	−0.8	−0.8	0.3	0.2	−0.7	−0.3	−0.9	−0.8	0.9	−0.4	0.7	−0.2	0.8	0.4	1.0					
drif	−0.1	−0.2	−0.1	−0.1	−0.3	−0.5	0.3	−0.1	0.0	0.8	0.3	0.3	−0.1	0.0	−0.3	1.0				
drit	−0.9	−0.9	0.2	0.2	−0.9	−0.6	−0.8	−0.9	0.9	0.0	0.9	−0.1	0.7	0.4	0.8	0.2	1.0			
cmrm	0.7	0.7	−0.5	−0.5	0.9	0.8	0.5	0.8	−0.7	−0.3	−0.8	0.2	−0.1	−0.1	−0.3	−0.6	−0.7	1.0		
cmrf	0.9	0.9	−0.2	−0.1	0.8	0.8	0.9	0.9	−0.8	0.1	−0.8	0.2	−0.3	0.1	−0.7	0.0	−0.7	0.6	1.0	
cmrt	0.9	0.9	−0.4	−0.3	0.9	0.9	0.8	0.9	−0.9	−0.1	−0.9	0.3	−0.2	0.1	−0.6	−0.3	−0.8	0.8	0.9	1.0

Appendix C: Ranking Analysis

			2004	2005	2006	2007	2008	2009	2010	2011	2012	2013
LEB	**M**	pos.	52	31	29	30	29	18	17	12	16	15
		n.	110	110	110	110	110	110	110	110	110	110
		m.v.	0	0	0	0	0	0	0	0	0	0
		dis. %	**53**	**72**	**74**	**73**	**74**	**84**	**85**	**90**	**86**	**87**
	F	pos.	23	23	22	10	5	10	14	11	29	10
		n.	110	110	110	110	110	110	110	110	110	110
		m.v.	0	0	0	0	0	0	0	0	0	0
		dis. %	**80**	**20**	**81**	**92**	**96**	**92**	**88**	**91**	**74**	**92**
INM	**M**	pos.	82	53	103	91	72	40	52	8		
		n.	110	110	110	110	110	110	110	110		
		m.v.	7	7	3	3	3	3	0	0		
		dis. %	**21**	**49**	**4**	**15**	**33**	**63**	**53**	**94**		
	F	pos.	13	56	29	56	19	59	80	45		
		n.	110	110	110	110	110	110	110	110		
		m.v.	7	7	3	3	3	3	0	0		
		dis. %	**88**	**46**	**74**	**48**	**83**	**45**	**28**	**60**		
	T	pos.	50	52	83	80	49	46	64	14		
		n.	110	110	110	110	110	110	110	110		
		m.v.	7	7	3	3	3	3	0	0		
		dis. %	**52**	**50**	**23**	**25**	**55**	**58**	**42**	**88**		
TIM	**M**	pos.			34	8	23	77	60	81		
		n.			110	110	110	110	110	110		
		m.v.			3	3	3	3	2	3		
		dis. %			**69**	**93**	**79**	**28**	**45**	**25**		
	F	pos.			72	7	67	na	60	9		
		n.			110	110	110	na	110	110		
		m.v.			15	23	30	na	32	28		
		dis. %			**24**	**93**	**16**	**66***	**23**	**90**		
	T	pos.			49	6	38	57	78	71		
		n.			110	110	110	110	110	110		
		m.v.			3	3	3	3	1	2		
		dis. %			**55**	**95**	**65**	**47**	**29**	**35**		

(continued)

(continued)

			2004	2005	2006	2007	2008	2009	2010	2011	2012	2013
DRI	**M**	pos.			39	12	46	13	18	1		
		n.			110	110	110	110	110	110		
		m.v.			3	3	3	3	0	0		
		dis. %			**64**	**90**	**58**	**89**	**84**	**100**		
	F	pos.			33	33	9	44	66	27		
		n.			110	110	110	110	110	110		
		m.v.			3	3	3	3	0	0		
		dis. %			**70**	**70**	**92**	**59**	**40**	**76**		
	T	pos.			36	14	18	12	31	3		
		n.			110	110	110	110	110	110		
		m.v.			3	3	3	3	0	0		
		dis. %			**67**	**88**	**84**	**90**	**72**	**98**		
CMR	**M**	pos.			62	73	100	83	61	97		
		n.			110	110	110	110	110	110		
		m.v.			3	3	3	3	0	0		
		dis. %			**42**	**32**	**7**	**23**	**45**	**12**		
	F	pos.			71	74	65	53	105	101		
		n.			110	110	110	110	110	110		
		m.v.			3	3	3	3	0	0		
		dis. %			**34**	**31**	**40**	**51**	**5**	**8**		
	T	pos.			75	73	87	71	95	103		
		n.			110	110	110	110	110	110		
		m.v.			3	3	3	3	0	0		
		dis. %			**30**	**32**	**19**	**34**	**14**	**6**		

References

Abrams, M. (1973). Research on subjective social indicators. In M. Nissel (Ed.), *Social trends* (Vol. 4, pp. 35–50). London: HMSO.

Adler, A. & Seligman, M. E. P. (2016). Using well-being for public policy: Theory, measurement, and recommendations. *International Journal of Well-being*, 6(1), 1–35.

ASTAT, (2014). La salute degli altoatesini – 2013. Astat info n.56. Bolzano.

ASTAT, (2015). Soddisfazione dei cittadini nei confronti dei servizi pubblici – 2015. Astat info n. 50. Bolzano.

Campbell, A., Converse, P., Rodgers, W. (1976). *The quality of American life*. New York: Russell Sage Foundation

Diener, E., Lucas, R. E., Schimmack, U., Helliwell, J. F. (2009). *Well-being for public policy*. Oxford/New York: Oxford University Press

Dolan, P., Layard, R., Metcalf, R. (2011). *Measuring subjective well-being for public policy; recommendations on measures*. Special paper No. 23. Centre for Economic Performance.

Dolan, P. & Peasgood, T. (2008). Measuring Well-Being for Public Policy: Preferences or Experiences?, *The Journal of Legal Studies*, 37, 5–31

Dolan, P. & White, M. P. (2007). How Can Measures of Subjective Well-Being be Used to Inform Public Policy?. *Perspectives on Psychological Science*, 2, 71–85

Duncan, G. (2010). Should happiness-maximization be the goal of government?. *Journal of Happiness Studies*, 11(2), 163–178.
Forgeard, M. J. C., Jayawickreme, E., Kern, M., Seligman, M. E. P. (2011). Doing the right thing: Measuring well-being for public policy. *International Journal of Well-being*, 1(1), 79–106
Frey B. & Stutzer A. (2002). What can economists learn from happiness research?. *Journal of Economic Literature*, 40(2):402–435
Frey B. & Stutzer A., (2010). Happiness and Public Choice. *Public Choice*, 144, 557–573
Helliwell, J. F. (2006). Well-being, social capital and public policy: what's new?. *Economic Journal*, 116, 34–45
Helliwell, J. F., Layard, R., Sachs, J. (Eds.). (2012). *World Happiness Report*. New York, NY: The Earth Institute, Columbia University
ISTAT (2015). URBES Il benessere equo e sostenibile nelle città. Rapporto SISTAN
ISTAT, CNEL, Città di Bolzano, (2015) Rapporto URBES 2015, Bolzano, http://www.istat.it/storage/urbes2015/bolzano.pdf. Accessed 1st November 2017.
Kahneman, D., Krueger, A. B., Schkade, D. A., Schwarz, N., Stone, A. A. (2004). A survey method for characterizing daily life experience: the day reconstruction method. *Science*, 306, 1776–1780
Kroll, C., & Delhey, J. (2013). A happy nation? Opportunities and challenges of using subjective indicators in policymaking. *Social Indicators Research*, 114(1), 13–28.
Layard, R. (2011). *Happiness: Lessons from a New Science* (2nd ed.). New York, NY: Penguin Press.
Noll, H. H. (2008). European survey data: Rich sources for quality of life research. In V. Møller, et al. (Eds.), *Barometers of quality of life around the globe social indicators research series* (Vol. 33, pp. 1–21). Dordrecht: Springer
Noll, H. H. (2013). Subjective Social Indicators: Benefits and Limitations for Policy Making—An Introduction to this Special Issue. *Social Indicators Research* 113, 1
OECD. (2013). *OECD guidelines on measuring subjective well-being*. OECD Publishing
Seaford C. (2013). The Multiple Uses of Subjective Well-Being Indicators. *Social Indicators Research*, 114: 29.
Stiglitz, J. E., Sen, A., Fitoussi, J. P. (2009). *Report by the Commission on the Measurement of Economic Performance and Social Progress*. OECD
Veenhoven R. (2001), Why social policy needs subjective indicators. Discussion Paper Series Social Science Research Center Berlin, Berlin.

Food Styles and Well-Being of Italian People: A Contribution from Official Statistics

Carolina Facioni, Isabella Corazziari, and Filomena Maggino

Abstract The work focuses the relationship between well-being and Italian lifestyle related to food, as it emerges from the National Institute of Statistics' data. The work highlights how the official statistics can help both common citizens and decision-makers to better understand the current state of eating habits in our country. There were used different approaches to data analysis, both using time series analysis about the body mass index distribution and also a gender and generation approach. Multidimensional data analysis – in particular, the dynamic factor analysis – was used to better highlight some possible criticalities related to food habits in Italy and the citizens' well-being. The results inspired some reflections: first of all, that food habits cannot be only considered a simple life domain. It's a complex aspect with political implications. Food not only concerns the individual's well-being: it involves both the society and the environment's well-being as a whole.

Introduction

The 2015 Expo in Milan, completely dedicated to the topic of food, highlighted the central role of it in the promotion of a sustainable well-being for human societies and environment. The theme of food has always been present in the reflection of scientific disciplines, from philosophy (Carrara 2007) to the physics (McGee 1984). However, it was only in the second half of the twentieth century that the scientific community started analyzing food in a complex perspective, linking phenomena apparently far between each other.

C. Facioni (✉) · I. Corazziari
Italian National Institute of Statistics, Rome, Italy
e-mail: facioni@istat.it

F. Maggino
"Sapienza" University of Rome, Rome, Italy

A. Bianco et al. (eds.), *Italian Studies on Quality of Life*, Social Indicators Research Series 77, https://doi.org/10.1007/978-3-030-06022-0_13

Indeed, food is not "only" an indispensable resource for the survival of all biological species. Food is civilization (Braudel 1979), and it is a distinctive feature of social life (Poulain 2002). Not least, the consumption of food has an impact on the environment. The consumption of food is a topic that's clearly connected with the still unclosed debate the Club of Rome started in the late 1960s, especially regarding to the famous MIT report on the limits to growth (Meadows et al. 1972). The Report demonstrated how eating habits too had a complex fallout on the Earth resources. It may be interesting to note that the food resources were identified, in some graphs in the 1972 Report, as "quality of life." Indeed, eating habits have an effect on the quality of life, both in the short and in the long term – and this aspect does not only concern individuals but the human race as a whole (Petrini 2010).

The present work[1] aims to focus the relationship between Italians' well-being and their lifestyles related to food, as it emerges from some recent data produced by the Italian National Institute of Statistics (ISTAT). In the paper there were used time series analysis and also a gender and generation approach. The emerging criticalities will also be described by multidimensional data analysis techniques. In particular, in this context there were used the 2015 CNEL-ISTAT report on Equal and Sustainable Well-being (BES) indicators.

A Half Empty or Half Full Glass? Some Puzzling Aspects Related to Food Style(s) in Italy

Italian food and its quality are worldwide appreciated. It should be stressed immediately that speaking of Italian food only in terms of "Mediterranean diet"[2] is quite reductive. Indeed, Italy has to be meant as an incredible context of different food cultures, as first emerges from the fundamental 1891 book by Pellegrino Artusi, who first illustrated the incredible richness of Italian[3] cuisine (Artusi 1891). This "biodiversity of food" is not only due to very specific historical reasons but also

[1]The paper should be considered as the fruit of the work of the authors as a whole. However, Paragraphs 1 and 2 must be attributed to Carolina Facioni, Paragraph 3 should be attributed to Isabella Corazziari, and Paragraph 4 to Filomena Maggino. The views expressed in the paper are to be considered solely by the authors and do not necessarily reflect the institutions they are members of.

[2]The concept of Mediterranean diet, and the theory about it, is based on the studies of Angel Keys, an American physiologist who in the XXth Century Fifties inspired and directed a famous research project on food habits in the world: the Seven Countries Studies. Although the agreement on the effectiveness of the Mediterranean diet on cardiovascular disease and cancer prevention is not entirely unanimous, in 2010, after long negotiations, this nutritional model has been inserted by the UNESCO intergovernmental Committee in the list of UNESCO Intangible Cultural Heritage, recognizing the heritage as belonging to Italy, Morocco, Greece, and Spain. In November 2013, the heritage has been extended to Cyprus, Croatia, and Portugal.

[3]Indeed, it is the first book on art of cooking where the adjective "Italian" is properly used. In fact, Italy became a nation in 1861.

to the fact that the various Italian regions do not produce the same raw materials. Even talking about Italian food culture in terms of a dichotomy, a sort of "Northern Italy's food vs. Southern Italy's food" is an oversimplification. Indeed, there are Northern regions (e.g., Liguria) where olive oil is used for cooking – just as in Southern Italy. Furthermore, in many Italian regions (e.g., Veneto), many different cooking traditions coexist, and some famous Italian recipes seem to be the result of various contributions throughout history. A valid example of a food developed by an evolutionary process is the Sicilian cake *cassata* (Scarpinato 2004). Social sciences have long been aware of the importance of food as a key element in building cultural and territorial identity (Di Francesco 2006). This is enough to illustrate how talking about a single Italian food style means making a no sense generalization. However, Italian official data[4] can tell us a lot about the consequences of different food styles in Italy – and some puzzling surprises, too. The data related to the body mass index (BMI below) distribution are very important for a better knowledge of well-being related to food in Italy. We have to stress that BMI can be defined as an *imperfect indicator*: in fact, official statistics do not collect data on waist size. However, the fat mass has a specific weight much lighter than the muscle mass. So, if the BMI data are not integrated with the waist measurement data, we could face an apparent paradox. Indeed, an overweight person can have the same BMI as a person who practices many sports. Figure 1 illustrates the evolution of adult individuals[5] BMI main categories (underweight, normal weight, overweight, obese) from year 2005 to 2015.

In 2015, normal weight adult people in Italy are over 26 million (51.8%); nearly 18 million people are overweight (35.3%). Obese adult people are nearly five million (9.8%), while the percentage of underweight people (about 1500 thousand people) is 3%. All percentages seem to be stable over time. The fluctuations in data over the years are negligible. So, the substantial data stability is the fundamental element emerging from the time series, and it leads to further considerations – corroborated by the stability of data itself. The first is that more than half of adult Italians are normal weight people. A further consideration is that almost half of the adult Italians are mostly overweight; five million Italians are obese; and a minority – which still exceeds one million people – is underweight. If the aim of the official statistics is to better know the citizens' life for building adequate policies, it should be better to analyze the Italian BMI distribution from the "half empty glass" perspective. The phenomenon of BMI distribution can be analyzed in a gender approach. Figure 2 clearly illustrates how, in Italy, the control of weight to be a typically feminine cure. Male and female distributions are substantially different.

[4]This paper reviews and analyzes the data produced by the Italian National Institute of Statistics. The main data sources are the Survey on Everyday Life of Citizens – year 2015, and the 2015 Report on BES (Equal and Sustainable Well-Being) indicators.

[5]We chose to limit our analysis to adult people only, as it may be very complicated to define exactly the BMI categories regarding the population under the age of 18, especially for children. With regard to this theme, and in particular on the prevention on obesity in children, interesting contents can be found on ISS (Italian Health Care Institute) website.

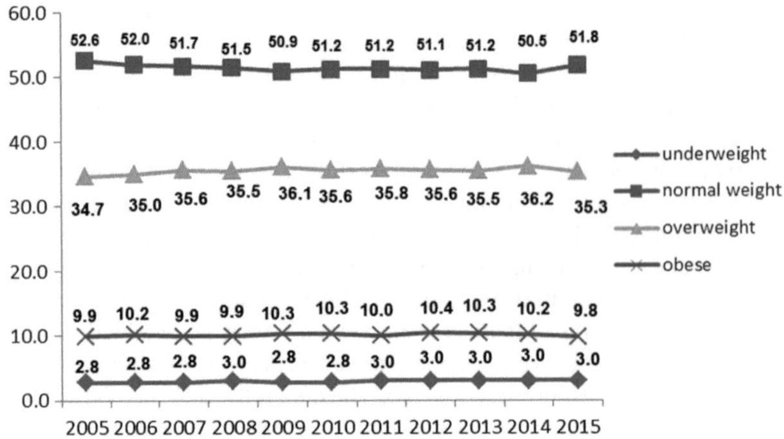

Fig. 1 Time series of adult people BMI percentage distribution in Italy. Years 2005–2015. (Data source: ISTAT)

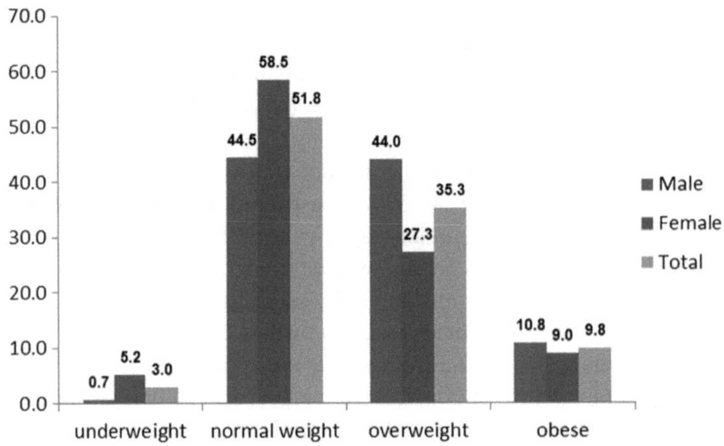

Fig. 2 Italian adult people BMI percentage distribution per sex. Year 2015. (Data source: ISTAT)

In 2015, women with normal weight have 14 percentage points more than men's values in the same condition: 58.5% in front of 44.5% of normal weight men. Considering the control of weight as a good practice to reach longevity (Veronesi 2013; Longo 2016), we might hypothesize that this feminine attitude to maintain a normal weight can be one of the factors that justifies the longer life expectancy of women, especially in Italy.

Considering underweight individuals, we can consider this (negative) phenomenon as exclusively feminine, and the absolute data clearly explain it. On 1527 thousand underweight people, 1354 thousand are women. Indeed, underweight men

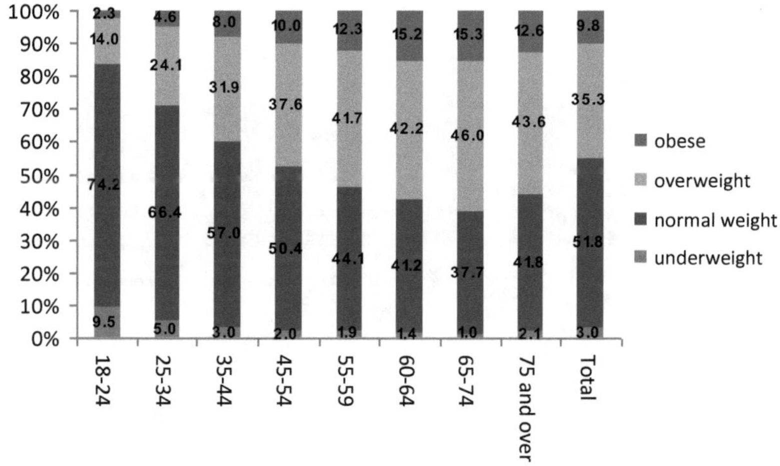

Fig. 3 Italian adult people BMI percentage distribution per class of age. Year 2015. (Data source: ISTAT)

are representing a very residual entity of a context, sometimes of pathological kind, which is practically related to women only.

Considering a generation approach, it's clear that there are more normal weight people between young adult population than between elderly one. Figure 3 well explains the composition of BMI classification per class of age. Considering 100 people aged between 18 and 24, the 74.2% are normal weight. This percentage gradually decreases as the age class grows – although the lowest value (37.7%) belongs to the 65–74 year old class. However, it should be noted that 14.2% of Italians aged 18–24 are overweight, and 2.3% of them are obese. Above all, in this age class, we find the highest number of underweight people. In this age class, the percentage of underweight people (mostly women, as we have seen) is 9.5%. Since percentages of both normal and underweight people are significantly decreasing from the age of 25, while overweight and obese people are increasing, we need to consider what habits of life interfere with a proper weight control over time. Maybe that policies are needed to reduce the risks for wealth due to obesity and overweight (Petrick et al. 2017).

In particular, the control of weight seems to be strictly related both to the level of education and to aspects related to family habits. Figure 4 clearly illustrates how the level of education can influence the BMI distribution. We stress that BMI can be considered as the complex consequence not only of genetic factors but also of good practices, such as following a healthy diet and exercising a regular weight control.

Data clearly show how a high level of education contributes to making people more sensitive to the issue of weight control: graduate and postgraduate people have the highest percentages of normal weight (63.6%). At the same, they have the lowest percentage of overweight (27.4%) and obesity (4.7%). Although, this class shows also the highest percentage of underweight people (4.3%) in Italy. So, the lower the

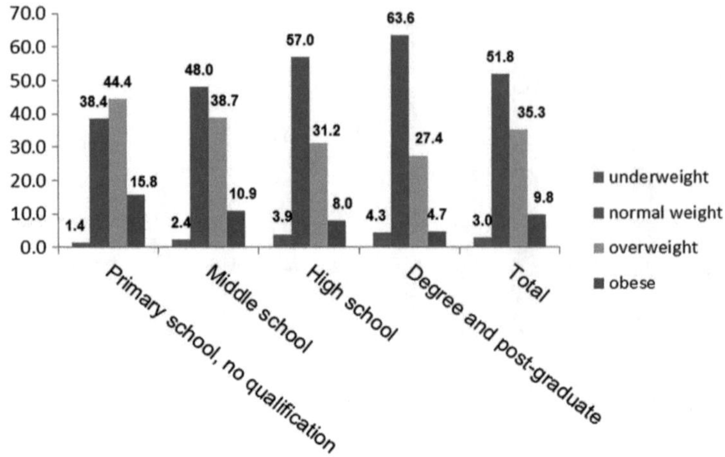

Fig. 4 Italian adult people BMI percentage distribution per level of education. Year 2015. (Data source: ISTAT)

Table 1 BMI percentage distribution in Italian territory. Year 2015 (per 100 individuals in the same territorial breakdown)

Italian territorial breakdowns	Underweight	Normal weight	Overweight	Obese	Total
Northwestern regions	4.5	54.5	32.1	8.9	100.0
Northeastern regions	2.8	53.5	34.5	9.2	100.0
Central Italy	2.6	52.4	35.5	9.6	100.0
Southern regions	2.1	47.5	38.6	11.8	100.0
Sardinia and Sicily	2.9	50.4	37.3	9.5	100.0
Italy	3.0	51.8	35.3	9.8	100.0

Data source: ISTAT

level of education, the higher the percentage of overweight or obese people. This relationship can explain one puzzling aspect of BMI distribution across the regions of Italy (Table 1). Indeed, in the South of Italy – where the Mediterranean diet is more practiced than in the North – there are more overweight and obese people. In Southern Italy obese people percentage is 11.8%, while the lowest percentage is in the Northwestern regions (8.9%). Indeed, this is an only apparent contradiction: it is likely to be attributed to the stronger percentage of individuals with high levels of education in Northern Italy, compared to Southern Italy. The food styles are strictly related and influenced by the level of education. So, the higher the level of education, the more careful is the weight control.

There is, however, a further fundamental factor that directly involves the role of Italian women in influencing the family's eating habits and therefore the distribution of BMI. Considering young adults aged 18–25 who live in families with their parents, it is evident that there is a direct relationship between overweight and obesity of parents and overweight and obesity of their children: 21.3% of young

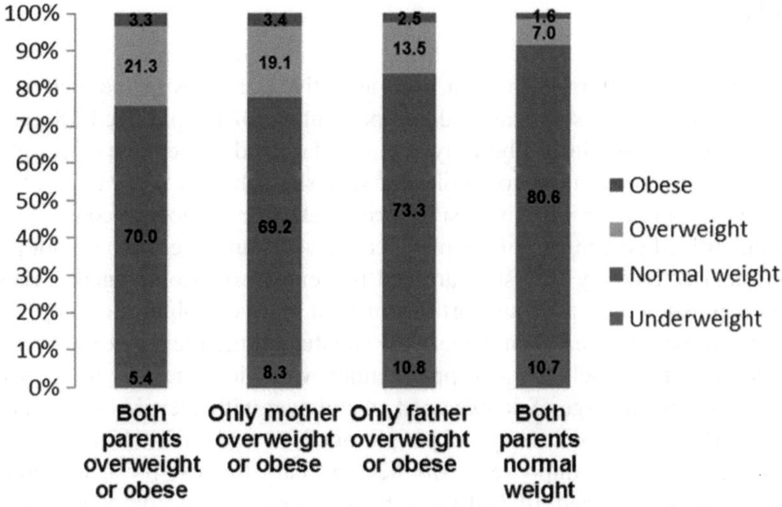

Fig. 5 BMI percentage distribution of Italian young adult people aged 18–25 and living with parents per BMI percentage distribution of parents. Year 2015. (Data source: Italian National Institute of Statistics)

adults are overweight when both parents are overweight or obese, while the percentage is only 7% (one third less!) between young adults whose parents are both normal weight. In particular, when only the mother is overweight or obese, the overweight and obesity rates of children are higher with respect to when only the father is overweight or obese: 19.1% vs. 13.5%. No doubt, Italian mothers' food styles matter (Fig. 5).

Materials and Methods: The Dynamic Factorial Analysis of Some Well-Being Indicators

In order to provide a very raw description of Italians' lifestyles and their relationships with personal well-being, a multiway analysis on some well-being indicators about health, life satisfaction, and lifestyles (from ISTAT BES reports), has been performed.

The Data

The following indicators have been used as active variables in the analysis[6]: life expectancy at birth by sex; standardized percentage of people aged 18 years and over who are overweight or obese by sex; standardized percentage of people aged 14 years and over declaring to smoke by sex; standardized percentage of people aged 14 years and over with at least one risk behavior in alcohol consumption by sex; standardized percentage of people aged 14 years and over who do not practice any physical activity by sex; standardized percentage of people aged 3 years and over who consume at least four portions of fruit and vegetables a day by sex; and percentage of people aged 14 and over very satisfied of their leisure time by sex. The following have been included as supplementary variables[7]: healthy life expectancy at birth by sex; percentage of people aged 14 and over with a level of life satisfaction from 8 to 10 by sex; percentage of people aged 14 and over which believe their personal situation will improve in the next 5 years by sex; physical component summary for people aged 14 and more by sex; and mental component summary for people aged 14 and more by sex (Figs. 6, 7, 8, 9).

Indicators are at regional level, to identify differences in well-being related to different lifestyles in different areas in Italy (Fig. 10). The analysis has been developed considering simultaneously years 2007–2015 and years 2005 and 2006 as supplementary times (2015 being the last year for which well-being indicators are available at the time of the research).

The Method

Since the 1970s, many methods have been developed to analyze multidimensional phenomena providing multiway or multimode data or data which can be classified according to more than the classic two dimensions unit time variables (Coppi and Bolasco 1989; Coppi 1994). Sequences of matrices referring to set of variables and units over different occasions, allowing both variables and units to be missing on some occasions, provide an array of data classified according to the three criteria *unit x variable x time* (Law 1984).

[6]Active variables, units, and in the above method times are used for the determination of the factors; supplementary units, variables, and times scores on the factorial plane are predicted using only the information provided by the performed factorial analysis on active variables/individuals/times, according to the usual connotation of supplementary for units, variables in ordinary factorial, or principal component analysis (Principal Component Analysis, Abdi and Williams 2010).

[7]For the meaning of supplementary, refer to the note above.

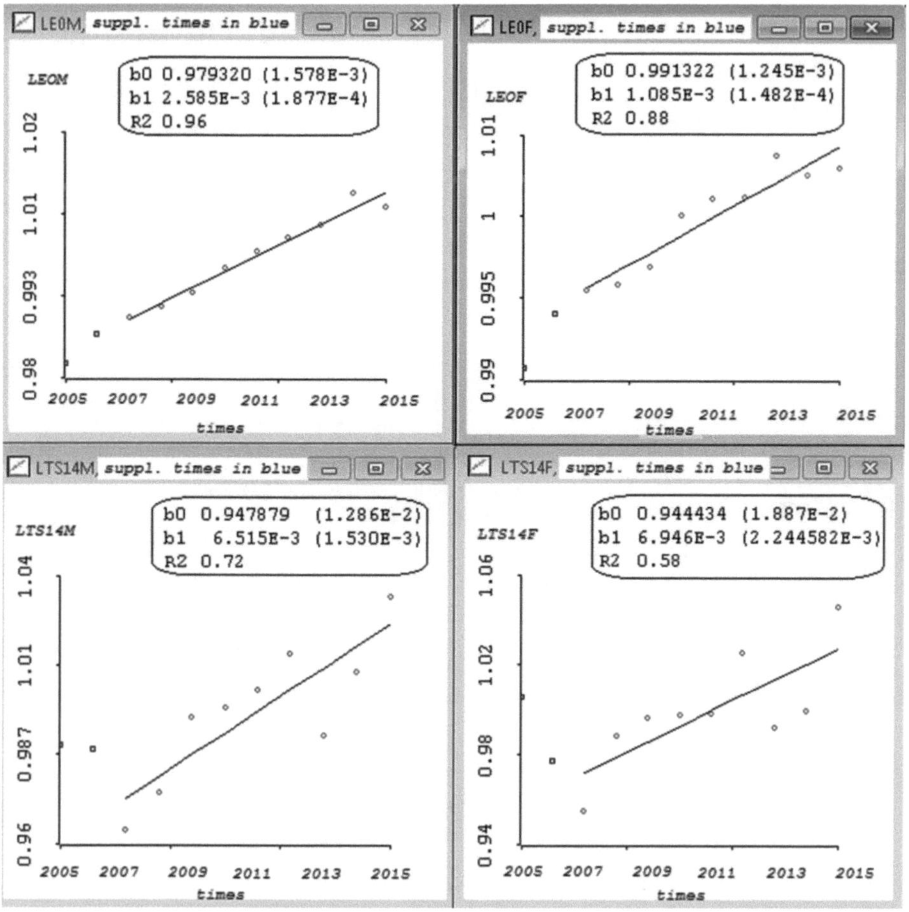

Fig. 6 Regression of indicator centers over time: life expectancy at birth; leisure time satisfaction

Dynamic factor models were originally proposed by Geweke (1977) as a time-series extension of factor models previously developed for cross-sectional data.

In the same period, Coppi and Zannella proposed the dynamic factor analysis (DFA Coppi and Zannella 1979) according to the French school of Analyse des donnèes for multivariate data that provides description of data represented in vectorial spaces and does not refer to probability models for the generating process of data. The DFA model, improved in the 1990s by Corazziari (1999), handles data classified according to different dimensions (multiway data, when the same variables and units are observed over time, so potential missing data have to be imputed). The method is based on the joint application of a principal component analysis and regression over time to centers calculated along specific mode of the

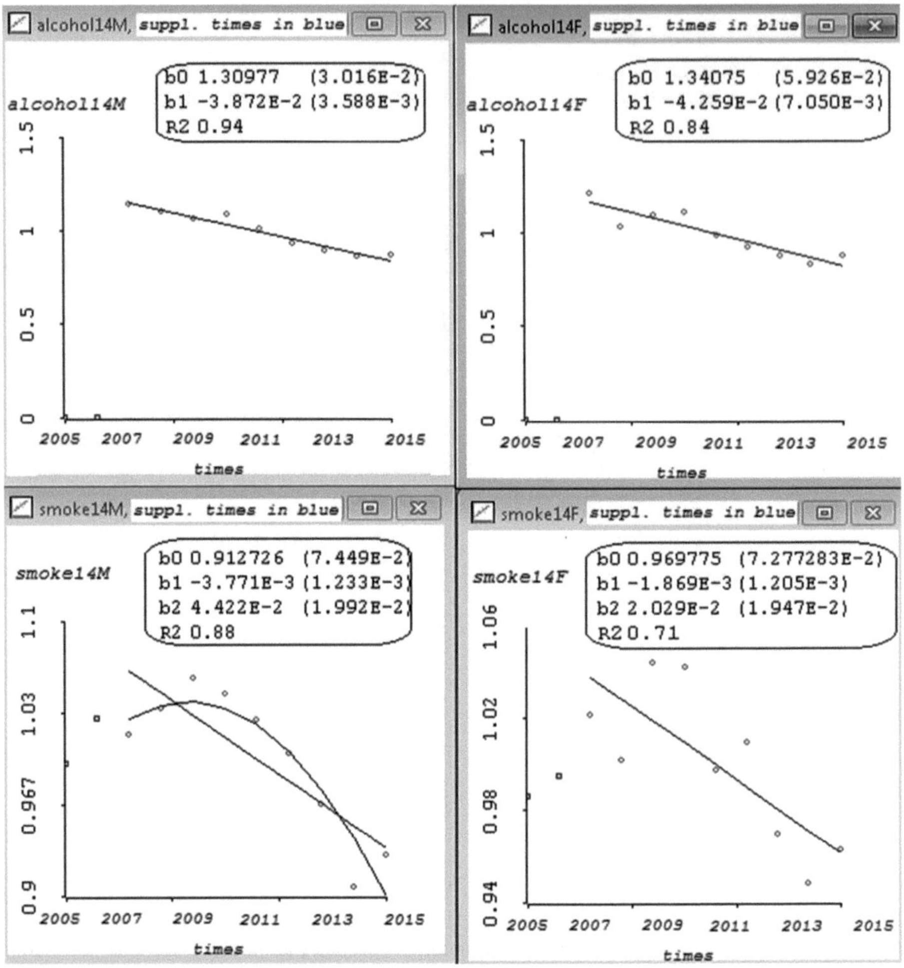

Fig. 7 Regression of Indicators centers over time: alcohol consumption; smoking

data (mode unit or time or variable). It can easily provide a first look at the global structure and dynamic of data, without requiring assumptions whose reliability could be questionable in very complex sets of data.

DFA considers quantitative array of the type "units × variables × times,"

$$X(I, J, T) = \{x_{ijt}\}, i = 1, \ldots I, j = 1 \ldots J, t = 1 \ldots T$$

where i is the unit (region) index, j the quantitative variable (indicator), and t the time (year).

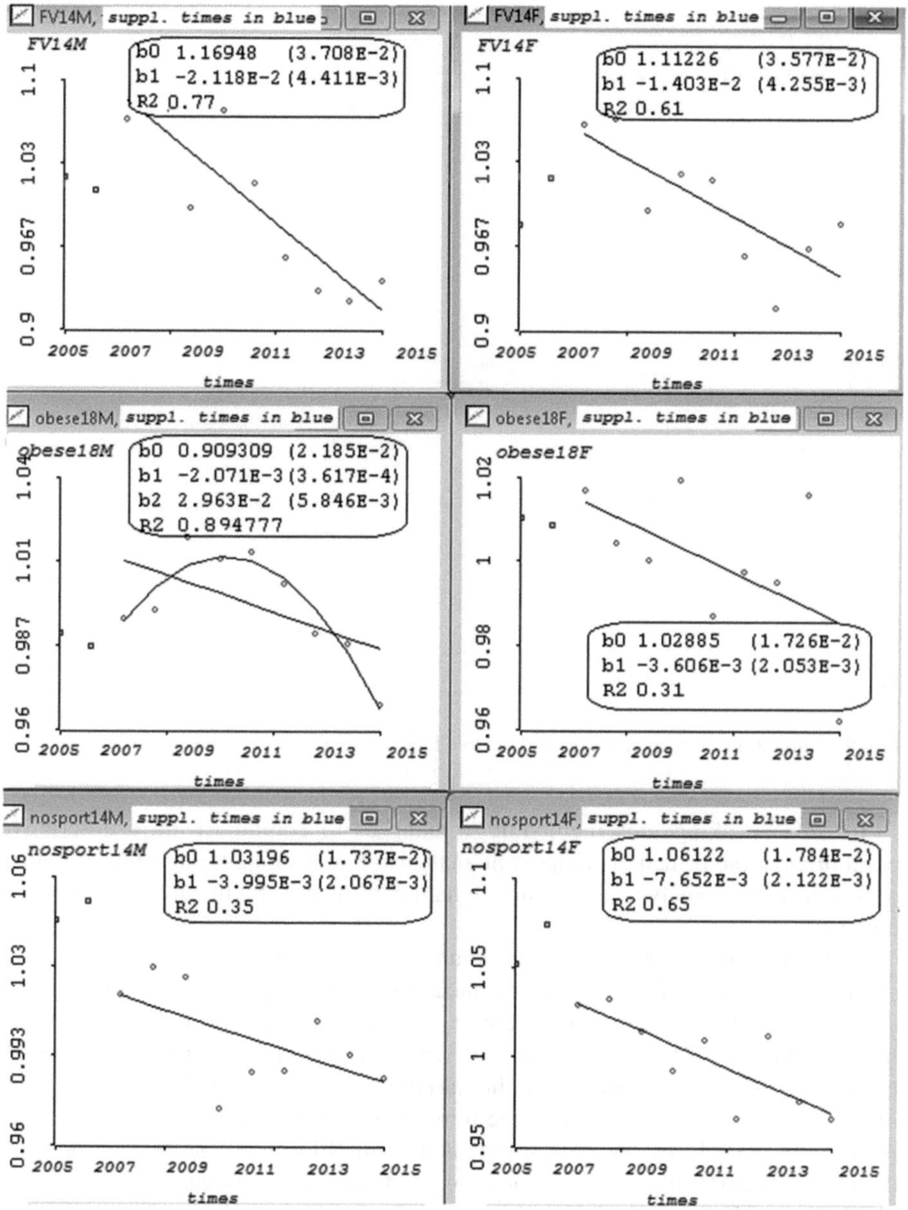

Fig. 8 Regression of indicators centers over time: fruit and vegetables consumption; overweight; no sport

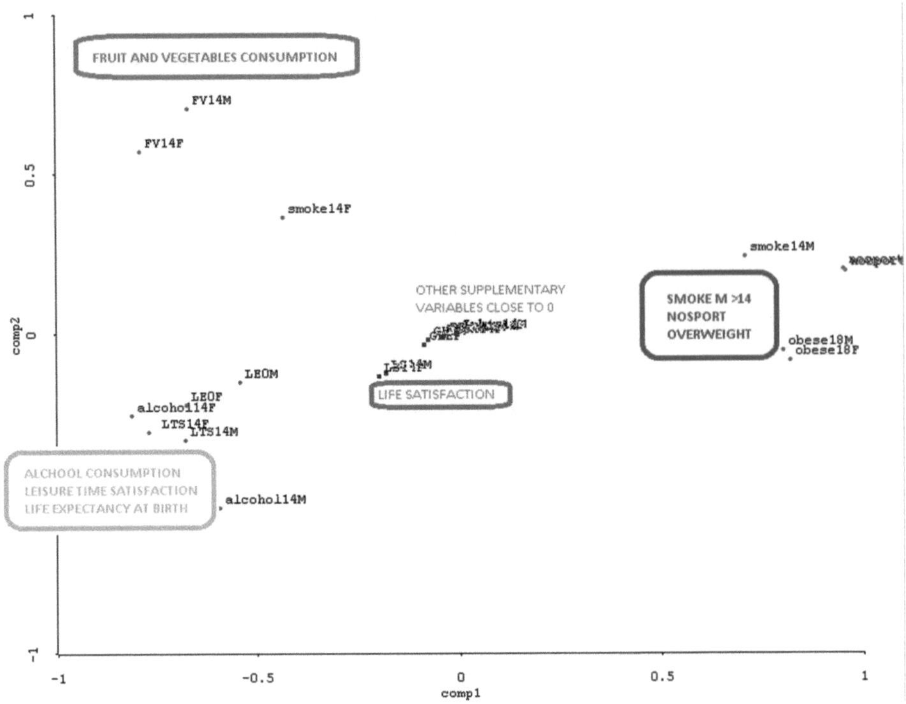

Fig. 9 Correlations among variables and the two PCs solution

Broadly speaking, this methodology manages to combine from a descriptive point of view the principal component analysis of an average (compromise) matrix over time and the analysis of the time dynamic of the data by linear time regression models.

In the cubic matrix $X(I, J, T)$, three sources of variation can be modeled. The first source of variation refers to the covariances between the quantitative indicators, on average over time. It can be considered a structural (or static) variability, provided by the centers $x_{ij.}$. The second source of variation refers to how time interacts with the indicators and is measured by the variability over time of the means of each indicator over the units ($x_{.jt}$), and the third source of variation refers to how time interacts with each region; such source is measured by the dynamic variability of the regions' center (obtained as a mean of all the indicators for each region: $x_{i.t}$).

The goal of the methodology is to linearly decompose the overall variability described by the covariance matrix of $X(I, J, T)$,[8] in the three sources of variability outlined above: the static variability ($x_{ij.}$), the variability of the indicators over time

[8]In Corazziari (1999), it has been shown that the overall covariance matrix of $X(I,J,T)$ is the covariance matrix of the two-way matrix $X(IT,J)$ obtained collapsing the single matrices $X(I,J)_t$ in each time, over time.

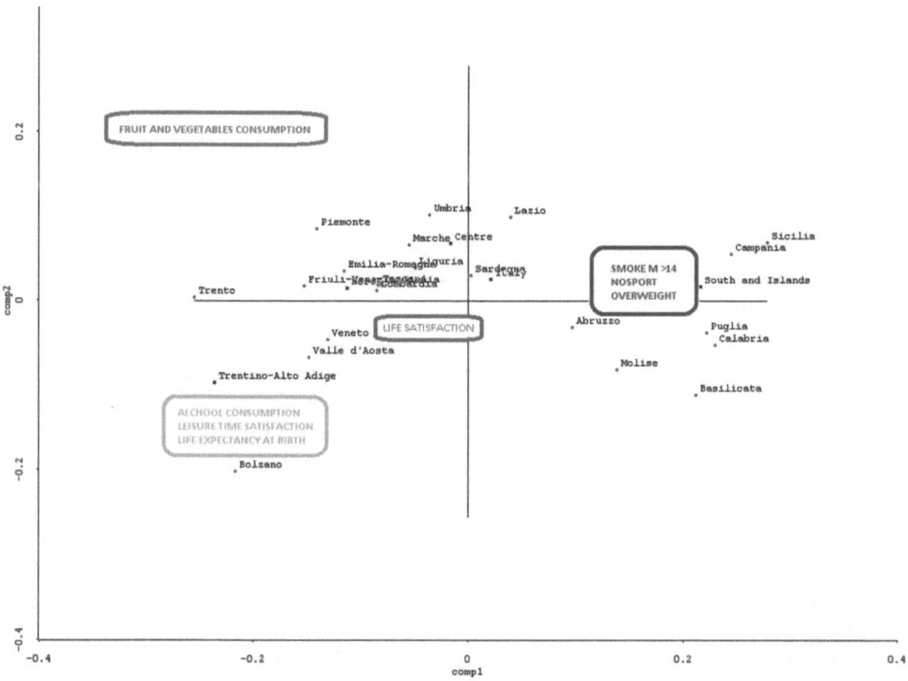

Fig. 10 Regions plotted on the factorial plane identified by the two PCs solution

($x_{.jt}$), and the differential dynamic of regions (residual dynamic of regions when controlling for the mean dynamic of indicators $x_{i.t}$). It has been shown (Coppi and Zannella 1979; Corazziari 1999) that the overall covariance matrix can be decomposed into the sum of three covariance matrices, with each of them describing one of the above sources of variation:

$$S = {}^{*}S_i + {}^{*}S_t + S_{it}$$

where S is the overall covariance of the cubic matrix $X(I, J, T)$, collapsed in two dimensions (see note 9), $^{*}S_i$ is the covariance matrix of the indicators means $x_{ij.}$ representing the mean structure over time, $^{*}S_t$ is the covariance matrix of $x_{.jt}$, to study the variability of the indicators over time, and S_{it} is the covariance matrix representing the differential dynamics of regions.

The DFA consists of four models, each of which employs a specific strategy in approaching the three sources of variation (Corazziari 1999). In this work we use the first model which allows us to focus on the variability of the indicators and their interaction with the other two dimensions of the data: regions' peculiarities and changes over time.

With regard to the time evolution of the centers indicators' $x_{.jt}$, the considered DFA model uses a linear (simple or polynomial) regression model for each indicator j, where the independent variable is time. The parameters are obtained by ordinary least squares, with the classic assumptions about residuals $e_{.jt}$: $\mathrm{cov}[e_{.jt}, e_{.j't'}] = w_j$, if $j = j'$ e $t = t'$, and zero otherwise.

The multivariate variability of the indicators among units is analyzed by a factorial analysis of the covariance matrix $S_t = {}^*S_i + S_{it}$, where $^*S_i$ is the covariance matrix of $^*X_i$, the matrix of the centers $x_{.jt}$, and S_{it} is the covariance matrix of the residuals $x_{ijt} - x_{ij.} - x_{.jt} + x_{.j.}$ describing the net dynamic of regions. It can be easily shown that $\mathbf{S_t}$ is also obtained as the sum of the covariance matrix of variables in each occasion, divided by the total number of times.

By projecting the matrices $^*\boldsymbol{X_i}$, $\boldsymbol{X_t}$ $t = 1,\ldots,T$, after centering, we obtain the factorial representation of each region center and region trajectory (i.e., their dynamic), and the comparison of the projected trajectory of each region on the factorial plane, with their corresponding averaged over time position (region center) on the plane, allows us to evaluate their differential or net time evolution.[9]

The interpretation of our results on the factorial plane is based on the correlation coefficients between the variables and the axes of the factor plane. If one region moves toward the center of the plane (which characterizes the overall dynamic of the system of data), homogeneity among units is increasing, by contrast, if the region move away from the center, its differential dynamic is to be interpreted according to its direction on the plane.

Indexes of the goodness of fit of each source of variation in each models are also provided. They are calculated as the ratio between the trace of the modeled covariance matrix of the specific source of variation, and the corresponding observed trace, for each of the covariance matrices described above.

The Results

Considering the first source of variation, due to the overall time dynamic of variables averaged over units for each time, few variables show an increasing trend: life expectancy at birth (LF0) and satisfaction for leisure time (LTS) both for males and females (the fit to the simple regression model is very good for LE0 with an

[9]The projected trajectories of the units on the factorial plane can be better described by applying a Cluster Analysis of trajectories (Carlier 1986; Coppi et al. 2010). When studying trajectories, two types of distance between couple of countries can be considered: a mean of the comparison (differences) between the two countries in each year (mean instantaneous distance) and a mean of the comparison of the variations between adjacent years of each country (mean unfolding distance). In this article a mean of the two above distances has been considered, and the Ward method of Cluster Analysis has been applied. The results of this last method have been confirmed by a final K-means Cluster Analysis based on the barycenter of the clusters of the better Ward partition (Kaur 2013). The obtained clusters are homogeneous in terms of the levels and of the dynamics of the considered quantitative indicators.

R-squared close to 0.9 or over) and good for LTS (showing more variability over time) (in red active times, in blue supplementary ones).

All the other active variables show decreasing trends, with different variability over time.

For example, considering variables describing attitudes as smoking and alcohol consumption addressing health, both show comparable decreasing trends.

Also the other variables describing lifestyles associated to worst potential consequences on health, but also fruit and vegetables consumption, show a decreasing trend over time in the considered period. Smoking among males shows a stronger decreasing trend over time, more accentuated in the last years (polynomial of order two regression).

The overall goodness of fit for the regression analysis is 0.88, only few variables show a fit not so good due to high variability of data over time: overweight for females and no practice of sport for males (maybe an outlier in 2010).

The factorial analysis of the static source of variability provided two principal components (PC) explaining 83.7% of total variance measured by St trace, where St is the mean of the covariance matrices by year (2007–2015). The following graph shows correlations of variables with the two principal components considered.

Three situations can be identified: the first is characterized by the consumption of fruit and vegetables but also higher levels of smoking for women aged more than 13 (on the left up side of the graph); the second shows higher levels of satisfacion for leisure time and better life expectancy at birth, but also higher levels of alcohol consumption (on the left bottom side of the graph); and the third characterised by overweight, male smoking, and lower if not sport practice for both males and females (right side of the graph).

Considering the plot on the factorial plane of regions' center over the considered period, South Italian regions share the most critical situation from the health point of view, with no regular sport, overweight, and male smoking (aged more than 13); north regions share better lifestyles in terms of fruit and vegetables consumption, higher levels of life expectancy at birth, more regular sport, but higher levels of alcohol consumption for females joined to higher levels of leisure time satisfaction for both males and females, while Bolzano seems to be characterized by higher levels of alcohol consumption for males.

Central regions show higher levels of fruit and vegetables consumption than South regions but also higher levels of female smoking (aged more than 13).

Also each year is well represented by the factorial plane identified by the two PCs: the best represented time is 2015, the worst one is 2011 (Table 2).

The variability of the regions' centers over time is well fitted by the factorial plane, being explained at 90%. The differential dynamics of units, which can be analyzed comparing regions' trajectories with the corresponding centers, is explained at 38%, a good result considering that it is residual, so characterized also by what is not linearly explained.

No regions show significant differential trajectory compared with the overall dynamic of indicators means; indeed trajectories show very not linear dynamic, around the corresponding region center. Few exceptions are Bolzano showing

Table 2 Variance explained by the PC solution, by year (*St)

Year	% of total variance explained
2007	0.834329
2008	0.821280
2009	0.812041
2010	0.825050
2011	0.784936
2012	0.849327
2013	0.859225
2014	0.868333
2015	0.880259

increasing levels of alcohol consumption for males; Emilia-Romagna increasing levels of leisure time satisfaction, life expectancy, and female alcohol consumption; Molise, Campania, Puglia, and Basilicata worsening their lifestyles, attitudes and behaviors; while Sicilia seems to improve its overall situation.

Conclusions

The topics here discussed inspire some reflections. First of all, food and all its aspects cannot be considered a simple life domain. It is complex aspect with political implications. In fact, food not only concerns the individual's well-being but that of the whole society. Moreover, food relates to the citizens' conscious sense of belonging to a territorial, and cultural, context. It is important to understand that every change in food style, for better or worse, always implies cultural aspects. The entire food chain implies choices at different levels whose effects do not only relate to the present time but also to the medium and long term. Data show, for example, that even an imperfect indicator like the BMI index can tell us a lot about individuals and their lifestyles. Our exercise suggests how the multidimensional analysis of the BES indicators may provide many suggestions to improve the citizens' lives (ISTAT 2016).

Moreover, the analysis and interpretation of official not only give us a picture of the present situation but are able to grasp the emerging critical elements in social life, helping citizens and policy makers in finding the best practices to overcome the emerging criticalities.[10] In this perspective, official data can be seen as a precious tool in making a very specific practice in future studies: the so-called anticipation (Appadurai 2013; Arnaldi and Poli 2012) that is finding what can be done, in the present time, in order to create better possibilities for possible futures. Food is a challenge of contemporary social complexity and a topic that involves the role of

[10]The present work is focused on adult population. For this reason, there is no mention of the critical issues related to the behavior of minors with regard to food styles.

social sciences (Maggino and Facioni 2016). Indeed, choosing a food style rather than another affects not only the individuals' health but also the environment and resources available on the planet. In this sense, the Milan Charter[11] – a document proposed during the opening of Expo 2015 (1 May – 31 October 2015) and entrusted to the Secretary General of the United Nations, Ban Ki-moon, on 16 October 2015 – makes clear that the policies about food are of a multidimensional kind. Indeed, the policies about food concern the well-being of humanity and the health of the planet. So, every citizen should be aware that every time he sits at a table to have a meal, he/she is making an important political act. So, the fundamental culture of food in any country should have to be considered an indispensable tool for building the quality of life for all.

References

Abdi, H., Williams L J. (2010). *Principal Component Analysis*, Wileys Interdisciplinary Reviews, Computational Statistics, volume 2 issue 4 Pages: 433–459.

Appadurai, A., (2013). *The future as Cultural Fact. Essays on the Global Condition*, Arjun Appadurai first published by Verso.

Arnaldi, S., Poli, R., (2012). *La previsione sociale. Introduzione allo studio dei futuri*, Carocci, Roma.

Artusi, P., (1891). *La scienza in cucina e l'arte di mangiar bene. Manuale pratico per le famiglie*, i tipi di Salvadore Landi, Firenze.

Braudel, F., (1979). *Civilisation matérielle, économie et capitalisme* (XVe-XVIIIe siècle). *La structure du quotidien: le possible et l'impossible*, Librairie Armand Colin, Paris.

Carlier A. (1986). *Factor Analysis of Evolution and Cluster* Methods *on Trajectories*, Compstat 1986.

Carrara, G. (2007). *Per una filosofia dell'alimentazione con un excursus sul peccato di gola. Suggerimenti teorici ed ipotesi didattiche*, su "Comunicazione filosofica. Rivista telematica di ricerca e didattica filosofica" n. 18.

Coppi, R., D'Urso, P., Giordani, P. (2010). *A Fuzzy Clustering Model for Multivariate Spatial Time Series*. Journal of Classification March 2010, Volume 27, Issue 1, pp 54–88

Coppi, R., Zannella, F. (1979). *L'analisi fattoriale di una serie temporale multipla relativa allo stesso insieme di unità statistiche*, Atti della XXIX Riunione della SIS.

Coppi, R., (1994). *An Introduction to Multiway Data and their Applications*. Computational Statistics and data analysis, 18 (4), pp. 3–13.

Coppi, R., Bolasco, S. (1989). *Multiway Data Analysis*. Amsterdam, North Holland.

Corazziari, I. (1999). *Analisi di Dati Longitudinali Multivariati*, Tesi di Dottorato XI ciclo, Napoli aprile 1999.

Di Francesco, G. (2006). *Armonie di baccalà*, Ce.R.I.S., Sant'Omero.

Geweke, J. (1977). "The Dynamic Factor Analysis of Economic Time Series," in Latent Variables in Socio-Economic Models, ed. by D.J. Aigner and A.S. Goldberger, Amsterdam: North-Holland.

ISTAT (2016). *Rapporto BES. Il benessere equo e sostenibile in Italia,* Istat, Roma.

[11]http://carta.milano.it/wp-content/uploads/2015/04/English_version_Milan_Charter.pdf (website visited on January 31, 2018).

M Kaur, (2013). *Clustering Approaches Using K-Means Algorithm.* International Journal of Advanced Research in Computer Science and Software Engineering vol. 3 issue 5, pp 861–864. Research Paper Available online at: www.ijarcsse.com

Longo, V., (2016). *La dieta della longevità*, Vallardi, Firenze.

Law, H.G. (1984). *Research methods i multimode data analysis Praeger Special Studies,* AbeBooks.co.uk

Maggino, F., Facioni, C. (2016). The *complex relationship between well-being and resources; the Italian studies contribution*, in Olah S., Roseanu G., Bodogai S., Coturbas L. , *Current challenges in Social Sciences*, Presa Universitara Clujeana, pp. 17–26

McGee, H., (1984). *On Food and Cooking*, Scribner, U.S.

Meadows, D.H., Meadows, D.L., Randers, J., Behrens, W.W. (1972). *The Limits to Growth: A Report for the Club of Rome's Project on the Predicament of Mankind*, Club of Rome, Ginevra.

Petrick, J.L., Kelly, S.P., Liao, L.M., Freedman, N.D., Graubard, B.I., Coo, M.B. (2017). *Body weight trajectories and risk of oesophageal and gastric cardia adenocarcinomas: a pooled analysis of NIH-AARP and PLCO Studies,* British Journal of Cancer (2017) n. 116, pp. 951–959, Nature Publishing Group, UK

Petrini, C. (2010). *Terra madre. Come non farci mangiare dal cibo*, Slow Food, Bra.

Poulain, J.P. (2002). *Sociologies de l'alimentation. Les mangeurs et l' espace social alimentaire*, Presses Universitaires de France, Paris.

Scarpinato, R. (2004). *Marilyn Monroe e la cassata siciliana*, in: *Il cibo e l'impegno*, I quaderni di MicroMega, Roma, (pagg. 66–73).

Veronesi, U. (2013). *La dieta del digiuno. Perdere peso e prevenire le malattie con la restrizione calorica*, Mondadori, Milano.

Food, Eating Behaviors, and Quality of Life of University Students

Gabriele Di Francesco

Abstract The essay aims to analyze the relationship between food, feeding behavior and a healthy lifestyle with other conditions and habits, such as a sedentary lifestyle, poor sports activity, stress and anxiety, while also trying to deepen the possible strategies of food-related coping, as well as the use of "doping" substances and products (intellectual doping) not only for recreational purposes, but also for the reduction of emotionality (e.g. anxiolytic), or for improving study performances (e.g. dietary supplements, energizing drinks, etc.). The analysis is a reflection of research carried out on a sample of university students in some European universities, including Rouen, Dunkerque (France), Cluj Napoca (Romania) and Chieti-Pescara (Italy), regarding their eating habits, their life styles, habits of study, and propensity to physical inactivity. Such dimensions often correlate with problematic food behaviors, with compulsive consumption of foods and beverages, and the acquisition of uncritical eating patterns.

Food and Quality of Life

Scholars of social sciences started only relatively recently to deal with phenomena related to eating practices. In classical sociological production, authors who have studied this subject in a "direct" way are rare; the raids of the social sciences in the food-culinary field have been subordinated to an order of discussions considered more "rightfully" proper to sociology and anthropology, such as social groups, commensality, rite, sacrifice, etc. The most obvious reasons for this snobbery of food are probably two: 1) the importance of food and food practices was such and so daily in the eyes of all, that the study of these phenomena and practices did not appear necessary; 2) food belonged to the domestic sphere and was therefore linked, in particular, to the role of woman; this relegated the topic to an inferior status to that

G. Di Francesco (✉)
Italy Department of Business Administration, University of G. d'Annunzio Chieti-Pescara, Chieti, Italy
e-mail: gabriele.difrancesco@unich.it

A. Bianco et al. (eds.), *Italian Studies on Quality of Life*, Social Indicators Research Series 77, https://doi.org/10.1007/978-3-030-06022-0_14

of the study of activities of the public sphere, which have always been considered male dominance, such as economics and politics, which were, in fact, abundantly studied (Mennell 1993).

Food and eating practices, lifestyle and the way to eat and consume, conviviality and commensality are on the other hand ongoing processes, though not always perceptible. They change in function of social changes and have changed, altered and innovated in almost continuous iteration and appear to represent also the social imprinting of each age, its cultural identity in food and wine terms. For example, it is the introduction of new foods, the contact with other cultures and civilizations that creates many food taboos or puts new ones on them, the introduction of new productive techniques that all affect the lifestyle of people and change their social costumes, beliefs and traditions. One of the historical references is the introduction of products from America that have had such an impact on our culture to be considered today as part of Mediterranean culture and diet. In this respect, eating habits, the link between man and food move between excesses and privations, hunger and satiety, prohibitions and remedies, balance and imbalances, pursuit of well-being and hunger, in building a harmony of resources and taste, for building that gastronomic capital that is the food culture and which is also necessarily a health culture. The relationship between humans and human groups with food also assumes the valence that reveals the notions of use and abuse, the criticalities, the disturbances caused and the psychosocial difficulties that arise, highlighting therapeutic responses to the overcoming pathological manifestations and tending to reestablish or improve a lost equilibrium.

The theme of nutrition and well-being, understood as physical and psychosocial health, is very complex and intrinsic to a variety of variables and indicators linked to physiological, bio-nutritional and psychological phenomena, on the one hand, and to the culture of eating and drinking, eating habits, customs, as well as social change and the influence of such lifestyle changes. Discrimination is nevertheless represented by the relationship between food and health, nourishment of the healthy man and the sick, according to a line of evolution that in the use of foods is the founding element of the same medicine.

"Medical art would not have been discovered," wrote Hippocrates in the Ancient Medical treatise, "nor would it have been sought if it had the same benefit to the patient as the ingestion of the same substances that are eaten and drunk by healthy individuals" (Vegetti 1998, p. 45). As a result of this necessity, men became enthusiastic about transforming and producing food: "They boiled, felt, mixed, and tempered the strong and intemperate substances with the weaker, conforming them all to the nature and power of man" (Di Francesco 2015a, p. 314).

"The importance and close bond between" nutrition and good health "is underlined by the World Health Organization (WHO), which considers adequate nutrition and health fundamental human rights. Nutrition is one of the factors that most affect the development, productivity and productivity of people, the quality of life and the psycho-physical conditions with which aging is concerned" (INRAN 2003).[1] WHO itself, in the very beginning of its Constitution,[2] refers to the concept of "complete physical, mental and social well-being", thus focusing on further variables that go beyond the simple "absence of illness or illness" well-being which include, on the one hand, "the improvement of nutrition" and the other factors having to do with hygiene of the environment', but which, on the other hand cannot include those elements of subjectivity which contribute to the outline of lifestyle and food style of individuals and social groups, where the life of relationship takes place. The concept of quality of life in relation to food, and food is therefore primarily related to health and, above all, to the prevention of infirmities and illnesses that result from inadequate, erroneous or harmful conduct and eating habits.

However, these dimensions do not exhaust the range of possible options and should be further specified in their conceptual content, for example referring to the health of foodstuffs, their production methods, their preservation, processing and preparation, their condiments, the circumstances, the times and places of consumption, the balance of the same and the variety (production and recruitment). It is also necessary to mention the traditions, the differences and diversity of taste, the psychological, sociological, cultural, ritual, philosophical, political, economic, norms and religious content of the food that affect the taste or edibility of a product, such as an animal or preparation in certain historical moments and territorial contexts (Di Francesco 2015b).

By way of example, the indications and the prospectus relating to the factors related to the quality of life contained in Fernández-Ballesteros et al.'s (1996) Cubrecavi (Short Course of Calidad de Vida), which identifies ten variables: to enjoy good health, to be able to rely on social support and therefore mutual aid, to do business not only physical, leisure, to have satisfactory economic conditions, to be personally satisfied, to refer to efficient health and social services, to socialize, to live in a healthy environment of high quality, have practical skills and a satisfactory culture. It is also in this regard that all the complex factors that can be applied to the analysis of systems and feeding processes are included (Di Francesco 2015b).

You could continue by referring to many other paradigms, exemplifications and perspectives, to different ways of determining and analyzing the subject. Twenty years ago some work in the medical field identified 159 different instruments for

---

[1]To make things worse, then there is the sedentary lifestyle. WHO estimates, in fact, that about 41% of Europeans do not carry out any kind of moderate physical activity over the course of the week and this increases the risk of chronic illness (INRAN, 2003).

[2]The Constitution of the WHO (RU, 1948, 976) states: "States participating in the present constitution declare, under the Charter of the United Nations, that the basis of happiness of peoples, their harmonious relations and their security are the The following principles: Health is a state of complete physical, mental and social well-being, it does not consist only of the absence of illness or infirmity. (...) Encourages, where necessary, other specialized institutions, improving nutrition, sanitation, best use of rescue intervals, improving economic and working conditions, including all other environmental hygiene factors" (WHO Constitution, Chapter II, Article 2, letter I, RU, 1948, 976).

measuring it (Gill, Feinstein 1994). In recent years, attention to the issues of quality of life has widened, extending it to more disciplinary disciplines and to different contexts, both scientific and non-existent. This testifies to a great deal of interest, but it can also be seen that there is not much difficulty in easily reaching a consensus on how to deepen the study, the variables to be taken into consideration, and so on. The reasons for this multiplicity of approaches and readings can be attributed to various explanatory hypotheses, which can be related, for example, to the vastness of the subject, to the difficulty of capturing its intrinsic nature, to the possibility of giving different interpretations (Majani 1999, pp. 103–104).[3] However, it is now widely recognized that there is a close connection between food, or rather quality of food, and quality of life, which is related to the issues of health and well-being. "In the past," one observes, "a conception was predominant that was limited to assessing the quality of food referring to the direct relationship with the individual consumer. By exemplifying: food must feed those who eat it; must be sure of who eats it; it should please those who eat it, and so on" (Vienna 2008, p. 35). This concept of quality, limited only to the health of the individual consumer, has now been overcome in a broader vision that tends to include in the concept of food quality the promotion of a real improvement in widespread food health.

New Food Models

It is, however, wise to wonder how this model is practicable in an era of rapid transformations and parallel changes in our lives, in which it is the daily experience of both individual and group (up to the family-group) to fracture and discontinuity with traditional socio-cultural contexts to admit that the majority of the models, both in the family context and outside them, is a libertarian and anomalous model until anarchy, both for the spaces involved and the set scenarios, both for related symbols, for time scans, for modes and content for their own consumption. In fact, a new pattern of transnational food consumption is imposed, which puts no emphasis on what is eaten but where it is bought, where it is eaten and the rhythm of how it is eaten, in the face of a gradual retrenchment of the holding of traditional cultures of local foodstuffs (Frudà 2009).

[3]This is how Giuseppina Majani speaks of the quality of life associated with health: "When a subject attracts so much attention, but there is no easy consensus on how to study it, several explanatory possibilities are given. Some of these seem more likely. The first is that it is such a big topic that any part of it is considered to be an aspect to be measured with a specific instrument. A second is that nature is not yet understood, and every detection method has the same rights as any other to be applied and the same probability of being appropriate. A third possibility is that this is an indefinite subject, which can be given many different interpretations, each corresponding to a detection tool. The quality of life is probably all this: it is a vast subject, of which it is difficult to comprehend completely the nature and passable to individual interpretations. And it is, however, of current interest" (Majani 1999, p. 103).

Faced with various eco-sustainable movements that enhance quality and taste, slowness, traceability, supply chain, and so on, and which are attentive to the health effects of food, since in the last 20 years of the twentieth century, also in Italy, an evolutionary path of dietary styles with their progressive modernization and increasingly marked adherence to innovative models, values and behaviors, were not always positive and healthy. Almost a sort of meal decontamination has occurred, with the abandonment of the traditional Italian first dish, second dish and fruit or sweet tripartite, to make room for a much simpler everyday style of consumption (Vercelloni 2002). It has also been noted that the replacement of traditional meals intended as meals, becoming more and more of the transitory, commercial and passage places, without identity, of real non-places, where you can quickly and easily eat attractive food for the color, preparation and application, ready for screening, but made with products that do not always ensure the origin, quality and sometimes genuineness.

These changes have been recorded by a series of surveys on Italians' habits and eating behavior. The research carried out between 2000 and 2008 (Ismea-Abacus, ANGEM – National Association of Catering Companies) shows that only 35% of Central-North Italians eat their lunch at home; the remaining quota uses canteens, bars and the like, or arrange them in the workplace. The Ismea-Nielsen survey carried out in July–December 2004 notes that during the period considered, 75% consumed at least one meal out of the home. More generally, it is estimated that extra-domestic food consumption now accounts for 30% of total food expenditure (Frudà 2009).[4] From the multiscope survey on the aspects of everyday life of Italian families, referring to 2009, emerges, in addition that "lunch continues to represent the main meal for most of the population. 67.9 percent of people aged 3 and over, in fact, have lunch as the most important meal of the day, while only 22.1 percent consider dinner as their most important meal. However, between 2001 and 2009 there is a gradual and slow decline in the share of the population for which lunch is the main meal, in fact this figure was 72.2% in 2001" (Orsini 2010, p. 55).

The data seem emblematic of a scenario that sees rhythms and patterns of nutrition in lively transformation in parallel with changing work needs and individuals, consequently, changing lifestyles, adapting to stimuli and offers of an increasingly complex and diversified world. Electronic communication, on the other hand, is growing in parallel with enormous consumption of goods, a heavy workload and the "distractions of the home foyer". Apart from the great occasions, home cooking is limited to just heating the dishes (Goody 1982: 308).

In the Internet society there is the most extreme food freedom, the possibility of access to a variety of foods, styles and nutritional patterns that are unthinkable, but where they are more and more often eaten alone or in the company of their own

[4]The data found in various surveys and various research institutes, behaviors and eating habits are not always consistent in identifying homogenous trends. In fact, they highlight many differences between the country's areas and some basic conditions and variables. With reference to the cohort of Italians who have a stable occupation, it seems to be always a habit to eat lunch outside the walls of home, also, traditionally, bringing the meal straight from home.

tablet or smartphone (Di Francesco 2015b, pp. 105–109). The concepts of lifestyle and eating styles (which refer to a system of individual or collective behaviors to read and interpret on the basis of values, beliefs and attitudes, as well as the constraints deriving from variables such as gender, age, status) can be an instrument of great utility for knowing, analyzing and highlighting what a person, a social group, a group of people think or feel or what habits it has in everyday life.

Particularly in contemporary society, where demarcation between the age classes has become rather rigid compared to a recent past, knowing ways of living, styles of relationships, social and intimate lives of people, groups and segments of the population – distinct based on specific variables – becomes essential for a variety of reasons, including: (1) addressing health and choosing the best possible options by recognizing current behaviors; (2) to put in place interventions to promote health and well-being, understood as a subjective and social dimension (together with the possibilities of being in the relationship with oneself and/or with others); (3) to expose risk behaviors that may affect physical and mental health; (4) to allow the spread of "virtuous" knowledge and behaviors, especially in the youth universe (Di Francesco, 2015a).

The study of young people's food and lifestyles is therefore in a multiple dimension: (a) as an option of knowledge of a world, such as youth, today more than ever liquid, to say it with Baumann, and more and more elusive; (b) how to act to reduce complexity of life and achieve better quality in everyday life; (c) as a health orientation for the youth population.

Lifestyle and Food Models of Italian University Students

In light of this premise it is possible to state that there is a close connection between food styles and quality of life. This is a relationship conditioned by different factors mainly of an environmental and economic nature, but also of social and cultural character. It is a very particular variable of quality of life in relation to food, which seems to be mainly related to health. It is interesting to analyze the relationship between food, food and a healthy lifestyle with other conditions and habits, such as sedentary, poor sports, stress and anxiety, while also trying to deepen the possible strategies of food-related coping, as well as the use of "doping" substances and products (intellectual doping) not only for recreational purposes, but also for the reduction of hemostility (e.g. anxiolytic) or for improving study performances (e.g. dietary supplements, energizing drinks, etc.).

The reflection in this respect leads to the desire to analyze the lifestyle of young people about some of the major variables (behaviors, attitudes, values, etc.) as well as trying to understand how and why certain lifestyles and values have changed.

The reference to deepening the topic of food, food styles and quality of life of university students is the source of some extensive national and European research. This refers in particular to the research on the social and economic conditions of university students at Community level (Finocchietti 2015)[5]; to the one conducted on some university services and among them the canteen services (ADSU Abruzzo Survey Survey – Right Survey on the Study of Palermitani Universities, etc. 2011–2014); analysis of the lifestyle and nutrition of university students (SELFI and SELFI2 survey of the Universities of Rouen – University of Littoral – Côte d'Opale – Institut Pasteur de Lille 2013–2015); and finally to the correlations that have been conducted in recent years (2013 to 2017) among the students of the "G. d'Annunzio" University in Chieti-Pescara.

The starting point, following the Eurostudent survey, is, however, the analysis of some of the essentially socio-economic variables that affect students' university life, especially students living outside the home, the so-called out-of-school students who live outside of the family, alone or in co-habitation with other students. It is believed that they are more capable of quantifying the financial implications of their study experience. Studying "out of the house" costs students about 9000 Euros/year. Housing expenditure is the largest item, accounting for more than one third of the total; while food is in second place, weighing about one fifth of the total cost and is followed by University fees, transportation and book expenses and other teaching materials.

To have an overall amount of how much it is costly for a family to keep an out-of-school student out of the expense for an annual rent has been added to university tuition fees (about 1000 euros annually for Italian public universities), the purchase of textbooks (About 500 euros a year in Italian public universities) and about 2400 euros per year (Indagine Movimento Consumatori 2012).[6]

Commuting has grown considerably since the post-reform era of the last decade. Commuters are currently 50.1% of students who attend classes regularly and are even greater among those who come from families in unfavorable socio-economic conditions (Finocchietti 2015). The consequences of this situation are rather heavy, as there is a drastic reduction in expenditure (from study materials and teaching aids), and from a nutrition point of view, the tendency to orient itself towards real "food bricolages", in the form of strategies of resistance to a general situation of social and economic disadvantage. Homemade self-made meals with family food supplies add high-quality foods that are mainly bought in discount stores with "cheap" or "on-demand" foods. There is the substitution of traditional Italian meals with "aperitif aperitifs" or "apericena" that allow you to combine your meal times with the loisirs.

[5]"Eurostudent V 2012–2015 Seventh report – Social and economic conditions of student life in Europe" has involved, beyond Italy, 28 European countries and ended with the publication of the Report" Eurostudent V 2012–2015 Synopsis of Indicators", presented during the Conference "The Social Dimension in European Higher Education" (Vienna 25-27-2-2015), http://www.eurostudent.it/files/2368_rapporto_vii_indagine_eurostudent-it-it.pdf

[6]http://www.consumersforum.it/voce-ai-soci/1930-indagine-movimento-consumatori-crisi-affitti-in-ribasso-for-gli-studenti-fuori-sede.html and http://www.studentpass.it/content/i-costi-dei-fuori-sede

"Food bricolages" are characterized by unbalanced meals with excess carbohydrates (pasta, pizza, sausages, etc.) and with scarcity of vegetables and fruit, minimized. The kitchen is slightly varied and with low quality food. Accentuate gastro-anomalous phenomena with compensatory periodic excesses and excessive use of alcoholic beverages (beer). They are alongside the "bricolages" of life, which manifest themselves with the tendency to sedentaryness, the lack of constant physical activity and a hyper-movement of the past (the soccer game, the outbreak of jogging), the irregular scanning of the hours of the day and especially the night, the loss of sleep and the little time spent on rest, tobacco smoke and the use of cannabis, coupled with inadequate coping strategies to solve stressful situations.

Orientation to Well-Being: An Open Conclusion

It is in this context that the study of the dietary styles of Chieti and Pescara university students is based on the analysis of the target population of students who, 2014/2015, he recourse to the canteen service of the University Law Firm (ADSU) of the Abruzzo Region at the "G. d'Annunzio" University.[7] The methodology adopted is consistent with the statistical methodology in customer satisfaction survey (Zeithaml et al. 2000; Parasuraman et al. 2007). The sample of 1009 respondents, with an average age of 22, represented 23% of the universe of 4367 students using the canteen service. Administration was carried out through the Surveymonkey platform and statistical representativeness is guaranteed by post-stratification proportional to gender, age and faculty of belonging.

The analysis of research data highlights the frequent use of university tuition by students and their use only for lunch for a majority share of 30.4%, for whoever it serves both for lunch and for lunch for dinner (27.0%) and who serves only for dinner (12.7%). Lunch is therefore the main meal consumed by students, with a minimum deviation compared to those who eat and dine there. Most of the students attending the canteens are Abruzzi (37.8%) and Apulia (29.2%), followed by other regions of the South (Apulia, Molise, Basilicata and Campania) with an almost homogeneous average of 8, 00%. Canteens are the most widely used service offered by ADSU, such as scholarships, sporting services, language courses, and so on.

Students for 66.2% consume meal meals, 19.7% in the home, 9.0% at the bar at the University, and 5.0% in hot tables outside the university. 29.2% consumes table meals by necessity, 39.8% for convenience, 29.6% for comfort, and only 0.5% for quality. A share of 85.5% of students consumes the whole meal versus 12.4%, which is limited to a single dish. The overall rating of the perceived quality is not high, but it is still on the line of sufficiency. Judgment is more positive among those who attend the service more assiduously.

[7] A survey carried out by ADSU by Dr. Riccardo Di Nisio.

Table 1 Body mass index found in a sample of Italian high schools students distinguished by gender. Survey 2016/2018 – absolute values and percentages

Body mass index	M	F	Total	M%	F%	Total%
Seriously underweight (< 16.00)	0	0	0	0.00	0.00	0.00
Underweight (16.00–18.49	8	36	44	6.90	17.14	13.50
Normal weight (18.50–24.99)	92	138	230	79.31	65.71	70.55
Overweight (25.00–29.99)	12	20	32	10.34	9.52	9.82
Obesity degree 1 (30.00–34.99)	2	5	7	1.72	2.38	2.15
Obesity degree 2 (35.00–39.99)	0	0	0	0.00	0.00	0.00
Obesity degree 3 (≥40.00)	1	0	1	0.86	0.00	0.31
Missed answer	1	11	12	0.86	5.24	3.68
Total	116	210	326	100	100	100

Table 2 Body mass index found in a sample of Italian university students according to sex – Survey 2016 – absolute values and percentages

Body mass index	M	F	Total	M%	F%	Total%
Seriously underweight (< 16.00)	0	1	1	0.00	0.85	0.61
Underweight (16.00–18.49)	2	12	14	4.26	10.17	8.48
Normal weight (18.50–24.99)	30	79	109	63.83	66.95	66.06
Overweight (25.00–29.99)	13	23	36	27.66	19.49	21.82
Obesity degree 1 (30.00–34.99)	1	1	2	2.13	0.85	1.21
Obesity degree 2 (35.00–39.99)	1	0	1	2.13	0.00	0.61
Obesity degree 3 (≥40.00)	0	0	0	0.00	0.00	0.00
Missed answer	0	2	2	0.00	1.69	1.21
Total	47	118	165	100	100	100

The judgment on the canteen service therefore appears to be a positive one. However, quality measurements should not only take account of canteens, but be extended to all students enrolled in university courses. Eating on a meal, however, ensures a balanced and controlled meal, different from the meals eaten at the many dining outlets around the university campus and which are very popular with most students for the food diets that characterize student life and produce. It has been noted that during the first year of university there is a tendency to be fatigued by subtle quotas of students.

From the study Students Evaluation Lifestyle Feeling Inventory (Selfie UdA) conducted in parallel with the "G. d'Annunzio" University of Chieti-Pescara and among the students of a High School in 2016 on a significant sample of students found that in passing to the university is a higher student rate that has a significant weight gain measured through the body mass index. In the case of overweight individuals in high school, 10.34% for males and 9.52% for females account for a rate of 27.66% for students and 19.49% for students. Overweight people are up from 9.82% to 21.82%. Young males considered to be high-grade fell from 79.31% to 63.83%, while high-school girls increased from 65.71% to 66.95%, with a parallel decrease (from 17.14% to 10.17%) underweight students (Tables 1 and 2).

Table 3 Nutrition status of Cluj-Napoca University students, according to their BMI (Body mass index) – V.A. is %

Nutritional status		BMI Intervals	Subjects	Proportion (%)
Under weight	Severe	<16	1	0.45
	Moderate	16–16.9	5	2.24
	Low	17–18.4	31	13.9
Normal weight		18.5–24.9	162	72.65
Overweight		25–29.9	19	8.52
Obesity	Degree I	30–34.9	4	1.79
	Degree II	35–39.9	1	0.45
	Degree III	>40	0	0

Bromboiu et al. (2016:38–39)

The transition from high school to university seems to have detrimental effects on the weight gain of young people. This is probably due to the changes that this step requires and the adoption of a lifestyle less regulated by family rhythms. Exiting from the home with the forced adoption of a different food style, at least for those who face the study far from the families, and the greater sedentariness that the college study imposes are probably the main causes of this weight gain. According to data from other researches conducted in other countries, we must, however, note that the Italian situation seems less robust than other countries. Data obtained between French and Romanian students using the same analytical tools in fact show significant differences.

Regarding the body mass index, 70% of French students are considered normal-grade, 11% in slightly underweight, 9% overweight, and 2% obese. Among students, 18% claim to have already followed one or more diets to lose weight. In the general population, young people between the ages of 18 and 24 show the most significant percentage of lean corpulence (10%) which ranges from 2% to 5% for other age classes (Inserm 2012, p. 60). For Romanian students the nutritional status was precarious for 16.6% of students, but 10.76% were overweight and 0.45% with a second degree obesity (Table 3).

The proportion of underweight (16.6%) was significantly higher ($z = 2.81$; $p = 0.004$) than the total overweight and obesity rate (10.76%). Together, underweight and overweight represented 27.35% of students. Much of the students (87.44%) admitted several issues with regard to their eating behavior. Particularly among problems loss of control over the amount of ingested foods emerges (2.35%) and perception of overweightness (Bromboiu et al. 2016, pp. 38–39).

Lifestyle and eating behaviors also affect exposure to risk factors or can cause pathological conditions. Since the appearance of morbid states can be observed after long periods of time, the causal exposure-disease relationship is perceived more difficultly. Without it we realize the style of food heavily affects the quality of life.

For society, the impact of a chronic illness is the sum of the losses attributable to the reduction in economic income and the loss of earnings due to inability to work, destabilization or the impossibility of exercising its own productive and social role, but also to the cost of care and premature deaths of the individual. For a company, the resource economy is of particular interest, the possibility of preventing diseases with the aim of reducing costs is based on knowledge of risk factors. The study of these risk factors, especially for the prevention of chronic diseases, is mainly through the study of behaviors and lifestyles (Adam and Herzlich 1994).

Inadequate street styles and foods seem to lead to contiguity with other substances or drugs, reading as addictive behavior (e.g. alcohol consumption), adversely affecting students' life expectancy, affecting academic achievement, and causing serious damage both in the present and in future prospects.

These aspects seem to correlate with other uses and consumption of university life, such as excessive use of social networks, breakdown of the sleep/wake cycle with disfiguring effects, inappropriate forms of sporting activity (irregular and defamatory) and overall, a mental habitus sometimes little inclined to consider the risks and consequences of unhealthy behaviors on psycho-physical well-being. To this end, it is also appropriate to evaluate, in the context of eating habits, the weight of cultural, environmental, daily life variables, etc., which can play a protective/preventive role for harmful effects (e.g. obesity, bulimia, addiction) by developing appropriate training strategies for learning healthy lifestyles and improving the quality of life.

The study of the factors that lead to the improvement of the nutritional status of the population, especially young people, in this regard, takes on a fundamental importance in guiding well-being and allowing information and prevention measures that constitute a bet for public health policies national, European and global.

References

Adam P, Herzlich C.: Sociologie de la maladie et de la médecine. Nathan, Paris (1994)

Bromboiu I. Mougin S., Cazacu I., Mogosan C. I., Porrovecchio A., Ladner J., Tavolacci Ma. P.: Les caractéristiques des étudiants participants à la première étude sur le style de vie et le comportement, fait à Cluj, Roumanie. Ratio Sociologica, 9, n. 2, (2016)

Di Francesco G.: The soul in a plate. In Azienda Speciale della Camera di Commercio di Imperia Promimperia (eds.) Food as identity/social value. Dieta Mediterranea/Mediterranean diet. FrancoAngeli, Milano (2015a)

Di Francesco G.: Stili alimentari e qualità della vita. In Corvo P., Fassino G. (eds.): Quando il cibo si fa benessere. Alimentazione e qualità della vita. FrancoAngeli, Milano (2015b)

Fernández-Ballesteros R., Zamarrón M.D., Maciá A.: Calidad de vida en la vejez en distintos contextos. Ministerio de Trabajo y Asuntos Sociales, Instituto Nacional de Servicios Sociales, Madrid (1996)

Finocchietti G. (eds.): Settima indagine Eurostudent. Le condizioni di vita e di studio degli studenti universitari 2012–2015. Universitas Quaderni n. **29**. AsRui editore, Roma (2015)

Frudà L.: Alimentazione, famiglia e stili di vita. In Cavanna D., Stagi S. (eds.): Sul fronte del cibo. Salute e Società, anno **VIII**, n. 3 (2009)

Gill T.M. e Feinstein A.R.: A critical appraisal of the quality of quality of life measurements. Journal of the American Medical Association. **272**, pp. 619–626 (1994)

Goody J.: Cooking, Cuisine and Class: A Study in Comparative Sociology. Cambridge University Press, Cambridge (1982)

Vegetti M. (ed.): Hippocrates. Antica Medicina: giuramento del medico. Rusconi, Milano (1998)
Indagine Movimento Consumatori. http://www.consumersforum.it/voce-ai-soci/1930-indagine-movimento-consumatori-crisi-affitti-in-ribasso-per-gli-studenti-fuori-sede.html (2012). Accesed September 2017
INRAN: Linee guida per una sana alimentazione italiana. Ministero delle Politiche agricole e forestali, http://www.salu-te.gov.it/portale/documentazione/p6_2_2_1.jsp?id=652 (2003). Accesed September 2017
INSERM: Enquête épidémiologique nationale sur le surpoids et l'obésité. Obépi, p. 60 (2012)
Majani G: Introduzione alla psicologia della salute. Erickson, Trento (1999)
Mennell, S.: The Sociology of Food: Eating, Diet and Culture. Thousand Oaks: Sage Publications (1993)
WHO: Constitution, RU, 1948, 976
Orsini S.(ed.): Gli stili alimentari, in La vita quotidiana nel 2009. Indagine multiscopo annuale sulle famiglie "Aspetti della vita quotidiana", Anno 2009. Informazioni. **5**, ISTAT, Roma (2010)
Parasuraman, A., Grewal D., Kishnan R. (eds.): Marketing research, Houghton Mifflin Co., Boston (2007).
Vercelloni L.: Le abitudini alimentari in Italia dagli anni Ottanta agli anni Duemila. In Fabris G., Codeluppi V. (eds.): Consumi e organizzazioni. Franco Angeli, Milano (2002)
Vienna A.: Ben... Essere: coinvolgere le scuole per educare ad una corretta alimentazione. Scuola & Ambiente. Educazione ambientale: un impegno condiviso. RAS-Rassegna dell'Autonomia Scolastica, **9**, pp. 48–49 (2008)
Zeithaml V. A., Parasuraman A., Berry L.L. (eds.): Servire qualità. McGraw-Hill, Milano (2000)

Food Waste and Quality of Life

Paolo Corvo

Abstract FAO affirms that food waste includes every health-safe edible substance which instead of being destined to human consumption is wasted, lost, degraded or consumed by parasites in every step of the food chain. The first arena of waste is agriculture: food is wasted when it is not grown to be harvested, but to obtain subsidies and other financial support instruments from national governments or global organizations. The second step of waste takes place within the processing and packaging industries. This happens because a proportion of the product decays before being processed, or because just some parts of the product are appreciated by the market (meat of fish fillets, chicken drumsticks, etc.), while the rest automatically becomes waste. The waste chain continues at supermarkets, where every product which is not impeccable is removed, even if still perfectly suitable for consumption. The last stage of waste creation takes place in eateries and consumers' homes.

Introduction

The world of food is undergoing profound transformations both in the spheres of production and consumption, due to the influence of the processes of economic globalization and individualization of society. In this article we will focus on food consumption, taking into account that in today's Western countries only a minority of the population is suffering from hunger and malnutrition problems. In this context eating no longer represents the simple satisfaction of a basic need, or a moment of break from work, but it becomes experience, enjoyment and adventure. Every restaurant dish becomes qualified as an artwork, deserving to be accurately photographed and visually shared with friends and acquaintances. In contemporary society, chefs acquire an importance similar to that given to intellectuals: they

P. Corvo (✉)
Director of Sociology Laboratory, University of Gastronomic Sciences, Pollenzo, Italy
e-mail: p.corvo@unisg.it

A. Bianco et al. (eds.), *Italian Studies on Quality of Life*, Social Indicators Research Series 77, https://doi.org/10.1007/978-3-030-06022-0_15

are expected to deliver their own vision of the world, together with a masterly-cooked meal. These are phenomena that are likely to be excessive and that not always contribute to the improvement of gastronomic culture (just think about the proliferation of TV cooking shows which are purely based on the dramatization and 'spectacularization' of food and its preparation, often referred to as 'food porn').

Nonetheless, food can translate into well-being for every individual and improve people's quality of life. Each one of us is given the chance to eat in order to experience pleasure, especially if we can to enjoy a dimension of conviviality and follow 'slow food' principles. The happiness we receive from food is combined with the responsibility we must undertake towards those who face difficulties in accessing food or still suffer from hunger, in every part of the world. The stark contrast between our plentiful tables and the food poverty suffered by some people cannot be treated with indifference. Food waste is a wound for humanity, and it is paradoxical that in Western countries food is left to waste whereas elsewhere people still die of starvation (Corvo 2015).

In the wealthiest part of the world we witness a massive waste of edible products, with enormous quantities of food being thrown away because of manufacturing flaws or just because not consumed. In addition, waste is often functional to the productive system, because the greater the waste, the higher the incentive to produce more (Poulain 2005). On a related note, it's worth acknowledging that the whole Western lifestyle system is characterized by a wastage of natural resources, as simple yet important practices can sadly testify: we make an excessive use of tap water, we leave the lights on at home even in empty rooms.

The Forms of Waste

FAO affirms that food waste includes every health-safe edible substance which instead of being intended for human consumption is wasted, lost, degraded or consumed by parasites in every step of the food chain. It also states the difference between food losses and food waste, the former affecting the food chain stages of agricultural production, harvesting and food processing, and the latter regarding the downstream segments of food distribution, retail and final consumption. Food losses are due to logistical and infrastructural shortcomings, while food waste depend of social actors' behavior (FAO 2015). For Stuart (2009) also every product which is suitable for human consumption but is voluntarily destined to animal consumption fits the definition of food waste, as well as any edible by-product coming out of human food manufacturing processes.

FAO estimates point out that every year one third of global food production – 1.3 billion tons – is wasted: 54% of it concerns the upstream stages of the chain, while 46% affects downstream stages. From 1974, global food waste increased by 50%. Of 1.3 billion tons of global waste, 400 tons wasted during consumption. For every European citizen, a total amount of 840 kg of food is produced every year; of this, 560 kg is consumed (an average of 1.5 kg a day), while 185 kg is eliminated before the consumer can access it, and 95 kg is wasted within the household (i.e. 260 g a day, 1.8 kg a week). Plus, this doesn't take into account the waste generated in restaurants, cafés, hospitals, and canteens. In North America, out of an availability of 900 kg of food, 600 are consumed, 180 are lost before consumers' purchase, and 120 are wasted within the household. People living in Sub-Saharan Africa and South East Asia are markedly less wasting: Africans waste 6 kg, and Asians waste 11 kg, but their food availability is half the Western, 460 kg (Fao 2011, p.5).

Around 180 kg per capita of food goes missing along the food chain, every year. These are impressive figures, that spur our thinking and make us worried. The food waste problem is connected to the dominance of the food processing industry (Belasco 2006; Guptill et al. 2013), which is currently conditioning the method of production, distribution and purchasing of products. As a matter of fact, food waste doesn't only concern the consumption stage, but it affects the whole productive process.

The first arena of waste is agriculture: food is wasted when it is grown not to be harvested but to obtain subsidies and other financial support instruments from national governments or global organizations. It is not infrequent, indeed, that contributions are granted on the basis of the extension of the cultivated area, and not on the actual crops harvested, whose market value is irrelevant. At times the product is not harvested due to price collapses, which are caused by financial speculation or over-production, making labor costs higher than the expected revenues. In addition, cosmetic problems have to be considered, since, as an example, consumers are not willing to purchase fruit spoiled by hail. In less economically advanced countries, many fields are abandoned because of drought or lack of irrigation equipment. In order to effectively operate on agricultural fields, adequate technical, structural, financial and management competences are required.

The second step of waste takes place within the processing and packaging industries. This happens because a proportion of the product decays before being processed, or because just some parts of the product are appreciated by the market (fish fillets, chicken drumsticks, etc.), while the rest automatically becomes waste. Other percentages of production are eliminated after quality checks. In addition, during the process, part of the production becomes damaged, and even small flaws prevent it from being sold. A similar destiny characterizes fruit and vegetables with non-standard shape and color is, as well as damaged packaging, which is thrown away along with its contents. Further problems relate to errors in weight count or label printing, to seasonality, to product or product's image variation strategies operated by companies, to weather events (a cold summer entails a lesser consumption of refreshing beverages), to errors in production planning, or to cancellations of orders from foreign markets.

Transport and distribution operations embody new opportunities for waste, especially since the distance between places of production and places of consumption has recently undertook a significant growth.

The waste chain continues at supermarkets, where every product which is not impeccable is removed, even if still perfectly suitable for consumption. In these cases, the winning strategy to attract and keep customers is to provide an image of infinite wealth, displaying large quantities of food, desirable and always available (Conner and Armitage 2002). Corporate retailers and fast food chains often consider the share of unsold and wasted food as an inevitable aspect of their business. Marketing strategies consider the lack of availability of a certain product as a worse failure than over-stocking it. Corporate retailers' data is not always easy to read, making the accurate calculation of purchased and wasted food a complicated task.

I recently supervised the thesis of a student who was actively involved in the freeganism movement, whose followers adopt an anti-consumerism and anti-capitalist lifestyle, aimed at minimizing traditional purchasing methods and centered on salvaging still edible food from waste bins, especially near large supermarkets. The student's work demonstrated that – somehow surprisingly – a large quantity of food which is still in good condition is wasted, such as pasta, bread and rice, and that freegans are able to feed themselves on a daily basis by plunging into waste. In fact, not only defective products are regularly binned, but also food that is about to expire or that must be replaced by a new product is often likely to be thrown away (Barnard 2016).

The last stage of waste creation takes place in eateries and consumers' homes (Hawkins 2006). This can be due to excessively large portions, food over-purchasing (also caused by retailers' promotional offers), inability to consume food within expiry date, or difficulties in understanding label's indications for a correct conservation of the products (Koch 2012). As already mentioned, in poorer countries the waste at the end-step of the chain is reduced, because the limited disposable income makes food waste socially inacceptable. In developed countries, on the other hand, the propensity to waste food is markedly higher. Sometimes, a limited knowledge of the methods to consume more efficiently comes into play, together with a lacking awareness of the entity of waste and of its economic and environmental impact (Alexander et al. 2013; Holm 2013).

The Reactions Against Food Waste

This twisted commercial mechanism, generated by the spiral of consumerism, makes every object a disposable item, and the possibility of reusing and recycling is not even taken into account (Pollan 2008; Stuart 2009). As a reaction, during the last years, many movements and associations have been set up in different countries, with the aim of tackling the negative effects of such orderings engendered in the food economy. These organizations periodically retrieve about-to-expire or other no longer sellable foods from supermarkets and shopping centers, to donate them to food banks or support centers for poor and elderly people. In Italy, the Banco Alimentare has been operating for many years now, collecting and distributing otherwise wasted food to as much as 8000 associations. In case of cooked meals, leftover from canteens or buffets, the delivery to those in need is immediate.

The Banco Alimentare Foundation makes a connection between the agri-food chain and the welfare associations. Large distribution and the companies involved give their production surpluses to the Banco Alimentare which provides storage and redistribution to the benefiting entities. The Banco Alimentare activity determines various types of positive externalities: firstly, it increases the efficiency and efficiency of the use of available resources. It is able to create a network between profit and non-profit actors. A second positive externality is the consistency of the results achieved with the declared goals (Segrè and Falasconi 2011). The purpose is to facilitate the collection of food surpluses created throughout all the agri-food chain, improving its redistribution to the network of territorial subjects. Moreover, Banco allows an increase in the capacity to produce social capital. The organization of food collection is based on reciprocity, that is, on an exchange that can create utility on all sides of the chain. Companies that give their food surpluses minimize transaction costs related to the need to dispose of them and increase their credibility in terms of social responsibility. Receiving organizations get more resources available that can be allocated to persons under conditions of poverty, with a minimum level of expenses about organization and management.

Another interesting case is the Waste & Resources Action Program (Wrap). This non-profit company was created in 2001 and is active in United Kingdom with the purpose of promoting practices of waste reduction, sustainable products development and resource efficient use. The program's purposes consist in the reduction of CO2 emissions and biodegradable waste in landfills, primary resource saving and the least waste of food. In the specific food sector, the program aims at saving, from 2017, 4 million tons per year of equivalent CO2 emissions, linked to the 'avoidable' waste of food and beverages. To achieve this goal, Wrap collaborates with manufacturers and distributors, provides suggestions to individuals on how to reduce food waste, and collaborates with the packing industry to optimize packaging design and functionality (Barilla Center 2013).

Significant is also the initiative created in one of the suburbs of Oakland, in United States. The City Slicker Farms is a consortium of seven community farms that manage a 100 yards and gardens, offering fresh products to the local community at affordable prices. The consortium also collects food donated by the local distribution network. The beneficiaries of these products are mainly poor or low-income families. In addition to the simple reduction of food waste that dumps in the landfill, the recovery programs for agricultural waste link the food waste of a single family to the food production of the whole community (Barilla Center 2013).

Initiatives like these are important demonstrations of the reaction of civil society to an economically dangerous and ethically despicable phenomenon, especially if taking into consideration that in other parts of the globe, people suffer from hunger. And by saying this, we don't think we are just repeating a trivial or rhetorical statement.

The movements fighting food waste advice to go food shopping frequently during the week, for a better management of home food storage, and to avoid buying products which we still have in our fridges. The best choice is to buy directly from producers, seeking the closer farmers' market. It's a matter of giving one's preference to those who produce following the principles of sustainable agriculture, while employing less natural resources and limiting emissions and pollution (Counihan and Van Esterik 2006).

Of high importance is also to learn to cook with scraps and leftovers. Traditional cuisines, in fact, feature a wealth of recipes which are meant to reduce waste. Let's think of meatballs, omelettes and quiches, salads, or stale-bread-based recipes. Though, unfortunately, the memory of the peasant tradition, which tended to reuse scraps and leftovers to create new and tasty recipes, is slowly fading. Nowadays, food is treated as any other consumer good, without even envisaging a further and equally pleasurable use. In addition, this is happening albeit refrigeration and other technologies enable a much longer conservation of food than in the past (Carolan 2012; Abbots and Lavis 2013; Evans 2014).

Furthermore, if we extend our scope to include cafés and restaurants, we immediately notice the huge amount of wasted and binned food, being it discarded during the preparation of dishes or left in the plate by customers. Nevertheless, it is fortunately true that in this sense the recovery of traditional recipes and the use of typical products increasingly operated by chefs is beginning to change the situation.

Food waste is a plague that must be vanquished or at least reduced. In this sense, the economic crisis is currently bringing about a re-modeling of food consumption, spurring people to save money and reduce waste. Novel and unexpected facts are occurring – which were unthinkable in the pre-crisis period – like the noticeable number of people in big cities buying 'bread from yesterday', which is sold half-price. In European restaurants, the practice of giving customers their leftovers in 'doggy bags' to take home is becoming established, as it has been for some time in the US. Evening suppers at home are being more frequently made with leftovers from mid-day lunch, in order to minimize waste. In some contexts, more moderate and frugal consumption practices are diffusing, not only for economic reasons, but also with the aim of adopting an alternative lifestyle (Stuart 2009; Campbell et al. 2013).

Food waste is not just a matter of food. To produce our daily food we employ and consume many natural resources and severely impact the environment. By food wasting we also waste resources like water, fertilizers, soil, fossil fuels, and energy resources of any kind. To this we should also add the waste of economic and human resources. The majority of world's water demand is due to food production, for which reason food waste and water waste are synonyms.

Noticeably, food waste is strictly linked to problems relating to the right to food and the right to a healthy nutrition, because it is largely depending on the behaviors of the main social actors of the global market, both on the level of the food industry and of simple consumers. The same social and economic mechanisms causing food waste are at the origin of malnutrition and hunger (Brown 2012). Every political and commercial institution, as well as every citizen, should engage in enacting the principle contained in the 25th article of the Universal Declaration of Human Rights: "Everyone has the right to a standard of living adequate for the health and well-being of himself and of his family, including food, clothing, housing and medical care and necessary social services".

The Role of Food Policies

In 2004, FAO Council published a set of guidelines to make the right to nutrition an enforceable fact. In this occasion, for the first time, the nations of the world found an agreement on the full meaning of this right. The document consists of a coherent corpus of strategic recommendations to governments and civil society. The nineteen guidelines relate to economic development, legal and institutional issues, food and agricultural policy, nutrition, food safety and consumer protection, education and awareness-raising, social and safety networks, emergency situations and international cooperation (FAO 2015). They represent a stepping stone for the integration of national policies towards food security.

A particularly relevant aspect relates to the food policies governments can adopt to regulate and limit the phenomenon of food waste (Coveney 2013). Recently, Italy approved an important law dealing with food waste (166/2016). It is composed of 18 articles that aim at making it easier for citizens and businesses (producers, restaurants, supermarkets, small shops) to donate food surpluses to associations and social enterprises involved in welfare activities. Municipalities can opt to reduce the fiscal imposition for those who act in this direction. The objective is to double the tonnage of surplus food collected. Law provides for a simplified bureaucracy for those who are willing to donate food. For those who do not donate, though, no sanction is applied, as instead happens in France: the valorization of best practices and the stabilization of long-lasting relation among involved social actors are deemed to be the desirable avenue. In fact, a legal enforcement could eventually create a situation where an excessive collection of food surpluses would become difficult to manage.

The law states the exact products that can be donated. Expired products cannot be sold, while past-best-before-date products can be consumed. For many, this law will be a success in tackling waste. It underlines that the food rescued is to be donated primarily to the poor, who in Italy exceed 4.5 million. We think it would be appropriate if every nation had effective legislation for addressing food waste in the various phases of production, processing, distribution and consumption, facilitating the recovery of food for the purpose of strengthening social solidarity and protecting the natural environment. Obviously not all food surplus is suitable for human consumption: in this case, it can be destined to animal consumption or to aerobic composting (Murcott et al. 2013).

An important part of policies against food waste deals with raising public and business operators' awareness of concerns related to food waste, the right to food, environmental impact, and consumption of natural resources (San-Epifanio 2015). Food waste problems are influenced by a multiplicity of social, cultural and economic factors, which are intertwined and often difficult to grasp. Undoubtedly, a primary role is undertaken by supra-national organizations (UN, EU, World Bank, IMF, WTO), which are called to profoundly transform the patterns of international cooperation, which has often shown its shortcomings and ineffectiveness (Belasco 2008). A set of rules of international law protecting poorer countries' food sovereignty is evidently needed. At the same time, the action of NGOs and civil society is not to be underestimated: they might represent a strong voice that could affect campaigning and decision-making against food waste (DuPuis et al. 2011; Clapp 2012). Individual action is fundamental as well, for it can testify the necessity to adopt a different, more moderate and sustainable lifestyle, one that is aware of the problems of nutrition (Nestle 2003; Corvo 2015). Only if the three social actors we highlighted (international and state institutions, movements and associations, individual citizens) play their part and cooperate, it will be possible to significantly reduce food waste and contemporarily defeat the plague of hunger (currently some 800 million people suffer from nutrition-related problems).

Some obstacles seem to hinder or delay such achievements, whose overcoming requires effort and determination. Specifically, supra-national institutions' action sometimes appears restrained by a too heavy bureaucratic apparatus and by the prevailing of different (if not opposed) interests. Such institutions would need to transform what are often just noble enunciations of principles into concrete and incisive intervention, able to modify long-established practices and dominant positions within the economic and financial world. We reckon it is not easy to counter act the concussive force of the food industry, but only international organizations have the power to intervene in such situation.

Undoubtedly, civil society can play a determinant role in stimulating institutions as well as the action of many players fighting food waste and food-related social injustice. To do so, movements and associations should be able to overcome what we call 'group individualism', i.e. the tendency to propose solutions without coordinating their own intervention with other groups, acting as if they had a monopoly on a certain subject. The more civil society will be able to find a univocal and solid orientation, the better it will express societal demands and serve its crucial function.

The Role of Consumers

We also deem important to underline the role of the individual, which is often overlooked within the current social and cultural context. The processes of globalization seem indeed to exclude the possibility of an individual intervention, because phenomena appear to overwhelm individual will. Everything looks too big and distant for our individual ability to make a dent in reality, even in our local daily surroundings. Actually this belief is objectively wrong, and it is determined by a common understanding which is heavily influenced by media, that in turn are conditioned by powerful economic interests.

The belief of being powerless brings about feelings of depression and resignation, causing individuals to underestimate the importance of their action. In the field of consumption this attitude is evident: as nicely argued by Fabris (2010), consuming is a political act and with their everyday choices citizens are able to affect market dynamics, but they are rarely aware of that. Preferring a product over another entails exerting a democratic right and can contribute to the modification of certain balances. It is not a case for boycotting, rather for practicing a 'buy-cott', i.e. buying ethically, environmentally, socially and culturally sustainable products. Consumers must realize their potential for agency, even in such a pervasive-looking global market. And if individual action is supported and represented by associations and movements, it can evidently become stronger and more effective. In this way, civil society can thoroughly fulfill its primary role as the tie that binds individuals and institutions.

In the field of food waste, individual responsibility is expressed through an increased attention towards food procurement, everyday meals, re-utilization of food, and through the adoption of more moderate and solidarity-oriented behaviors. Individuals must gain awareness that their action can change reality, maybe slightly but still significantly; without overlooking the possibility that such personal struggle against waste can have a marked proselytizing effect within their social circles. In this sense, nutritional education can be effective if supported by a consistent behavior.

A healthy and balanced nutrition, together with an endeavor to avoid or at least reduce waste, is the best way to obtain a good quality of life in relation to food. Who eats well lives well and longer, as is demonstrated by those who practice the Mediterranean diet. Fighting against waste makes us serene and aware, because it helps us fully accomplish our humanity. It is also a way to fight against the scandal of hunger.

Well-being is achieved also through sharing the pleasure of food with others, through a form of conviviality that characterizes the most important moments of our existence. While eating together, quality of life is expressed with simplicity and genuineness, and food is granted a renewed relevance. In this shared space, following the 'slow food' principles opens up a way to contrast food waste, for they aim at refocusing our attention on food and its chain. Eating becomes an important moment of the day, renovating the meaning we attach to time and nature and overtaking the 'fast' logic that privileges the dimension of quantity over quality.

In essence, fighting food waste means changing our lifestyle, going beyond the logics of exasperated consumerism and stressful frenzy, to favor a soberer and serene existence. A better relationship with food and nutrition represents a guarantee of a better quality of life. Physical and mental well-being can make us feel pleasurable emotions and live moments of happiness: without ignoring the joy of other human beings, happiness derives from the awareness of our ethical responsibility towards the problems of the world.

References

Abbots, E.J., Lavis, A. editors (2013). *Why We Eat, How We Eat. Contemporary Encounters between Foods and Bodies*. Farnham: Ashgate.

Alexander, C., Gregson, N., Gille, Z. (2013). Food Waste. In A. Murcott, W. Belasco, P. Jackson (Eds), *The handbook of Food Research* (pp. 471–483).s London-New York: Bloomsbury.

Barilla Center for food and nutrition (2013) Lo spreco alimentare: cause, impatti e proposte (Bologna: Barilla).

Barnard, A.V. (2016). *Freegans: Diving into the Wealth of Food Waste in America*. Minneapolis: University of Minnesota Press.
Belasco, W. (2006). *Meals to Come: A History of the Future of Food*. Berkeley: University of California Press.
Belasco, W. (2008). *Food. The key concepts*. Oxford-New York: Berg.
Brown, L. R. (2012). *Full planet, Empty Plates. The New Geopolitics of Food Scarcity*. Washington: Earth Policy Institute.
Campbell, H., Murcott, A., Evans, D. (2013). *Waste Matters: New perspectives of Food and Society*. Hoboken: Blackwell Publisher.
Carolan, M. (2012). *The Sociology of Food and Agriculture*. Abingdon: Routledge.
Clapp, J. (2012). *Food*. Cambridge: Polity Press.
Conner, M., Armitage C.J. (2002). *The Social Psychology of Food*. Buckingham- Philadelphia: Open University Press.
Corvo, P. (2015). *Food culture, consumption and society*. Basingstoke: Palgrave MacMillanp.
Counihan, C.M., Van Esterik, P. (2006). *Food and Culture. A reader*. New York: Routledge.
Coveney, J. (2013). *Food*. Abingdon: Routledge.
DuPuis, E., Harrison, J, Goodman, D. (2011). Just Food?. In A. Alkon, J. Agyeman (Eds), *Cultivating Food Justice: Race, Class and Sustainability* (pp. 283–308). Cambridge MA: MIT Press..
Evans, D. (2014). *Home Consumption, Material Culture and Everyday Life*. London, New York: Bloomsbury Academic.
Fabris, G. (2010). *La società post crescita. Consumi e stili di vita*. Milano: Egea.
FAO (2011). *Global Food Losses and Waste. Extent, Causes and Prevention*. New York: Fao.
FAO (2015). *Global Food Losses and Food Waste*. New York: Fao.
Guptill, A.E., Copelton, D.A., Lucal, B. (2013). *Food & Society. Principles and Paradoxes*. Cambridge: Polity Press.
Hawkins, G. (2006). *The ethics of Waste: How We Relate to Rubbish*. Rowman and Littlefield: Lanham.
Holm, L. (2013). Sociology of Food Consumption. In A. Murcott, W. Belasco, P. Jackson (Eds), *The handbook of Food Research* (pp. 324–337). London-New York: Bloomsbury.
Koch, S.L. (2012). *A Theory of Grocery Shopping. Food, Choice and Conflict*. London: Berg.
San-Epifanio, L.E. (2015). *Envisioning a Future Without Food Waste and Food Poverty: Societal Challenges*. Wageningen: Academic Publisher.
Murcott, A., Belasco W., Jackson P. (Eds) (2013). *The handbook of Food Research*. London-New York: Bloomsbury.
Nestle, M. (2003). *Food Politics: How the Food Industry Influences Nutrition and Health*. Berkeley: University of California Press.
Pollan, M. (2008). *In Defense of Food: An Eater's Manifesto*. New York: Penny Press.
Poulain, J.P. (2005). *Sociologies de l'alimentation. Les mangeurs et l'espace social alimentaire*. Paris: Presses Universitaires de France.
Segrè, A., Falasconi L. (2011). *Il libro nero dello spreco: il cibo*. Milano: Edizioni Ambiente.
Stuart, T. (2009). *Waste: Uncovering the Global Food Scandal*. New York: Norton.

Culture, Creativity and Quality of Life in Old Age

Carlo Cristini and Marcello Cesa-Bianchi

Abstract Older people's culture represents a synthesis of many existential problems and a basic universal factor. Psychological researches show that all people possess creative skills, up until the end of life. Culture and creativity may facilitate aging and help develop a model for cross-generational relationships. In old age, many people may discover the desire to explore new creative, affective and relational spaces. Creativity qualifies many elders' lives. For many famous artists, creativity contributed to improve their quality of life in the last years. On the edge of life, ultimate creativity may find peace, not as the end of struggling, but as its absence. So, it may bring up memories and biographical stories, opening new perspectives for the new generations. The relationship between grandchildren and grandparents seems to reconcile nature and culture, develop creativity, clarify and separate technological knowledge and human knowledge and improve the quality of life itself.

Introduction

In old age, culture and creativity represent an important opportunity for improving the quality of life.[1] Neuroscientific researches have shown that brain plasticity may compensate for any deficit, and the onset of certain diseases may be used also as a

This chapter was written with Marcello Cesa-Bianchi who, unfortunately and sadly, passed away on March 15th 2018.

[1] This paper deals with the topic of creativity in old age only referring to western culture.

C. Cristini (✉)
University of Brescia, Brescia, Italy
e-mail: carlo.cristini@unibs.it

M. Cesa-Bianchi
University of Milan, Milano, Italy

A. Bianco et al. (eds.), *Italian Studies on Quality of Life*, Social Indicators Research Series 77, https://doi.org/10.1007/978-3-030-06022-0_16

developing tool, which is widely demonstrated by the artistic skills of people with neuropsychiatric syndromes (Kandel 2012).

The cultural knowledge of elderly people has often times stimulated the attention of the youngest, often focused on new technologies, toward social issues, by facilitating the dialogue between generations. Older people's culture is not an alternative to young culture, rather, it is proposed as a synthesis of existential problems and as a basic factor for universal convergence (Cesa-Bianchi 1998; Cipolli and Cristini 2012).

Psychological researches have shown that creativity – previously only recognised in childhood-adolescence and in geniuses – is present in every person, regardless of age and often even health and independence, up to the very last moments of life, like many great artists and many ordinary people have shown.

Creativity may make a major contribution to the realization of the self, also through its last expressions.

Culture and creativity may carry out different functions: (a) facilitate aging; (b) constitute a model for cross-generational relationships; (c) represent a therapeutic tool for elderly patients, including those with dementia.

In nursing homes, researchers have discovered creative trends in elderly people (Ploton 2010). Culture and creativity offer an innovative concept of aging and the elders; process and age must also be considered as humour, "the ability to smile about everything, even what you love, and yet continue to love it" and are able to offer optimal solutions, even to the less fortunate.

Nowadays people may experience aging not as decay, but as evolution towards self-realization and overall personal knowledge. Culture and creativity may be expressed until very late in life and give meaning not only to the quality of life during aging but throughout one's lifespan (Baltes et al. 1999). This is also in harmony with the results of so-called 'late creativity' (Cristini et al. 2011), which we often are unwitting carriers of and which enables a person to experience aging as an opportunity to continue to learn, grow and develop new ideas.

Late creativity promotes the development of 'elderly-thinking' (Cristini et al. 2014), which is perhaps the most evolved and free expression of thinking, or the richest with experiences, processing and synthesis; invaluable preconditions for improving the quality of life in old age.

Creativity and Aging

Creative skills are potentially present in everyone, regardless of age and often health conditions. They reflect the personality and identity of an individual and may be expressed in the various situations that women and men can experience. In old age, creativity may help people not to lose themselves in the existential void, to stave off decline or preserve cognitive skills. Creativity may promote the re-start of activities and functions, giving more sense to a period of life often overlooked by the modern world.

It is appropriate to discredit the false myths that have supported the concept of creativity in the past (Antonietti and Pizzingrilli 2011). Ancient people regarded creativity as something pertaining purely to the divine. Up to two or three centuries ago, the concept that individuals could be creative in thought and action was considered blasphemous (Anderson 1959).

Creativity – as a new opportunity of expressing oneself – was analysed by psychology around the middle of the last century. For several decades, it was considered as a prerogative of childhood and adolescence which was preserved afterwards only by exceptional individuals (Cesa-Bianchi and Antonietti 2003).

Nowadays, creativity is recognized as a skill that enables people to achieve positive aging and complete their individuality and biography (Cesa-Bianchi et al. 2004).

According to Rollo May (1959), creativity allows everyone to express and realise themselves, not as a product of a morbid state, but as a representation of the highest degree of emotional equilibrium.

Creativity may be enriched and enhanced over time. In old age, many famous characters were able to continue and refine their artistic style, and many common people were able to express their inventive and imaginative abilities. Furthermore, many old people with dementia, appropriately stimulated and involved, were able to activate their creative resources, sometimes surprisingly so (Cesa-Bianchi 2002, 2006; Peruchon 2011; Cesa-Bianchi et al. 2012; Cristini et al. 2012).

In old age, many people may discover or rediscover the desire and the pleasure to explore new creative, affective and relational spaces, take initiatives, activities other than the usual ones, seize other opportunities and paths of thinking, feeling and doing. According to George Minois (1987), age often allows one to rise above every kind of convention and expand creativity and genius at 70 or 80 years too.

Elderly people may express their creativity in various fields: reading and writing, painting and sculpture, music and theatre, crafts and cooking, photography and video recording, organizational activities and volunteering, intergenerational communication, game invention and pet care (Cesa-Bianchi et al. 2009; Cesa-Bianchi and Cristini 2012; Cesa-Bianchi and Cristini 2014; Cesa-Bianchi et al. 2014).

Many Universities of the Third Age have risen in Italy in recent decades. Many seniors have enrolled progressively. They have promoted, organised and participated in various cultural, creative and social activities and initiatives. Other spontaneous groups of elderly people – some composed of women only – have been organised and developed.

There are various cultural courses, craft activities, intergenerational meetings, cultural and artistic trips and initiatives to support the less fortunate elderly. The quality of life of elderly participants has improved.

The Ferrero Foundation represents another important model, made up of elderly volunteers who previously worked with the Ferrero company. Now they are retired members and perform various activities, have a strong sense of belonging and identity, maintain a better quality of life and enjoy a condition of well-being.

In some elderly people at the end of their life, studies have highlighted the expression of an innovative form of creative thinking which allows them to complete their own knowledge and self-realization and also to find a better conception of life for themselves, including through irony and self-irony (Cesa-Bianchi et al. 2013; Randall 2013). “Last Creativity” has been configured; a flash of light that precedes the darkness of death and conscience, the last stage of a journey towards self-realization.

Creativity qualifies the lives of many elderly as research shows (Sierpina and Cole 2004; Cohen 2006; Flood and Phillips 2007; Andolfi et al. 2016); it constitutes the essence of the human being, characterizes nature, learning, experiences, choices, behaviours, customs, culture and evolution (Sternberg 1999); it does not end at the threshold of an age. Age and experience encourage the search for new expressions, renewed models of thought and representation about what we have imagined, felt and learned.

Even in old age, it is always possible to learn, to be open-minded to news, to discover different itineraries of thought and feeling. Creativity allows one to renew, sometimes to invent life, even when one is very old.

With the passing of the years, what gives meaning and strength to existence often results in greater enrichment from experiences. Elkhonon Goldberg (2005) states that the *mind can grow stronger when the brain grows old*er; this is possible if people are able to maintain their interests, curiosity and desire to learn more and more, to be in charge and aware of their choices and life experiences, what is happening to their life and what surrounds, influences and characterises it.

Creativity is the main factor for better quality of life and positive aging continuing with confidence and serenity towards new experiences.

Quality of Life and Positive Aging: Last Creativity

In old age, famous artists rediscovered attitudes, resources and skills toward the end of their lives, the last moments of their lives, despite having health problems in some cases. Their creativity and their last creativity contributed to improving the quality of life in their last years.

In older people, the artistic experience often produces continuous refinement (Antonini and Magnolfi 1991; Paolucci 2000). An artist creates a certain idea and then, progressively with the passing of years, he deepens it more and more and may give the best of himself in the very last days of his life.

Even in the last moments, creativity may always surprise, offer gleams of light over one’s self-awareness and whole existence. The consciousness of dying may open the thought process, deliver to the individual the meaning of his existence and limits, the value and essence of who he is. The lights on the twilight roads often light up. The inscrutable ultimate creativity may appear (Cesa-Bianchi et al. 2002; Cristini et al. 2011; Cristini and Cesa-Bianchi 2011; Cesa-Bianchi et al. 2014). Which factors, meanings and ways set a path, its goal and realization?

The interaction, the confrontation or the conflict between to be or not to be, to become or to decline contend with each other in the life of a person, in the expectation and representation of one or the other. Lights or obscurity of old age and life. In the game of prevalence, between the one and the other, a biographical portrait is in the making. On the edge of life, ultimate creativity may discover inner peace, not as the end of struggling, but as its absence.

At 81 years, Henri Matisse confided the following to a friend: "My life followed a harmonious curve, with struggles and conflicts, but in any case a harmonious curve. So I want it to end", and with his hand slowly traced a curve in the air that ended with delicacy; a gesture that reminds us of *Moderate Slumber*, Kandinsky's latest creativity.

How can you know life if you do not consider its limitations and temporality? Perhaps the courage to live and think is also the courage to recognise and think about dying. The elaboration of temporality and the end of existence may promote and extend the creative process. Marcel Proust said: "Some face death with indifference, not because they have more courage than others, but because they have less imagination".

The last creative inspiration may offer the symbol and the effigy of a story such as that played by Molière during a performance by Argante in *The Imaginary Patient* or Charlie Chaplin in the role of Calvero in *Limelight*. Both characters die, Molière in reality, Charlie Chaplin only on film, giving to the public – who unaware applauds while the show continues – the allegorical, humorous and creative image of an end.

Many elderly people showed that they were aware of the end of their existence and they expressed adequate attitudes towards their end. Others maintained a detachment or were more involved by restlessness, anxiety, apathy or depression (Cristini 2007).

Perhaps last creativity may help one to live better the latest years, but also to experience dying with the imagination of the mind and not with the decline of the body. An elderly person may invent his own death through a creative expression that reworks the significant traits of his identity and biography in a new image. So he/she may discover the meaning of his/her life for the first time. By means of last creativity, an individual may find himself, after a life-long search, understanding that it is above all the development of a project that may be fully understood only after its realization. Or perhaps it is possible that an individual makes a work of art inventing one's own death, in the same way as Kandinsky said: "A masterpiece originates in the same way that the cosmos originated: through disasters that through the chaotic and loud noise of instruments form finally a symphony whose name is the harmony of the spheres. The creation of a work of art is the creation of a world", and it can be the end of an old individual. Moreover, it is the principle of his memory and his biographical story that may open new perspectives to new generations.

What was the last creativity of famous characters? What creative spirit is kept by history? How did they live, how did they grow old, how did they spend their last days and hours?

At 89 years, Michelangelo made his last masterpiece, his last creativity: *Pietà Rondanini*. As documented in a diary kept by his most devoted pupil – Daniele

Ricciarelli, known as Daniele from Volterra, but perhaps better known as the Braghettone for covering, on Pope Pius IV's mandate, some nakedness of the *Last Judgment* of the *Sistine Chapel* – Michelangelo, before dying, worked on *Pietà Rondanini* with his strength gradually waning. His last thoughts, his latest hammer blows were like a companion for his old age. Initially the body of Christ was all unbalanced, with his head collapsing on one side, our Lady standing and supporting the body of Christ, holding it in her arms. What did Michelangelo do before dying? He dropped the protruding parts, including Christ's head and afterwards he sculpted them again in his mother's chest. Christ is no longer detached from his mother, but physically enters "inside" her body. In this *Pietà* Christ's face is just sketched, embedded within the body of his mother. For Michelangelo, *Pietà Rondanini* became a reason for reflection on himself and life. When we say that at the very end of life, in old age, we may understand the essential, we must think about *Pietà Rondanini* and the deep reflection of the last Michelangelo: a window on infinity.

At 90 years old, Titian, almost blind, abandoned the paint-brush and dipped his fingers in colour to finish his last masterpieces. The artist burned the necessary technical tools to paint with his dominance of the chromatic expressive medium: the greatness of the last Titian (Paolucci 2000).

Donatello completed just before dying the bronze panels of the pulpit of the Church of S. Lorenzo in Florence. The pulpit is believed to be his absolute masterpiece, in which – despite the decline of his sight and the progressive physical weakness – the anti-classic, shortened and essential style was further developed and refined. Donatello was suffering from a late-onset parkinsonism, but he finished the last work of his life, the resurrection of Christ, in a completely innovative and revolutionary way. No longer a triumphant and glorious Jesus, but a suffering man, wrapped in bandages, comparable to a prisoner who comes out of a concentration camp, not very persuaded to return to those who have martyred him, but driven by a great feeling of love.

Francisco Goya, after recovering from a serious illness – evidenced by a picture dedicated to the doctor who cared for him – during his convalescence traced the famous *Black Paintings* on the walls of a room. Just after that, despite the progressive reduction of his sight, he made his last great paintings, such as *The milk-woman of Bordeaux*, at age 81. Baudelaire wrote about the Aragonese painter: "At the end of his artistic career, Goya's eyes were so weakened that somebody had to give him the tips of the pencils, so people said. However, at that time, he made great and very important lithographs, beautiful engravings, magnificent miniature paintings".

Claude Monet became almost blind towards the end of his existence; he developed monochrome tendencies, making masterpieces such as *The Rose House*, at 85 years, and *Clouds* at 86. At 85 years he wrote to his ophthalmologist who had prescribed a new type of lens: "When a singer loses his voice, he retires from the stage; a painter who has undergone cataract surgery should retire; it's just what I cannot do". And after a few months he wrote ironically to a friend: "From your last visit, my sight has improved completely. I work harder than before, I'm happy with what I do, and if the new glasses were even better I'd like to live until one hundred years".

Henri Matisse made some of his masterpieces in the last years of his life, including the stained glass window *The Tree of Life* in the "Chappelle du Rosaire" in Vence. He said to a friend: "In my Chapel, I became aware of the inexhaustible power of colour". And in the letter addressed to the bishop of Nice, he wrote: "I consider (the Chapel of Vence), despite all its imperfections, my masterpiece", at 82 years old.

Pablo Picasso was always a great artist, but he seemed to reach the peak of his creativity and skills to represent and give image to everything in his last years. He said that he did not seek, but he found. The ability to quickly find and transfigure what is found in true art is a privilege for very few individuals. Picasso takes everything, shreds and transforms it, and everything becomes a figure: this is his greatness expressed with particular effectiveness, intensity and lucidity in the last years of his long life. Among his last works we remember *The Musketeer*, made at 91 years old – a year before his death in 1973 – a fighting figure, ready to defy what life may bring still.

The process of aging leaves nothing to chance and does not seem to neglect the shadows and lights of a whole, singular human story. To die is not only the biological, passive and fatal act of a life that ends but represents again a creative experience of something about which little is known, like life in the early days.

Dying may be the last creative act in which the flow of the whole existential representation is often focused, clarifying its meaning and content. Life may express the essence of the plot in its final act, sometimes in an innovative and humorous way.

Intergenerational Dialogue on Culture, Creativity and Quality of Life

In rural and artisanal societies based on extended and multi-generational family structures, the relationship between old and young, grandparents and grandchildren, was part of daily domestic life. Private and professional knowledge was acquired through many years of experience. The elders were a reference for the transmission of traditions, customs, education and cultural models.

Rural societies usually kept intergenerational cohesion and continuity. Elderly people played and supported a recognised role and the general social attitude toward them was marked by respect. They were listened to for their knowledge and skills, people asked for their advice and guidance. The elderly were assisted at home when they were sick and/or no longer self-sufficient.

Social transformations have changed generational relationships. The industrialization process and rapid technological development have changed the hierarchy of professional skills, no longer requiring craftsmanship, sometimes complex and creative, but a rapid, mechanical and performative type of learning.

In modern society, especially in metropolitan contexts, the relationship between old and young people is gradually reducing. The one and the other sometimes go to the same places, live in the same buildings, without knowing each other, meeting or exchanging greetings.

However, big cities are generally able to offer greater social and cultural opportunities for every age group (Cesa-Bianchi e Cristini 2009).

Some researchers have documented that the elderly and children have rediscovered the affective, educational, cultural, playful and creative value of intergenerationality. During leisure time, among other occupations, elders prefer the role of grandparenting. Dialogue takes most of the time spent together with one's grandchildren (Cristini and Cesa-Bianchi 2001).

Implicit and explicit, conscious or unconscious thoughts, feelings and meanings pass through communication, narration and transgenerationality (Kaës et al. 1993; Cristini 2012). Grandparents want to know the interests and curiosities offered by school, games, friends and television. Grandchildren also ask their parents about their history and sometimes their absences. Story telling is preferred because it seems to favour the elaboration of their own experiences and to convey to their grandchildren their knowledge as a point of reference, security and confidence in a modern society that often creates confusion. Story telling is the most direct way to transfer emotions and experiences. Narrative shows the images of long gone times, aspirations and memories (Bruner 1999; Cesa-Bianchi 2012). Grandchildren are often fascinated and ask for questions, insights and want to hear more stories.

Grandmothers communicate much more than grandfathers. Grandmothers seem to be more inclined to approach their grandchildren's world and deal with it. They can grasp children's modulations and emotional difficulties. Grandfathers tend to adopt more directive and normative behaviour in order to protect their grandchildren from negative social conditions. Grandchildren seem to follow with greater attention and sensitivity the suggestions proposed by their grandparents, especially when these suggestions are characterised by propositional attitudes, dialogue, understanding and explanations about what was said and advised.

The interaction between elderly people and children may enrich both and constitute reciprocal references, curiosity and creativity. Grandparent speak about history and stories, a far world, old experiences, events that may be recalled as legends in the child's fantasy and represent a source of interests, stimulations and openness.

Grandparents' memories, heard by grandchildren, correspond to a distant time and to a more extended and longer concept of time that may reflect a temporal perspective of the future. Parental time seems more concentrated and shrunken in the present, and to be bound as though conditioned through the concept of now and immediately. Grandparents' time offers greater availability and it is for the mediation of thought, the development of fantasy and creativity.

Elderly people and children are often isolated from the adult world, the working society which determines the great social choices. They often are alone, each on their own, experiencing and also suffering from the same existential condition.

The relationship between elderly people and children may rediscover the sense of solidarity, aging, growing and learning, on the cognitive and emotional level. It is a relational context that educates the affections and prepares for more valid, proactive and creative development and aging.

Grandparents rediscover the rite and the meaning of narration and find the educational force of communication.

Not only do grandparents teach grandchildren, sometimes grandchildren help grandparents, like in the approach to technical innovations. Old people and children are an ideal conjunction that reinvents the affective plot and is often forgotten by the technocratic society; they return with their relationship to the continuity of transmission and exemplify the value of intersubjectivity.

The dialogue between grandchildren and grandparents seems to reconcile nature and culture, clarify and separate technological knowledge and human knowledge and reconstruct the sense of existence, without prejudice or profit.

The stories of many elders tell us about work and labour, sacrifices and sufferings, obligations and duties, but also experience, perseverance, strength in living and hoping, desire to know. Researches have described active, enterprising and creative elderly people, in charge of their choices and their lives (Cesa-Bianchi 1999, 2000; Cesa-Bianchi et al. 2006). These aged people were able to get themselves rid of the injury of time and age. Retirement did not result in a lost, empty state, but offered an opportunity for rebirth, revaluation and expressive freedom. Leisure time became the time to live, according to one's own needs and creative aspirations. Becoming and being a grandparent helps find motivation, rediscover the importance of communication and transmit educational references and models. It is possible to rediscover new interests, feelings and thoughts; in other words, a sense of well-being and a better quality of life.

References

Anderson, H. H. (1959). *Preface,* in H. H. Anderson (Ed.), *Creativity and its Cultivation* (IX–XIII). New York: Harper Row.

Andolfi, V.R., Valenti, C., Cesa-Bianchi, G., & Cristini, C. (2016). Creativity and leisure in the elderly: an investigation about the relationships between divergent thinking and hobbies. *Ricerche di Psicologia*, 4: 497–513.

Antonietti, A., & Pizzingrilli, P. (2011). Resilienza e creatività: nessi possibili. In C. Castelli (Ed.), *Resilienza e creatività. Teorie e tecniche nei contesti di vulnerabilità*, (pp. 31–50). Milano: FrancoAngeli.

Antonini, F. M., & Magnolfi, S. (1991). *L'età dei capolavori. Creatività e vecchiaia nelle arti figurative*. Venezia: Marsilio.

Baltes, P.B., Staudinger, U.M., & Lindenberger, U. (1999). Lifespan psychology: theory and application to intellectual functioning, *Annual Reviews Psychol.,* 50: 471–507.

Bruner, J. (1999). Narratives of aging. *Journal of Aging Studies*, 13(1): 7–9.

Cesa-Bianchi G., Cristini C., Solimeno-Cipriano A., & Aveni Casucci M.A. (2006). Diventare ed essere nonni: risultati di una ricerca, *Giornale di Gerontologia*, LIV, 5: 475.

Cesa-Bianchi G., Porro A., & Cristini C. (2012). Processo creativo e longevità, *Giornale di Gerontologia*, LX, 1: 3–7.
Cesa-Bianchi, G., & Cristini, C. (2012). Espressioni creative ed artistiche: oltre l'età e la salute. In C. Cipolli & C. Cristini (Eds), La psicologia e la psicopatologia dell'invecchiamento e dell'età senile: un contributo alla ridefinizione dell'arco di vita, numero monografico dedicato a Marcello Cesa-Bianchi, *Ricerche di Psicologia*, 2–3: 339–368.
Cesa-Bianchi, M., (1998). *Giovani per sempre? L'arte di invecchiare*. Roma-Bari: Laterza.
Cesa-Bianchi, M. (1999). Cultura e condizione anziana. *Vita e Pensiero, Rivista Culturale dell'Università Cattolica del Sacro Cuore*, 3: 273–286.
Cesa-Bianchi, M. (2000). *Psicologia dell'invecchiamento*. Roma: Carocci.
Cesa-Bianchi, M. (2002). Comunicazione, creatività, invecchiamento. *Ricerche di Psicologia*, XXV, 3: 175–188.
Cesa-Bianchi, M., Cristini, C., & Cesa-Bianchi, G. (2002). L'ultima creatività? In L. Pinkus & A. Filiberti (Eds.), *La qualità della morte*, (pp. 213–218). Milano: FrancoAngeli.
Cesa-Bianchi, M., & Antonietti, A. (2003). *Creatività nella vita e nella scuola*. Milano: Mondadori Università.
Cesa-Bianchi M., Cristini C., & Cesa-Bianchi G. (2004). Positive Aging. *Ricerche di Psicologia*, 7, 1, 191–206.
Cesa-Bianchi, M. (2006). Lectio. In *Laurea honoris causa in Scienze della Comunicazione*. Napoli: Università degli Studi Suor Orsola Benincasa.
Cesa-Bianchi, M., & Cristini, C. (2009). *Vecchio sarà lei! Muoversi, pensare, comunicare*. Napoli: Guida.
Cesa-Bianchi, M., Cristini, C., & Giusti, E. (2009). *La creatività scientifica. Il processo che cambia il mondo*. Roma: Sovera.
Cesa-Bianchi, M. (2012). *Sempre in anticipo sul mio futuro. Auto-biografia* [...], E. Mancino (Ed.), Napoli: Guida.
Cesa-Bianchi, M., Forabosco, G., Cristini, C., Cesa-Bianchi, G., & Porro, A. (2013). *Umorismo, creatività e invecchiamento*. Roma: Aracne.
Cesa-Bianchi, M., & Cristini, C. (2014). *Come invecchiare. Dalla psicologia generale alla psicogerontologia*. Roma: Aracne.
Cesa-Bianchi, M., Cristini, C., Fulcheri, M., & Peirone, L. (Eds.) (2014). *Vivere e valorizzare il tempo. Invecchiare con creatività e coraggio*. Torino: Premedia.
Cipolli, C., & Cristini, C. (Eds) (2012). La psicologia e la psicopatologia dell'invecchiamento e dell'età senile: un contributo alla ridefinizione dell'arco di vita. Numero monografico dedicato a Marcello Cesa-Bianchi, *Ricerche di Psicologia*, 2–3.
Cohen, G.D. (2006). Research on creativity and aging: the positive impact of the arts on health and illness. *Generations*, 30, 1: 7–15.
Cristini, C., & Cesa-Bianchi, G. (2001). Arte quale stimolo alla comunicazione negli anziani, *IKON – Forme e processi del comunicare*, 42–43: 143–194.
Cristini, C. (Ed.) (2007). *Vivere il morire. L'assistenza nelle fasi terminali*. Roma: Aracne.
Cristini, C., Cesa-Bianchi, M., Cesa-Bianchi, G., & Porro, A. (2011). *L'ultima creatività. Luci nella vecchiaia*. Milano: Springer.
Cristini, C., & Cesa-Bianchi, M. (2011). L'ultima creatività fra declino e recupero di sé. In C. Cristini, A. Porro & M. Cesa-Bianchi (Eds.), *Le capacità di recupero dell'anziano. Modelli, strumenti e interventi per i professionisti della salute*, (pp. 486–521). Milano: FrancoAngeli.
Cristini, C. (2012). Processo psicoterapeutico, relazione e cambiamento. In C. Cristini (Ed.), *Il cambiamento psicoterapeutico*, (pp. 151–168). Milano: FrancoAngeli.
Cristini, C, Cesa-Bianchi, G, & Guerrini, G. (2012). Espressioni creative e demenza: arte e cultura. *G. Gerontol.*, LX, 6, 411.
Cristini, C., Cesa-Bianchi, G., & Cesa-Bianchi, M. (2014). The "elder-thinking": towards the last creativity. *Ricerche di Psicologia*, 4: 521–544.
Flood, M., & Phillips, K. D. (2007). Creativity in older adults: a plethora of possibilities. *Issues in Ment Health Nurs*, 28, 4: 389–411.

Goldberg, E. (2005). *The wisdom paradox. How your mind can grow stronger as your brain grows older*. New York: Gotham Books.
Kaës, R., Faimberg, H., Enriquez, M., & Baranes, J.-J. (1993). *Transmission de la vie psychique entre générations*. Paris: Dunod.
Kandel E.R. (2012). *The age of insight*. New York: Random House.
May R. (1959). The nature of creativity, in H.H. Anderson (Ed.), *Creativity and its Cultivation* (pp. 55–68). New York: Harper Row.
Minois, G. (1987). Histoire de la vieillesse de l'Antiquité à la Renaissance: Paris.
Paolucci, A. (2000). La creatività artistica nella terza età, in *Il sapere nella terza età* (pp. 21–30). Bologna: Università Primo Levi.
Peruchon, M. (2011). Création picturales ou graphiques dans la maladie d'Alzheimer et dans la schizophrénie. Point de vue psychanalytique. *Gérontologie et Société,* 137: 131–150.
Ploton, L. (2010). *Ce que nous enseignent les malades d'Alzheimer*. Lyon: Chronique Sociale.
Randall, W.L. (2013). Aging, irony, and wisdom: On the narrative psychology of later life, *Theory & Psychology,* 23 (2): 164–183.
Sierpina, M., & Cole T. R. (2004). Stimulating creativity in all elders: A continuum of interventions. *Care Manag J.*, 5, 3: 175–182.
Sternberg, R. J. (1999). *Handbook of creativity*. Cambridge: Cambridge University Press.

The Past Empowering the Present: Intergenerational Solidarity Improving the Quality of Life

Laura Dryjanska and Roberto Giua

Abstract This chapter focuses on intergenerational solidarity towards older adults as one of the ways to improve the quality of life. The authors discuss the Train the Brain Protocol, which includes diverse practices, such as physical exercise, cognitive stimulation, diet, art-therapy, etc. The study evaluates the reminiscence approach within the theoretical framework of social representations, taking into account that younger generations are dependent on the memory of older people, but they do not always have the culture of preservation of cultural heritage. Thanks to the collaboration of centres for older adults in the city of Rome and young volunteers, it was possible to apply the reminiscence approach that concentrated on urban socially constructed realities through the memories of participants. Young people (age between 20 and 30) have engaged older persons in reminiscence activities discussing the memories of the city of Rome, places significant to participants and their daily practices in the urban setting.

Introduction: Intergenerational Solidarity Empowering Silver Universe

Intergenerational activities in the context of ageing often presuppose solidarity: the young are expected to help the old, often as an interpretation of reciprocity. We have decided to look at this issue concentrating on the old helping the young. By emphasizing how memories of the past can be valuable and useful to the new generations, we stress the older persons' potential to empower the present and thus the future. For example, the recall of urban entertainment 40 years ago may

L. Dryjanska (✉)
Rosemead School of Psychology, Biola University, La Mirada, CA, USA
e-mail: laura.dryjanska@biola.edu

R. Giua
Intergenerational Family Solidarity Across Europe COST Action, Brussels, Belgium

A. Bianco et al. (eds.), *Italian Studies on Quality of Life*, Social Indicators Research Series 77, https://doi.org/10.1007/978-3-030-06022-0_17

be an inspiration for the young people to find new ways of interaction with their neighbourhood, such as rediscovering certain areas (now largely touristy). In such a way, intergenerational solidarity may improve the quality of life of everyone involved by recognizing the value of older persons' memories and stimulating ideas among the youth. Such engagement is likely to affect self-esteem (feeling useful by the older and inspired by the younger), which in turn enhances wellbeing and thus the quality of life is enriched by a meaningful interaction with other generations.

In this chapter we discuss two examples of intergenerational solidarity from the Italian context of the city of Rome – interactions of older persons with young adults and interactions of older persons with children. We emphasize the role of culture, while tackling the question of appropriateness of implementing projects in diversified groups of older persons. To emphasize this heterogeneous character we have proposed a term "silver universe" (Dryjanska and Giua 2018), which purposefully does not include references to "old" or "ageing", but valorises the later stages in life, in the awareness of their multiplicity.

Theoretical Framework: Social Representations, Intergenerational Interaction and Quality of Life

The term "intergenerational solidarity" has been introduced by Bengtson in the late 1960s and 1970s in the context of family (Cruz-Saco 2010) and subsequently brought to the macro-social or group level (Bengtson and Oyama 2010). It has been defined as "intentional connection between two or more persons of different age groups" (Cruz-Saco 2010: 9).

Such relations can be seen from the paradigmatic perspective of social representations. The construct proposed by Moscovici (1961/1973) refers to the theory of social representations that defines the processes responsible for the order that exists between mental operations that cognitive theory describes, "just like sense introduces an order within the sounds, which could compose a word" (Moscovici 2014: 777). In this chapter we deal with processes, subtle aspects of reality that could not have been predicted or planned by the authors. While planning the research, they have initially concentrated on the cognitive assessment, but the subtle aspects such as interpersonal communication dynamics have emerged spontaneously. In other words, the focus here is on the form, rather than the content. Social representations of ageing deal with common sense knowledge, including both rational and irrational beliefs, as well as emotions that undergo changes. It has been found that social representations of ageing have a strong negative connotation with death, decay and illness (Contarello et al. 2011), although positive aspects include the value of wisdom and experience. According to Leone (2008), younger generations are dependent on the memory of the older people, but they do not always have the culture of preservation of cultural heritage, underestimating memories of older generations. Drawing on remote recall, reminiscence activities tend to focus on the processes (Bornat 2001; Butler 1963), which are the heart of the dynamic perspective of social representations. The activities include discussion of past events with others, often facilitated by tangible prompts such as photographs, artefacts, music or archival sound and video recordings, life review and life story work based on personal biographies (Westerhof 2017). Intergenerational interaction through reminiscence processes has the power to challenge stereotypes and prejudices (Desouza 2007) that constitute negative aspects of social representations that the two groups hold of each other. This process often involves emotions and building or strengthening the mutual sense of respect/admiration (Heyman and Gutheil 2008).

Over time, oral history interviews conducted by young people with older persons are stimulated during an intergenerational encounter. They may contribute to improving quality of life among older persons (Ligon et al. 2012) by positively affecting their self-esteem based on feeling useful and thus valuable to others rather than a burden. This is especially relevant since the quality of life is affected at early stages of cognitive decline (Barrios et al. 2013) that in many cases emerges during later years, for example in the form of mild cognitive impairment (MCI). Working specifically with adults affected by MCI, Xaverius and Matthews (2004) found that structured activities with children had a more significant impact than unstructured activities with children on levels of engagement and expressiveness of older persons. There are some distinctions within silver universe in relation to intergenerational interactions with youth. According to Reisig and Fees (2007), older adults in the Midwestern US agricultural communities in general perceived a heightened sense of wellbeing as a result of such interaction. In particular, adults aged 74–85 experienced significantly greater satisfaction and enjoyment than their older counterparts. This does not mean that the oral history interview should preferably take place at some particular age, but that the interaction with young people (particularly adolescents) tends to be more meaningful for this age group. However, not necessarily everyone likes children or young people and takes pleasure in interaction with them. At times, intergenerational activities may have a negative rather than positive impact on the quality of life, especially if they are a source of stress or frustration due to a factor such as mobility issues. Based on interviews with UK care home residents recruited from the UK My Home Life North-East care home network, Cook and Bailey (2013) concluded that organized intergenerational practice needed to be guided, time-limited, and purposeful. One may also wonder what the added value of interactions between generations is in comparison with any other planned activity that does not contemplate participation of younger people. In fact, Rotenberg-Shpigelman and Maeir (2011) have shown the potential utility of participation-centred treatment for the growing population of elderly with mild cognitive deficits in Israel. A significant factor that contributes to the quality of life of older persons, not necessarily related to intergenerational issues, seems to be a sense of control in line with the model proposed by Grewal et al. (2006) that identifies five attributes shown in Fig. 1.

Applying this model of attributes of quality of life, Koehn et al. (2016) have found that a sense of control was foremost for ethno-culturally diverse older persons at three different sites in Canada in British Columbia.

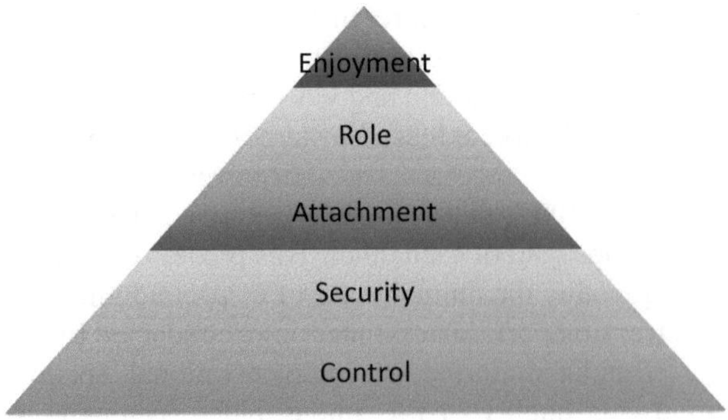

Fig. 1 Five attributes of the quality of life of older persons (Grewal et al. 2006). Adapted from "Developing attributes for a generic quality of life measure for older people: Preferences or capabilities?" by I. Grewal et al., Social Science & Medicine, 62(8), 1891–1901. (Source: Figure designed by Laura Dryjanska)

Not by chance we have chosen to discuss some examples from diverse cultures. The theoretical framework of social representations implies a particular sensitivity to the context on different levels. Concepts have various meanings across cultures assuming different shapes between groups, which means that the concept of enjoyment may mean essentially collective, relational activity in one society, while in another it may be readily associated with individual gratification and pleasure. For example, quality of life of older persons assessed in Italy, Portugal and Turkey (Arun and Çakıroğlu Çevik 2011) using data provided by the European Quality of Life Survey demonstrated differences based not only on the modernization process in each society, but also the cultural conditions such as household typology and education level. In other words, what would be considered crowded and unpleasant living conditions for someone from Western Europe appears as desirable for an elderly from Italy. Roos (2011) has described an intergenerational group reflecting technique as a culturally appropriate research method, used to obtain insight into how important information between grandparents and grandchildren is transferred and to cast light on the relational dynamics between the two generations. First, grandchildren sit in the inner circle (while the grandmothers sit in the outer circle) actively listening to the narrative; then, the positions are inverted. This technique respects cultural norming based on taking turns during the conversation with an older person speaking first. Considering the context, one has to pay attention to the fact that the technique was applied at a day care facility for older adults in a semi-urban historically disadvantaged community of Ikageng, just outside Potchefstroom in the North West Province of South Africa.

Methodology

This chapter uses qualitative methodology based on participant observation of two types of intergenerational activities that took place in Rome, Italy.

Living in the Eternal City of Rome

The specific urban context of Rome is embedded in the national and regional cultures. The living styles of older persons in Rome are marked by the urban infrastructure of a historic city. They live almost exclusively in apartments, without a garden or any personal green space, in an environment characterized by heavy traffic, smog, and presence of crowds, including residents, commuters and tourists. Many streets and buildings are challenging in terms of mobility, such as the lack of ramps and elevators. Thus, access to services may be difficult for an older person who often relies on the help of others. Very few older persons drive; they mostly use public transportation. Even if one can afford a car, parking it poses numerous challenges, as historical parts of the city do not have sufficient space. Moreover, Rome is known for fairly frequent strikes and large gatherings that further restrict urban traffic and access to services. Traditionally, inhabitants of the city tend to be known for their distrust and rather crude manners, yet fitting the overarching self-representation of Italians as "good fellows" (Leone and Sarrica 2012). Moreover, physical environment has implications for all citizens, in particular older persons. According to the World Health Organization (2007), an age-friendly city is one that "encourages active ageing by optimizing opportunities for health, participation and security in order to enhance quality of life as people age" (p. 1). Among many different issues, including transportation, access to healthcare facilities, architectonic barriers, a significant issue in the lives of many older persons tends to be religion and spirituality. This is especially true in Rome, with a very high number of churches and a significant involvement of religious persons in healthcare. Taking into account the religious dimension has proven successful in case of programs for older adults, such as the Health Promotion for the Mind, Body, and Spirit course that stimulates the mind, moving the body, and rejuvenating the spirit – providing needed purpose, meaning, and connection (Richeson et al. 2007). Among the centres for older adults discussed in this chapter, especially San Saba stands out as one run by nuns who constituted the majority of fulltime, onsite staff. Also, the activity at this location, focused on Christmas celebration with children, included numerous references to religious themes.

Intergenerational Activities

The first set of intergenerational activities took place with older adults, members of the centres in the neighbourhoods of Borgo Pio, Sabotino and Angelo Emo. Young adults supported by a local Rotary Club have engaged them in reminiscences about the city of Rome with the objective of producing a documentary that would valorise the cultural heritage (Dryjanska 2014). Prompted by the photographs and songs from their youth, the elderly were asked to share narratives about growing up in their city. The documentary included narratives of older persons and scenes from the past of the city as well as contemporary images further elaborated by an architect expert in urban studies. The purpose of the documentary was the promotion of intangible cultural heritage of Rome found through narratives of its elderly inhabitants.

The second set of intergenerational activities involved older adults from the centers in the neighbourhoods of San Giovanni and San Saba, with young children whose mothers turn to a Roman organization *Salvamamme Salvabebe* (Italian for "Save moms, save babies") for help with diapers, food, toys, etc. The encounters took place before Christmas, and the older participants had the task of talking to children (often of non-Italian descent) about local traditions during this period, singing carols together, and receiving gifts from the children provided by the organization. The outcomes of both encounters differed due to the age and ability of participants: the young people possessed skills necessary to produce a documentary, while the children could perform the tasks of listening, singing, and handing the presents. The shorter attention span of children and their more limited abilities compared with young people were the reasons to engage them in a different type of intergenerational activity.

The criteria for belonging to the municipal centres for older persons include age (at least 55 years old) or certified disability of at least 60% (in this case the age has to be at least 45 years old). This official rule stated by the urban authorities reveals the specificity of the Italian context, in which the minimum age of an older person is lower than in the literature.

Characteristics of Participants

The intergenerational activities described above took place in different settings in Rome, Italy: centres for older adults and a residential facility, in diverse historical areas of the city (Borgo Pio close to the Vatican, Sabotino and Angelo Emo in Prati neighbourhood, San Giovanni neighbourhood, and San Saba neighbourhood on a hill near the Coliseum). The centres constitute associations sponsored by the Municipality of Rome and have been identified after contacting the governing authority that authorized activities in these specific locations, following meetings with the city officials and governing bodies of each one of them. The convenience sample was thus based on the indications from the urban authorities and consents of first the leaders of the centres and then participants themselves. Altogether, 107 older persons participated in this research; see Fig. 2 below.

Reflecting the gender composition of the centres and the fact that women tend to live longer, in each context there were more female participants, as detailed in Fig. 3.

Age of participants varied significantly, from 49 to 97 (see the discussion above concerning the Italian centres for older persons), but the majority of them fell in the age cohort from 70 to 80 years old, as shown in Fig. 4. This wide range of age groups within the centres hints on the first challenge of performing intergenerational activities – who is actually the target? "Older persons" may be a very vague

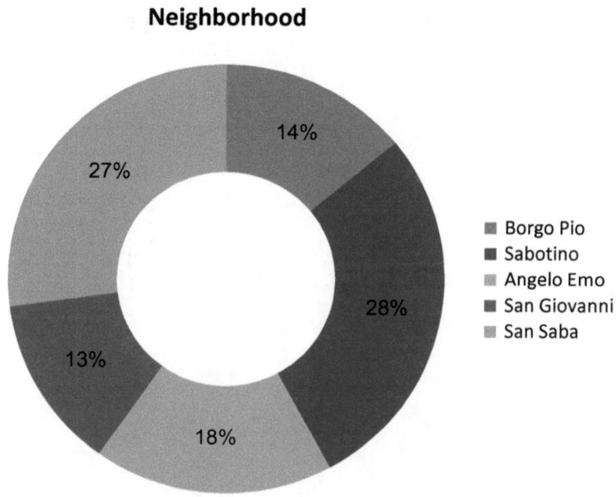

Fig. 2 Locations of participants in the city of Rome. (Source: data elaboration by Laura Dryjanska and Roberto Giua)

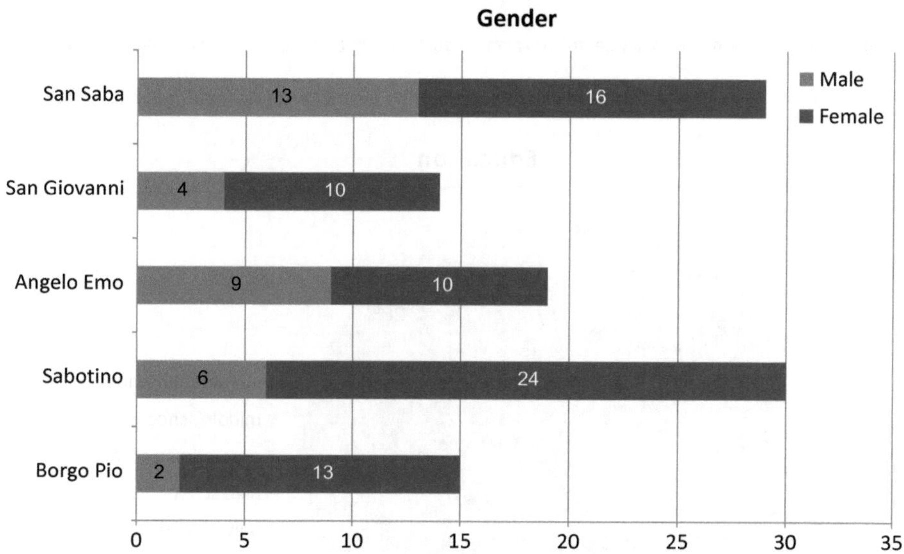

Fig. 3 Gender of participants by neighborhood. (Source: data elaboration by Laura Dryjanska and Roberto Giua)

term; although generally they are grouped together, very likely there are significant differences simply based on the age. To put it differently, in Italian centres for older people one may easily find representatives of two different generations, and this should be taken into account.

Another factor that contributes to the diversity of participants is their education. Interaction, way of expressing themselves, cultural preferences and intellectual interests have to do with the level and type of schooling, as detailed in Fig. 5.

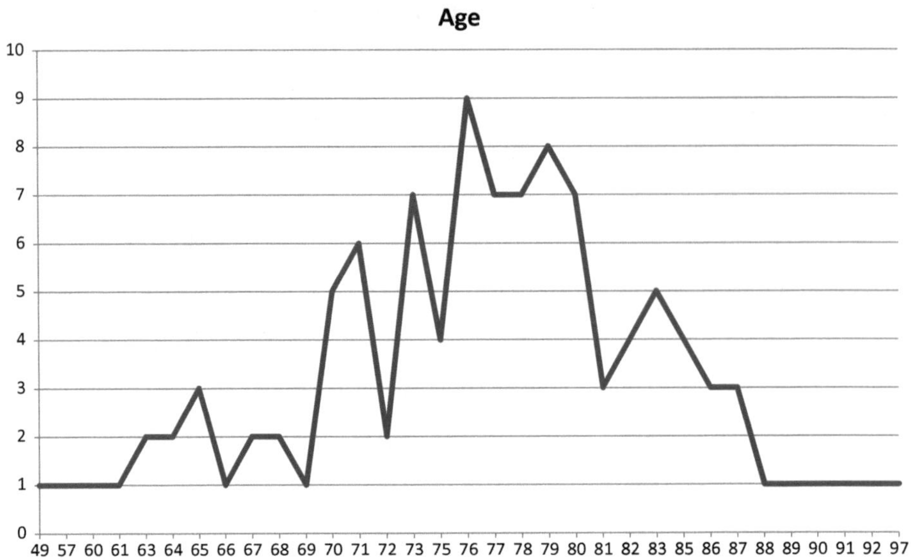

Fig. 4 Age of participants. (Source: data elaboration by Laura Dryjanska and Roberto Giua)

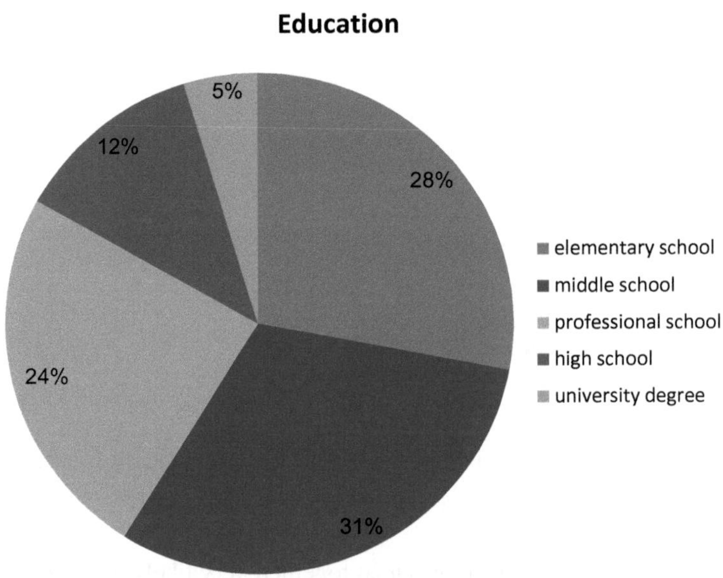

Fig. 5 Education of participants. (Source: data elaboration by Laura Dryjanska and Roberto Giua)

Finally, as a part of this research, qualified psychotherapists have applied the Mini Mental State Examination and Montreal Cognitive Assessment, paying attention to the conditions and immediate context, aware of the limitations of such

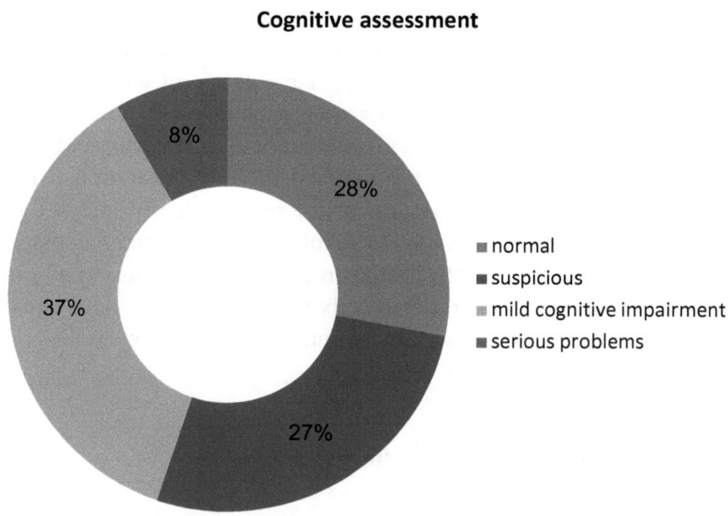

Fig. 6 Cognitive assessment of participants. (Source: data elaboration by Laura Dryjanska and Roberto Giua)

standardized testing (Dryjanska et al. 2017). The results have revealed that more than 60% of participants were already or very likely to be affected by mild cognitive impairment as defined by Feldman and Jacova (2005), which is shown in Fig. 6.

Research Design

Aware of the considerable diversity of participants concerning different factors, as demonstrated above, we have posed the following questions prior to conducting the activities:

- Is it proper to offer intergenerational activities to such a heterogeneous group? One could think that the chronological age typology of persons in their sixties as opposed to those in their nineties would affect and shape intergenerational relations. Would those older be left behind? Or would those with mild cognitive impairment be undermined by their peers or representatives of younger generations?
- What activities stimulate empowerment of the silver universe in interaction with younger generations? How does this empowerment occur?

Concerning the first research question, it should be noted that an ecologically valid study that took place in the natural context where participants usually meet and interact, required non-discriminatory treatment. Since among these groups diversified by age other activities occur without differentiation based on birth date, it would be perceived as unfair and strange to include only some and not others or to diversify the involvement. Upon consultation with the leaders of communities and municipality authorities, the authors opted for involving all willing participants in order to respect the group dynamics and need for inclusion.

A qualitative methodology of participant observation was chosen to address the questions above. The researchers have assisted the intergenerational interactions, also documented though photos and videos, first independently analysed by each of the two judges (a clinical[1] and a social psychologist), then jointly assessed to reach an agreement. The results, deeply rooted in the cultural context and community settings of two specific intergenerational activities (with young adults and children), are discussed in the sections below, concentrating on three case studies.

Results: Scenes Behind the Scenes

The analysis based on participant observation has revealed some stimulating, culture-specific nuances related to the heterogeneous characteristics of older persons involved. In the following sections, we discuss three "scenes behind the scenes" that feature intergenerational relationships not necessarily planned or meant ahead of time, in the light of the research question.

Case 1: Solving a Problem Together

The main goal of young people involved in the project was to produce a documentary based on the older participants' memories of Rome. Fresh professionals were supposed to come earlier to set up the equipment and to prepare the interview setting, ensuring proper light and sound. In their minds, this preliminary work did not constitute an intergenerational activity. However the older persons arrived first, curious to see *the entire* process, including the preparation. As often happens in Rome, due to logistic difficulties (traffic, buses coming late, etc.), young people reached the centre later and had to face the pressure of setting up closely watched by dozens of quite vocal observers who would comment on virtually every move. The first shortcomings, such as missing cables and inappropriate light, constituted a source of frustration. It seemed like everyone in the room had an opinion and was eager to share it. The young people initially did not take advice and tended to ignore the spectators, but eventually, when a few of them showed up with an extension cord or physically intervened, they started to work together. Older persons, familiar with

[1]The authors wish to acknowledge the role of Marzia Giua, a clinical psychologist who administered cognitive tests to participants and provided psychotherapeutic insight during the participant observation and subsequent discussion.

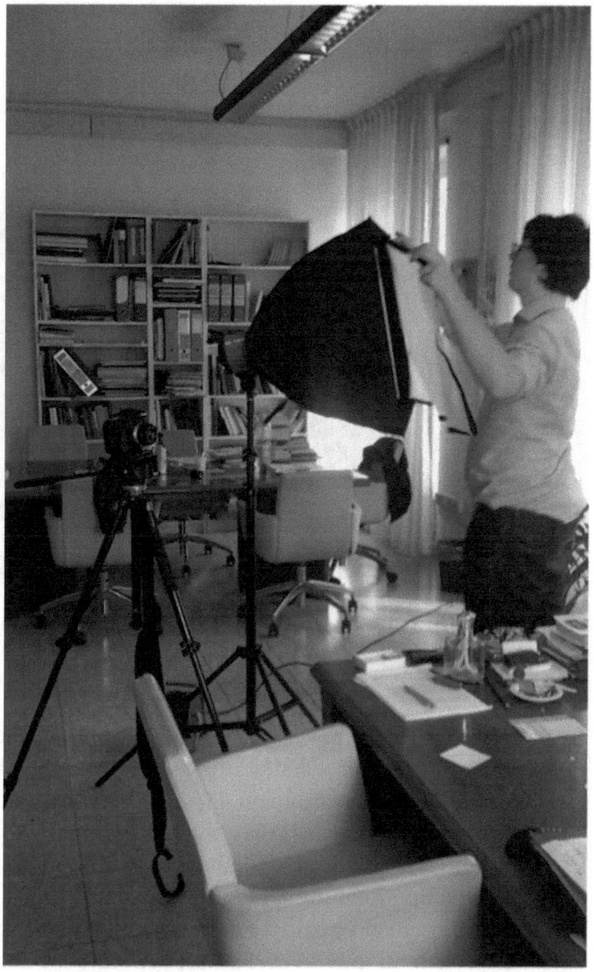

Photo 1 Young man preparing the interview setting. (Source: photo by Roberto Giua)

the centre, were able to actively contribute on this practical level of setting up. Those especially helpful turned out instrumental by encouraging other participants to speak about Rome in the later phases. Although their skills and know-how initially were not requested, this off-record encounter became an icebreaker through which the different generations got to know and appreciate each other (Photo 1).

Case 2: "You Don't Talk to a Girl Like That!"

In a later phase of the project, the young people had the task of stimulating memories of Rome with photos and other materials. One of the girls involved was supposed to bring them on a certain day, but she forgot to do so. This was a cause of

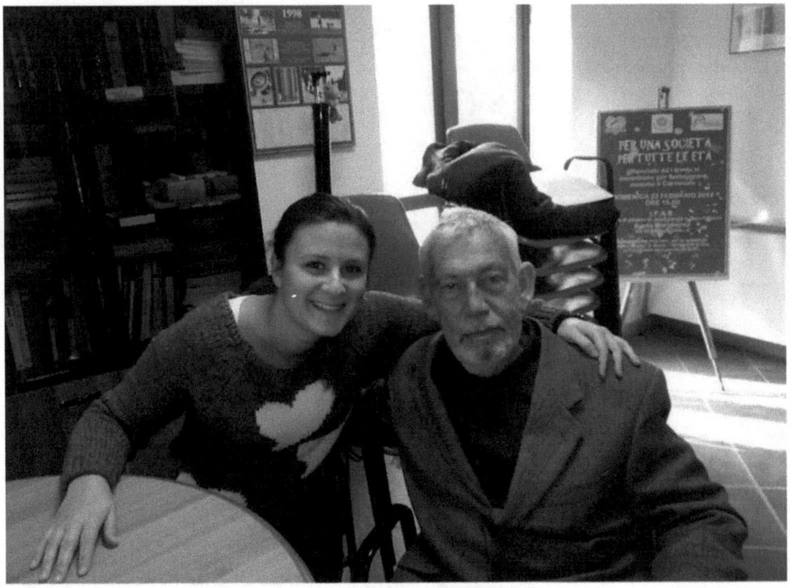

Photo 2 Young woman and older man who became bonded as a result of the discussion on gender. (Source: photo by Roberto Giua)

frustration and led to an intense argument among the young people. Also in this case, participants intervened: at first an older man shouted, "You don't talk to a girl like that!" After a moment of silence, a few older ladies started to whisper to one another. Eventually, they voiced their position, stating that young people nowadays did not differentiate between how one should treat a woman as opposed to a man. The young men immediately agreed, emphasizing that their quarrel actually demonstrated gender equality. On the other hand, the girls sided with the older men whose approach, in their eyes, had brought into the surface some forgotten qualities of courtship and being a gentleman. The controversial issue involved all participants, roughly divided in two groups based on their opinion on gender equality: boys and older ladies on the one hand, and girls and older men on the other hand. Although on that afternoon the video project did not advance, the intergenerational relationships became much stronger (Photo 2).

Case 3: Breaking the Rules Together

The intergenerational activity that involved a Christmas program for children was quite structured. The leading purpose was to facilitate intergenerational solidarity based on mutual respect and active roles of persons of different ages. The structure followed the purpose by involving the elderly and children in specific ways. The

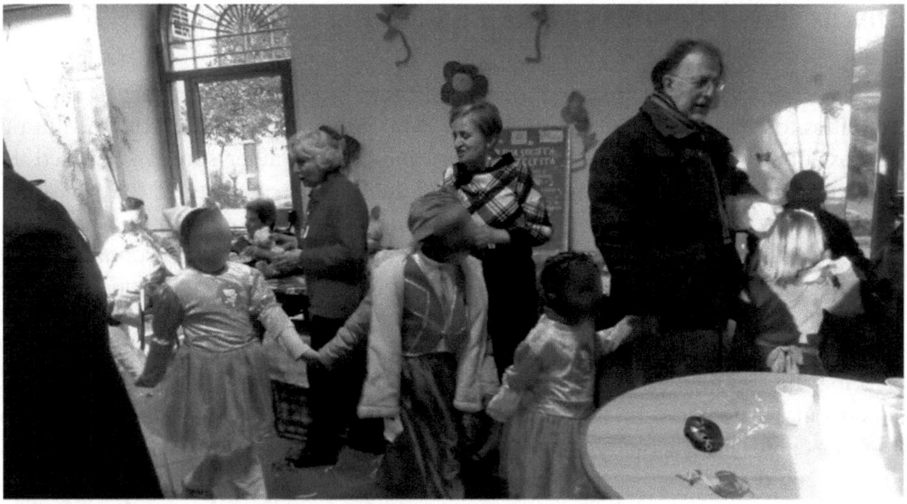

Photo 3 The author engaged in the unstructured activity with children. (Source: photo by Laura Dryjanska)

schedule included carolling (together by both generations), reading stories (performed by the older persons to the children), giving gifts (performed by the children to the older persons) and having refreshments (together by both generations); all led by some middle-age facilitators. The authors expected a smooth, guided sequence of activities in the atmosphere of respectful mutual exchange. It was their hope to observe giving and receiving by both generations, which would result in positive emotions that characterize intergenerational solidarity.

At first, the older participants were not very keen on actively contributing to the activity. In particular, those much older, beyond eighty, expressed some distrust related to "treating them like children". Not much interaction took place initially: the children stayed on one side, separate from the older people, each group watching the carolling and story-reading individually. Gift-giving presented some unexpected difficulties due to mobility issues in a crowded room. Things did not quite go as planned, as evidenced by the frustration of facilitators and amusement of older spectators. Children, anxious to get their gifts, started racing across ignoring the rules and order. Many of them did not want to give the gifts to older persons, but kept them to themselves. Shunned by their mothers, they easily convinced the older persons to forget the rules. The gifts got mixed up which caused some to end up with more and others with less. A general confusion of children playing and making noise while running around with their new toys, was a source of enjoyment to older participants who later stated that from that moment on it felt more like real Christmas with the family. The facilitators gave up and started serving drinks and treats in the seeming conditions of chaos, eventually appreciated by everyone(Photo 3).

Discussion of Findings in the Light of the Literature

The short answer to our research question ("Is it proper to offer intergenerational activities to very heterogeneous groups of older persons?") is "yes." In the cultural context of Rome, the proposed programs have proven rather successful based on the participant observation; which included subsequent analysis of reactions and behaviour by a clinical psychologist. Present during the activities, the clinical psychologist has confirmed the interpretation of participants' behaviour proposed by the authors, further elaborating emotions and reactions to ensure correct understanding of events that took place. However, the diversity aspects based on gender and education of participants were not indifferent; they have played different roles.

First, the immediate setting of each centre and its physical characteristics has stood out particularly in the first and third scene. The shortcomings related to missing cables have actually created an opportunity for a joint problem solving. This in turn could challenge stereotypes and prejudices (Desouza 2007) that constitute negative aspects of social representations, which young people may have had of their older counterparts as "useless". By helping out with practical difficulties in a critical moment of tension, the participants have demonstrated that they could be "useful". This process has also involved emotions and building the mutual sense of respect (Heyman and Gutheil 2008). In addition, during the experience of breaking the rules with children, the physical setting of a crowded room (although negative in objective terms) has stimulated interaction and contact. Contrary to findings of Xaverius and Matthews (2004), in this case, unstructured activities with children had a more significant impact. This could be due to cultural characteristics of Italians in general and Romans in particular. In Italian culture, described as affective by Trompenaars (1993), expressing emotions is legitimate and useful for action. Rome is known for the chaos and crowd, with short distances between persons in terms of territoriality. Such cultural factors may have contributed to the preference for unstructured activities, not in line with Cook and Bailey (2013) who concluded that organized intergenerational practice needed to be guided and purposeful.

Second, the gender differences have emerged during the second and third scenes. Interestingly in the former case, a conflict within the group of young people gave rise to intergenerational solidarity, an intentional connection between different age groups (Cruz-Saco 2010). Older men sided with young women, while older women sided with young men. This situation is a powerful reminder that each individual has multiple social identities which may be linked with gender, ethnicity, age, social status, convictions, etc. Intergenerational relations do not take place in a vacuum, just like social representations they are strongly rooted in a given context and prone to transformation (Moscovici 1963/1971). The ambivalent intergroup relations may change to positive ones also as a function of gender, when conflict gives rise to an intergenerational group reflecting process, similar to the one proposed by Roos (2011). On the other hand, it has been observed that during interaction with children some older men did not participate with the same intensity of older women. Lack of physical, direct contact with children in their past (for many Italians in previous generations the role of a man in the family was primarily the bread-winner, not a caregiver) had caused them to feel a bit overwhelmed.

Third, in terms of age the older participants constituted a very diverse group. However, in none of the activities the chronological age seemed to make a substantial difference. Unlike Reisig and Fees' (2007) conclusion concerning adults aged 74–85 who experienced significantly greater satisfaction and enjoyment than their older counterparts, the participant observation did not reveal any particular difference due to age. On the contrary, although the young participants could easily liken some of the ladies to grandmothers while other to great-grandmothers, no one deemed such distinction useful or necessary. It could be interpreted on a cultural level, since in Italian society the role of grandparents does not seem to differ much from great-grandparents.

As demonstrated by Arun and Çakıroğlu Çevik (2011), the quality of life of older persons is related to the education level, among other factors such as income level, health, accessing material sources, and social contacts. In the first two cases discussed above, both of them with the young people, education seemed to make a slight difference. From the one side, during the problem solving related to setting up the room, the participants with professional school training and thus some technical abilities had an advantage over others. On the other hand, the intergroup discussion concerning gender issues and in particular the emancipation of women, seemed to be an occasion for higher educated participants to emerge as more critical thinkers with a wider range of arguments. For instance, since the older persons were in general aware of one another's education status, they tended to give more credit to statements made by the few of them with a university diploma.

The final issue of cognitive capacities may seem especially sensitive. The participants with a mild cognitive impairment as defined by Feldman and Jacova (2005) paired with those in a suspicious condition (initial signs of mild cognitive impairment) have outnumbered the rest. In other words, the suspicion of cognitive decline is based on a specific score and requires a referral by the person who conducted the initial test. It was evident from the participant observation that serious cognitive problems often made intergenerational relations much more difficult, if not impossible, due to isolation of some of these individuals. However, the mild and suspicious impairment did not constitute a barrier to getting involved in reminiscence activities, which drew on memory of remote events (Bornat 2001; Butler 1963). Support of this was evidenced through, a woman who could not remember what they had for breakfast has shared very specific details of her childhood entertainment by the Tiber River in Rome, or a man unable to accurately state current date and time of the day has eloquently described how urban public transportation worked before the construction of the metro. In fact, some of the persons with quite serious problems have proven to be excellent narrators and top contributors when sharing the intangible cultural heritage of Rome with the young generations (Dryjanska 2014). As stated by Ligon et al. (2012), oral history interviews stimulated during the intergenerational encounter may have contributed to improved quality of life among older persons. Especially in the cases when the quality of life is negatively affected at early stages of cognitive decline (Barrios et al.

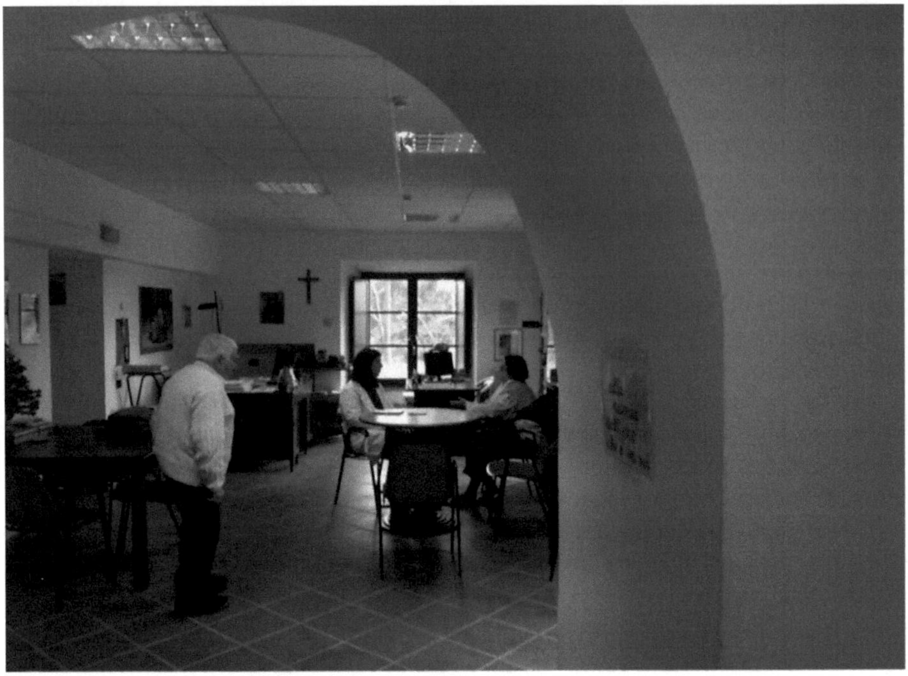

Photo 4 Psychotherapist administering MMSE test. (Source: photo by Roberto Giua)

2013), successful involvement in reminiscence-based intergenerational activity may, at least partially, restore a sense of control, security and enjoyment, factors identified by Grewal et al. (2006) as some of the attributes of quality of life. Moreover, the interaction with children also provided enjoyment and fulfilment to some of the participants with mild cognitive impairment. Their spiritual and relational needs have been fulfilled during the Christmas celebration, which at least in some cases had seemed to provide purpose, meaning, and connection (Richeson et al. 2007) (Photo 4).

Conclusion

The culturally sensitive assessment of intergenerational activities in Rome was based on participant observation and qualitative analysis of selected events that took place during the implementation of programs. Overall the structure of centres for older persons, very diversified in terms of the demographic characteristics of participants, seems to be appropriate for the local context. The Romans' flexibility, even later in life, paired with affective culture (Trompenaars 1993), gives them advantage when interacting with younger generations. The authors have not detected expressions of intergenerational discrimination. On the contrary, even situations of intergroup conflict that emerged quite often, seemed to be oriented to solve the problem and did not have lasting consequences.

References

Arun, Ö., and Çakıroğlu Çevik, A. (2011). Quality of Life in Ageing Societies: Italy, Portugal, and Turkey. *Educational Gerontology,* 37(11), 945–966.

Bárrios, H., Narciso, S., Guerreiro, M., Maroco, J., Logsdon, R., de Mendonça, A. (2013). Quality of life in patients with mild cognitive impairment. *Aging & Mental Health,* 17(3), 287–292.

Bengtson, V. L., and Oyama, P. S. (2010). Intergenerational solidarity and conflict: What does it mean and what are the big issues? In M. A. Cruz-Saco and S. Zelenev (Eds.), *Intergenerational solidarity: Strengthening economic and social ties* (pp. 35–52). New York: Palgrave Macmillan.

Bornat, J. (2001). Reminiscence and oral history: Parallel universes or shared endeavour? *Ageing and Society,* 21(2), 219–241.

Butler, R. N. (1963). The life review: An interpretation of reminiscence in the aged. *Psychiatry,* 26, 65–76.

Contarello, A., Marini, I., Nencini, A., Ricci, G. (2011). Rappresentazioni sociali dell'invecchiamento tra psicologia sociale e letteratura. *Revista Psicologia & Sociedade,* 23(1), 171–180.

Cook, G., and Bailey, C. (2013). Older Care Home Residents' Views of Intergenerational Practice. *Journal of Intergenerational Relationships,* 11(4), 410–424.

Cruz-Saco, M. A. (2010). Intergenerational solidarity. In M. A. Cruz-Saco and S. Zelenev (Eds.), *Intergenerational solidarity: Strengthening economic and social ties* (pp. 9–34). New York: Palgrave Macmillan.

Desouza, E. (2007). Intergenerational Interaction through Reminiscence Processes. *Journal of Intergenerational Relationships,* 5(1), 39–56.

Dryjanska, L. (2014). A social psychological approach to cultural heritage: memories of the elderly inhabitants of Rome. *Journal of Heritage Tourism,* 10(1), 38–56.

Dryjanska, L. & Giua, R. (2018). *Solidarietà intergenerazionale: Universo argento.* Rome: Aracne Editrice.

Dryjanska, L., Aiello, S., Giua, M. (2017). Social representations, ageing and memory: a holistic approach to cognitive assessment. *Ageing and Society,* 37(4), 804–822.

Feldman, H. H., & Jacova, C. (2005). Mild cognitive impairment. *The American Journal of Geriatric Psychiatry,* 13(8), 645–655.

Grewal, I., Lewis, J., Flynn, T., Brown, J., Bond, J., Coast, J. (2006). Developing attributes for a generic quality of life measure for older people: Preferences or capabilities? *Social Science & Medicine,* 62(8), 1891–1901.

Heyman, J. C., & Gutheil, I. A. (2008). "They Touch Our Hearts": The Experiences of Shared Site Intergenerational Program Participants. *Journal of Intergenerational Relationships,* 6(4), 397–412.

Koehn, S. D., Mahmood, A. N., & Stott-Eveneshen, S. (2016). Quality of Life for Diverse Older Adults in Assisted Living: The Centrality of Control. *Journal of Gerontological Social Work,* 59(7–8), 512–536.

Leone, G. (2008). Risvegliarsi alla storia. La memoria degli anziani come risorsa di sviluppo e di riconciliazione per la comunità. In F. Ruggeri (Ed.), *La memoria del futuro. Soggetti fragili e possibilità di azione,* (pp. 139–160). Milano: F. Angeli.

Leone, G., and Sarrica, M. (2012). Challenging the myth of Italians as "good fellows": Is clarity about in-group crimes the best choice when narrating a war to its perpetrators' descendants? *Papers on Social Representations,* 21(2), 1–28.

Ligon, M., Welleford, E. A., Cotter, J.J., Lam, M. (2012). Oral History: A Pragmatic Approach to Improving Life Satisfaction of Elders. *Journal of Intergenerational Relationships,* 10(2), 147–159.

Moscovici, S. (1961/1973). *La psychanalyse: Son image et son public.* Paris: PUF.

Moscovici, S. (2014). The new magical thinking. *Public Understanding of Science,* 23(7), 759–779.

Reisig, C. N., and Fees, B. S. (2007). Older Adults' Perceptions of Well-Being after Intergenerational Experiences with Youth. *Journal of Intergenerational Relationships,* 4(4), 6–22.

Richeson, N. E., Boyne, S., Brady, E. M. (2007). Education for Older Adults with Early-Stage Dementia: Health Promotion for the Mind, Body, and Spirit. *Educational Gerontology, 33*(9), 723–736.

Roos, V. (2011). "The Generational Other": The Cultural Appropriateness of an Intergenerational Group Reflecting Technique. *Journal of Intergenerational Relationships,* 9(1), 90–97.

Rotenberg-Shpigelman, S., Maeir, A. (2011). Participation-Centered Treatment for Elderly with Mild Cognitive Deficits: A "Book Club" Group Case Study. *Physical & Occupational Therapy in Geriatrics,* 29(3), 222–232.

Trompenaars, F. (1993). *Riding the waves of culture.* London: Nicholas Brealey.

Westerhof, G. J. (2017). Technologies to Remember or Forget? A Perspective from Reminiscence and Life Review. *The International Journal of Reminiscence and Life Review,* 4(1), 8–13.

World Health Organization. (2007). Checklist of essential features of age-friendly cities. http://www.who.int/ageing/publications/Age_friendly_cities_checklist.pdf Accessed 26 Sep 2017.

Xaverius, P. K., and Matthews, R. M. (2004). Evaluating the Impact of Intergenerational Activities on Elders' Engagement and Expressiveness Levels in Two Settings. *Journal of Intergenerational Relationships,* 1(4), 53–69.

Intergenerational Sustainable Tourism and Quality of Life

Antonietta Albanese and Elena Bocci

Abstract This paper is part of a long series of research and experimental projects in intergenerational tourism, which started in 2000 at the University of Milan. Study projects take a multi-methodological approach based on the principal theories of social psychology and recent studies on psychology of ageing.

The projects have been monitored by A.R.I.P.T.Fo.R.P, the University network which awards a certificate of "Manager in Environment and Intergenerational Tourism".

The contribution presents the results of the most recent research projects in Central Italy (Viterbo, 2010–2016). These results confirm the phases of communication development introduced by Albanese 2001, from "drawing close" to "group generative creativity', conducting to the creation of two urban intergenerational woodland areas and collaboration in Caritas "solidarity vegetable plots".

From the a.y. 2015–2016, A.R.I.P.T.Fo.R.P. has set up 'sandwich course' contracts with secondary schools to provide intergenerational holidays in North and Central Italy.

Research Background

For several years, research in psychological field has looked into the factors that affect the aging process.

A. Albanese (✉)
Department of Social and Political Sciences, Milan University, Association A.R.I.P.T. Fo.R.P. (Association of Interdisciplinary Research in Psychology of Tourism: Training, Research and Planning), Milan, Italy
e-mail: antonietta.albanese@unimi.it

E. Bocci
Department of Developmental and Social Psychology, Sapienza University of Rome, Association A.R.I.P.T. Fo.R.P. (Association of Interdisciplinary Research in Psychology of Tourism: Training, Research and Planning), Rome, Italy
e-mail: elena.bocci@uniroma1.it

A. Bianco et al. (eds.), *Italian Studies on Quality of Life*, Social Indicators Research Series 77, https://doi.org/10.1007/978-3-030-06022-0_18

Studies of the last 20 years show that constant work on cognitive, affective and motivational processes facilitates a positive life in elder age (Havighurst et al. 1969; Cesa-Bianchi and Cristini 2014; Giua 2015).

Social conditions and cultural context "accompany" and determine the different ways of approaching the elderly (Cesa-Bianchi 2002).

Recent psycho-social research has focused the transition from work to retirement as the time of retirement represents the critical state of the transition phase. The individual leaves an active life where professional identity is closely linked to the personal and social identity and enters a long-expected phase of "time free" from work. This leads to a loss of the professional role that strongly affects the individual identity.

For example, a research conducted in the years 2004–2005 for the Lombardy Region (Italy), "From Work to Retirement: Experiences, Projects", studied individual experiences related to retirement, pensioner's projects for the future and motivations towards voluntary activities in the provinces of the region (Albanese et al. 2006).

According to the research results, the age of retirement does not represent a decline phase, but rather "the" phase for setting up new projects regarding:

- intensifying family relationships;
- dedicating to volunteering;
- regaining the cultivation of neglected interests in working years – culture and tourism resulted as new interests or "renewed" interests –.

Based on the above-mentioned studies, Italian researches on tourism benefits for the quality of life in old age (Serino 1999; Corna-Pellegrini 2005; Nenci 2005) and on the recently diagnosed "generation network poverty" (Albanese and Bocci 2014), the 'Generational Encounters Study Group' at the University of Milan,[1] proposes innovative research/interventions (Lewin 1946) of intergenerational tourism (Albanese 1999). This is done in collaboration with the University network A.R.I.P.T.Fo.R.P. (Association of Interdisciplinary Research in Psychology of Tourism: Training, Research and Planning).

Because of the close relationship between research and training activities (Albanese and Bocci 2012a), the University network awards a certificate of Manager in Environment and Intergenerational Tourism (Albanese and Bocci 2012b, 2016b).

Theoretical Background

Intergenerational tourism forms an opportunity for knowledge, through a touristic-socio-cultural experience, called "Grandparents and Grandchildren", between participants of different generations – with no reciprocal family links.

[1] The 'Generational Encounters Study Group' has started its activity in 1998 at the Department of Social and Political Studies of the University of Milan. The activities are now continuing within the national research group coordinated by Prof. Roberta Maeran of the University of Padua.

The research/interventions are based on a well-constructed multi-theoretical model research/interventions that involves specific themes of intergenerational studies (Albanese and Bocci 2013):

- The Self Theory (Mead 1934; Markus 1977) suggests the existence of different types of Self: Private Self, Public Self, Collective Self. In a temporal perspective, it also suggests the presence of: the "past Self" -represented by the elderly within intergenerational tourism research/interventions-, the "present Self" -expressed by the young people teaching technological innovations– the "future Self"-expressed by the encounter/clash between generations, within intergenerational communication difficulties, mediated by new computer languages-. The integration between "past Self" and "present Self" leads to a rooted and prosperous "future Self" for the society.

Psychosocial studies also highlighted how each person tends to identify positive traits in his own group -in-group- and negative traits in the other group -out-group- (Brown 1988/2000; Sherif 1966; Tajfel 1978, 1981). The attribution of stiff features to groups and people can generate unsuccessful interactions or even cognitive and relational errors. Participants end up creating rigid stereotypes that take form of associations between a categorical label and an attribute they believe to share with most members of that category. Consider, for example, expressions like: "grandfather to be scraped" or "rude nephew". Instead, interaction between groups may help overcoming conflicts and create co-operation with a common goal.

- Concerning the Theory of Social Representations (Moscovici 1961/1976), in research/interventions attention is focused on:
- the "objectification" process that translates concepts into images also through the use of metaphorical lexicon in computer-mediated communication;
- the function of "familiarization" with social groups and physical-virtual spaces (for example, the use of internet environments for grandparents and the discovery of corners of highly cultural, historical and landscaping value for grandchildren);
- a relationship between "representations" and "practices", highlighting above all the role of practices in the evolution of social representations (Albanese and Bocci 2009).

Multi-methodological Approach

Tools and Participants of the Researches

In the framework of the research/interventions activated in Italy in the early 2000s – of a week period per year-, the present contribution will focus on the most recent studies carried out in Viterbo and province for the period 2010/2016.

The rich methodological instrumentation – as proposed by the 'Generational Encounters Study Group' – uses a multi-method approach (de Rosa 1990).

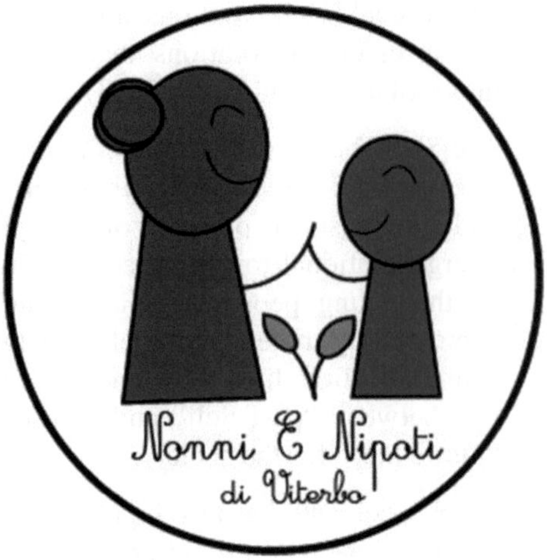

Fig. 1 Logo "Grandparents and Grandchildren" realized by Dr Sabrina Polimeni and voted among different proposals by "Grandparents and Grandchildren" on June 2012. (Albanese and Bocci 2014)

By using different tools adopted in social psychology -questionnaires, interviews, direct observations during leisure activities and in computer labs, focus groups and free associations around the logo – the present study intends to analyze modes of interaction between sub-groups of ten young and ten elderly people in a holiday setting.

The list of word evoked by the research participants in 2014 through the "associative network" technique around "Grandparents and Grandchildren" logo have been analyzed by the Lexical Correspondences Analysis. Afterwards, the information has been synthesised into five dimensions (Fig. 1).

Graphical representation of the factors enabled interpretation of the structure of associations among the lexemes. In this way aspects not directly identifiable through reading the individual factor tables were highlighted (Geometric-structural approach).

The data collected during the focus group have been analysed through the Descending Hierarchical Classification (Reinert 1993). This method "quantifies" a text by extracting the most significant, underlying semantic structures. Thus, the differences in vocabulary refer to the different shared representations.

The age range of the "grandchildren" is between 12 and 17 while "grandparents" are over 60s.

As motivations for the participation, grandchildren stress the "fun" and "the knowledge gained about villages and natural environments" in an enlarged social dimension: "the most significant experience is to be together with others, to socialize in broad terms, not just with peers."

In young people, tourist-socio-cultural nature motivations appear prominent, while for grandparents the motivation for volunteering prevails -as a form of pro-social action- characterized by a throughout-the-year active involvement in networked entities like Caritas, Acli Provinciali of Viterbo, Pro Loco and Elderly Community Centres.

They are also interested in local history and culture. Some of them have a good geographic competence and a good propensity to use new technologies (use of digital cameras, computers and the Internet, up to the creation of the web site www.nonnienipotiviterbo.com) (Albanese and Bocci 2016a).

Facilitative Strategies for Intergenerational Tourism

Learning the use of the computer and of the digital camera as well as the use of smartphones and their apps, or experimenting with the 3D printer, together with the tourist experience, are crucial during the holiday week. In relation to new technologies, the elder experiences the role of "pupil". Similarly, the young man experiences the "wisdom" of his "grandfather" in the tourist activities of meeting the cultural and historical heritage and the local communities.

This results in an "equality of status" that, together with institutional support, cooperation for a common purpose, adequate frequency, duration of meetings and the pleasure of interaction, (Allport 1954; Brewer and Miller 1984) contributes to the successful outcome of research/interventions.

Through the learning of the new technologies mediated by the one-to-one relationship (young/elder) and the activities on the territory, the expectation is:

- the progressive modification of stereotypes and negative attributions;
- to gradually establish, during the holiday week, an empathic communication between the young and elder, typical of the grand-niece's relationship.

Intergenerational tourism produced positive outcomes regarding: the participants (with the reduction of reciprocal stereotypes, evolution of intergenerational communication, group cohesion); the hosting communities (through "generative group creativity" -planning on socio/cultural and environmental sustainability-).

Main Results

Reduction of Stereotypical Negative Attributions Between the Intergenerational Groups

The use of questionnaire technique, with regard to the overcoming of barriers and erroneous attributions between different generational groups, resulted in:

- a substantial stability in the evocation of positive attributions by young people and the elderly at the beginning and at the end of the research/interventions, and in
- a drastic reduction in stereotypical attributes with negative connotation at the end of the project.

Negative attributions expressed by young people towards grandparents in the 2010–2013 Editions, such as the vision young people have to "ready-for-scrapping grandparents" or grandparents who prefigure boys as "rude", are reduced between 30 and 40% – comparing the beginning and the end of the four research/interventions.

Reduction of such stereotypical attributes is even more evident in the images grandparents have of grandchildren. The percentage of the decrease of negative attributions in the 2010–2013 Editions exceeds 50%, reaching at times 100% (2013) with a radical change in the evaluative dimension (in attitude, in the light of Social Representation Theory) of the elderly (Albanese and Bocci 2016a).

Diadical Emphatic Communication Mediated by the Technology

In addition to the reduction of stereotypes and categorizations, it was possible to model the evolution of intergenerational communication -through the observation grids of computer lab activities- in three phases: "Approach-Knowledge-Empathy".

Grandparent/grandchildren couples at first created a predominantly cognitive, task-oriented relationship with a rigid assumption of roles leaving little space for creative and empathic exchange.

Gradually a change in the couples' approach occurred which was favoured by the new self-image of grandparents in the process of learning new technologies. This has led grandparents to perceive grandchildren no longer as out-groups, but as active partners of interaction, with whom they could engage in a more dynamic and deep communication.

In 2010, it was possible to record a gap in progressive focus reduction of cognitive aspects of communication, towards empathic aspects (Albanese and Bocci 2016a).

During the explanation of the functioning of the digital camera and computer lab lessons, grandchildren – dressed up as teachers – sought to simplify the content by inventing a language made of rhetorical figures that translate concepts into images. Communication occurs through gestures, words, messages of esteem and affection, like that of a grandchild who, using the computer lexicon, wrote: "for me it is an infinite keyboard, like the moments I would like to pass with you. I love you".

Through the anchoring (to pre-existing categories) and objectification processes (according to Theory of Social Representations) young people encouraged grandparents' positive approach to new technologies, even to the newest possible.

Some of the photo manipulations and editing results made by grandparent-niece couples showed evidence of osmosis: with different technologies, such as laptop in 2002 and a smartphone in 2016, couples worked on a faces fusion effect process (Passafaro et al. 2017) (Fig. 2).

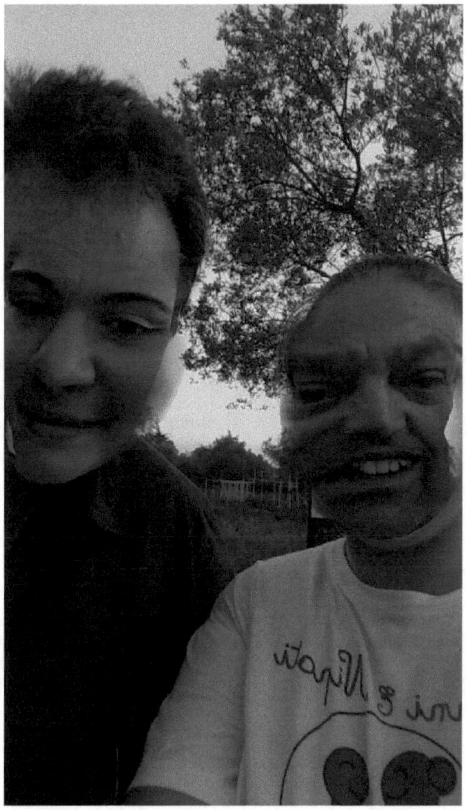

Fig. 2 The couple of participants spontaneously decided to use a specific app to produce pictures in which the facial characteristics of each one were mixed with those of the other

Group Cohesion in the Intergenerational Tourism

The rich and cohesive climate – as recorded with "associative network" technique (de Rosa 1990, 2003) around "Grandparents and Grandchildren" logo – emerges from the chart produced by the Lexical Correspondences Analysis which was applied to the list of words evoked by the research participants in 2014.

Elicited terms were subject to Lexical Correspondences Analysis.

The chart regarding the first horizontal and second vertical dimensions shows a number of references to specific elements of the 2014 experience program on the positive semi axis. This includes excursions to lakes, parks and spas close to nature where intergenerational popular games took place.

The central portion of the chart refers to those elements that characterize intergenerational tourism in general (memories, travel, nature, walks, experiences and friendly interactions).

The negative semi axis focusing on value references (communion, respect, sharing, integration, group, family, friendship, solidarity, collaboration) aimed to establish a solid and lasting intergenerational relationship.

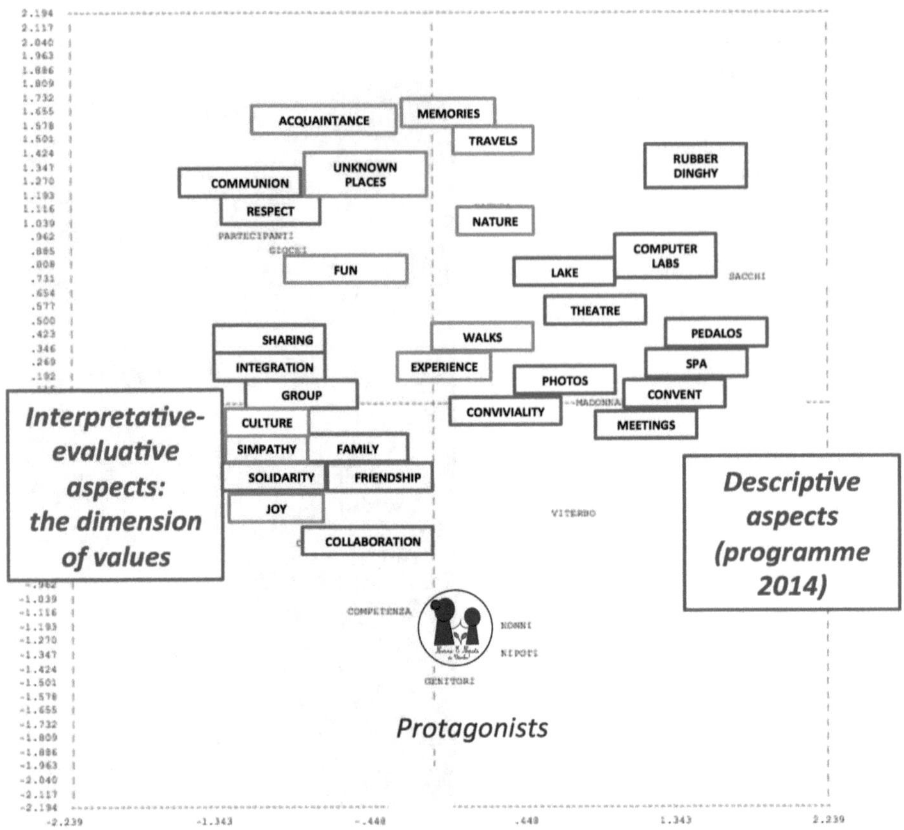

Fig. 3 Results of the Correspondences Analysis performed on the words associated to the logo by participants during 2014 Edition. (Albanese and Bocci 2014)

To summarize, it was possible to investigate the descriptive aspects of the holiday, as emphasized by young people with their preference to excursions, popular games and computer activities. Above all, it was possible to address the interpretative-evaluative component of the social representations of the logo that has mainly – but not exclusively – characterized grandparents' evocations (Albanese and Bocci 2014) (Fig. 3).

The value dimension, as the basis of integration of "present Self" of children with "past Self" of grandparents, towards a "future Self" for a better rooted and prosperous society, is also recorded through the focus group technique -as shown by the results of the 2015 Edition-.

A Descending Hierarchical Classification, applied to contents expressed by research/interventions participants during the final focus group, proposes a classification tree with four content classes.

First and third classes focus on the relationship between generations: deep values such as friendship, solidarity and fraternity persist over time and do not vanish during difficult times.

Second and fourth classes focus mainly on memories, by objectifying them through symbolism (such as a fishing net to recall activities on the lake), sharing them in poetry form or by expressing satisfaction for shared experiences.

Eventually, the act of remembering is an opportunity for appreciation towards a grandfather or a grandchild, met in the project: "I have no grandchildren by blood, but I hope and wish that, if my children give me at least one, they will be like her" (Albanese and Bocci 2016a).

Creativity and Sustainability for the Local Communities

Value and empathic elements detected by data collection techniques construct a fourth phase called "group generative creativity". Within research/interventions conducted in Viterbo those elements were expressed in terms of socio-cultural and environmental sustainability.

A few examples of deepening, reviewing and disseminating local history are:

- Participation at the short movie shooting on David Lazzaretti "The Christ of the Mountain", directed by Nicola Ragone;
- Historical re-enactment of the trial to Damiano Menichetti of Toscanella (2011);
- Theatre performances on the theme "Grandparents and Grandchildren: Tiburzi behind the legend" – with texts by Filippo Ottoni and Romualdo Luzi – staged in several cities in Northern and Central Italy from 2011.

An example of project implementations on the environmental side is the construction of two urban forests planted in Viterbo and in Cellere (Vt) in the year 2012. This was later followed up by ecological afternoons promoted by Acli Provinciali of Viterbo and was carried out by the group Grandparents and Grandchildren and other local Institutions.

The most recent challenge is the collaboration with "Solidarity Orchard" which was inaugurated in the city of Viterbo in 2016 (Passafaro et al. 2017).

"Solidarity Orchard" extends on a land of about 9000 square meters that Municipality of Viterbo has assigned to the Caritas Diocesana with the ambition of recovering and preserving a green urban area and, at the same time, create an opportunity for aggregation to favour integration, solidarity and sharing.

Within the "Solidarity Orchard" structure, Caritas has appointed the group "Grandparents and Grandchildren" to act as an active presence in terms of fraternity, friendship and collaboration with all gardeners.

This it may be concluded that on one hand the Group of Grandparents and Grandchildren uses the resources of the territory but on the other hand it contributes to the transition from "the welfare society to the welfare within the society".

This guarantees continuity to the project throughout the year and defines intergenerational tourism as "quality tourism" (Albanese and Bocci 2011) that contributed to the quality of life of the participants associated with the emotional, value and relational aspects (cfr inter alia: Schalock 1990; WHOQOL Group 1994; Cummins 1998; Shalock and Felce 2004).

Conclusions and Future Perspectives

The "Manager of Intergenerational Tourism" (post bachelor's Master as proposed by Albanese and Bocci 2012b and implemented from 2016 – Albanese and Bocci 2016b) is attentive to the dynamics of intergenerational communication and actively choose hosting communities. He is involved with studies on the quality of life in rural contexts where research/interventions occur (cfr. inter alia: Di Franco 1989; Ferrari et al. 2014; Knez and Eliasson 2017).

This innovative professional profile by designing quality research/interventions encourages the synergies in the territory. This is done in collaboration with other scholars from local communities and with local authorities, following the motto "Socialize Generations, Socializing Institutions" (Albanese 2000).

The Manager also makes use of the latest regulations, such as those referred to "Aree Interne" (National Strategy for Internal Areas) and to "Alternanza Scuola Lavoro" (School Work Alternation). From 2015/2016, the latter made it possible to enter Conventions with vocational, high and professional training schools in the hotel, tourism and agritourism sectors for intergenerational holidays in San Pellegrino Terme (Brignoli 2016) and in Val di Non (North of Italy) (Cattaneo and Fenili 2016).

In addition, intergenerational tourism research/interventions are planned for 2017/2018 in Central Italy which stimulate the internationalization of the "model" (introduced in Passafaro et al. 2017) for better quality of intergenerational communication in European contexts and encourage the dialogue among multidisciplinary inter-university network like A.R.I.P.T.Fo.R.P. and AIQUAV.

References

Albanese, A. (1999). *Prospettive e progettualità per gli anziani come strumenti di salvaguardia psicosociale*. In *I nuovi anziani e la città: scenari, prospettive e risorse*, Milano: AIM.

Albanese, A. (2000). *Linguaggi informatici e comunicazione intergenerazionale.* Milano: CUEM.

Albanese, A. (2001). *Nonn@nline.* Milano: Cuem

Albanese, A., & Bocci, E. (2009). Turismo intergenerazionale ed educazione ambientale tra ricerca e sperimentazione. Atti del XIII Congresso del Comitato Scientifico Nazione "Psicologia e Turismo" - IV Congresso Nazionale A.R.I.P.T. *Turismo e Psicologia. Rivista Interdisciplinare di Studi e Ricerche e Formazione*, 2, 117–155. (Padova: Padova University Press. ISSN: 2240-0443 (www.turismoepsicologia.it)

Albanese, A., & Bocci, E. (2011). Ricerche e sperimentazioni intergenerazionali e interculturali per un turismo sociale di qualità. Atti del XIV Congresso del Comitato Scientifico Nazionale "Psicologia e Turismo" – V Congresso Nazionale A.R.I.P.T. *Turismo e Psicologia. Rivista Interdisciplinare di Studi e Ricerche e Formazione*, 1. pp. 15. (Padova: Padova University Press. ISSN: 2240-0443 (www.turismoepsicologia.it)

Albanese, A., & Bocci, E. (2012a). Nuove strategie di ricerca-formazione manageriale: verso un turismo di qualità. Atti della Giornata di studi su "Turismo e psicologia. Dalla ricerca alla formazione per un'offerta di qualità". *Turismo e Psicologia. Rivista Interdisciplinare di Studi e Ricerche e Formazione,* 1. 117–122. (Padova: Padova University Press. ISSN: 2240-0443 (www.turismoepsicologia.it)

Albanese, A., & Bocci, E. (2012b). Il futuro manager del turismo intergenerazionale: aspetti psico-sociali. Atti della Giornata di studi su "Turismo e psicologia. Dalla ricerca alla formazione per un'offerta di qualità". *Turismo e Psicologia. Rivista Interdisciplinare di Studi e Ricerche e Formazione,* 1. 183–187. (Padova: Padova University Press. ISSN: 2240-0443 (www.turismoepsicologia.it)

Albanese, A., & Bocci, E. (2013). I modelli teorici di riferimento per un turismo intergenerazionale. *Turismo e Psicologia. Rivista Interdisciplinare di Studi e Ricerche e Formazione*, 25–35. (Padova: Padova University Press. ISSN: 2240-0443 (www.turismoepsicologia.it)

Albanese A., & Bocci, E. (2014) Dalla carente comunicazione tra le generazioni, alle ricerche/sperimentazioni di turismo intergenerazionale. *Rivista Interdisciplinare di Studi e Ricerche e Formazione,1*, 38–57 (Padova: Padova University Press. ISSN: 2240-0443 (www.turismoepsicologia.it)

Albanese, A., & Bocci, E. (2016a). Invecchiamento attivo e turismo intergenerazionale. In R. Giua e L. Dryjanska (Eds.). *Solidarietà intergenerazionale: Universo argento* (pp. 21–42). Milano: Edizioni Accademiche Italiane.

Albanese, A., & Bocci, E. (2016b). Ricerca e sperimentazione per l'orientamento alle professioni turistiche. Atti del Convegno su: "Il Counselling e l'Orientamento in Italia e in Europa". *Turismo e Psicologia. Rivista Interdisciplinare di Studi e Ricerche e Formazione*, 9, (2) 26–41 (Padova: Padova University Press. ISSN: 2240-0443 (www.turismoepsicologia.it)

Albanese, A., Facchini, C., & Vitrotti, G. (2006). *Dal lavoro al pensionamento. Vissuti, progetti*, Milano: F. Angeli.

Allport, G. (1954). *The Nature of Prejudice.* Cambridge: Addison-Wesley Publishing Co

Brewer, M., & Miller, N. (1984). Beyond the Contact Hypothesis: Theoretical perspectives on desegregation. In N. Miller e M. Brewer (Eds). *Groups in Contact: the Psychology of Desegregation.* New York: Academic Press.

Brignoli, M. (2016). La vacanza intergenerazionale a San Pellegrino Terme: nuove modalità di realizzazione finalizzate a rafforzare le sinergie interistituzionali e a rafforzare ruoli e funzioni dei Nonni e dei Nipoti. *Turismo e Psicologia. Rivista Interdisciplinare di Studi e Ricerche e Formazione*, 9, (2) 57–63. (Padova: Padova University Press. ISSN: 2240-0443 (www.turismoepsicologia.it)

Brown, R. (1988/2000). *Group processes: dynamics within and between groups.* Oxford, UK: Blackwell Publishers Ltd.

Cattaneo, G., & Fenili, C. (2016). Nonni e Nipoti a Sfruz –Val di Non (Tn): un'esperienza di vacanza intergenerazionale e alternanza scuola-lavoro. *Turismo e Psicologia. Rivista Interdisciplinare di Studi e Ricerche e Formazione*, 9, (2) 42–56. (Padova: Padova University Press. ISSN: 2240-0443 (www.turismoepsicologia.it)

Cesa-Bianchi, M. (2002). Comunicazione, creatività, invecchiamento, *Ricerche di psicologia*, n. 3, vol. 25, p. 175–188.

Cesa-Bianchi, M., & Cristini C. (2014). Come invecchiare. Dalla psicologia generale alla psicogerontologia. Roma: Aracne.

Corna-Pellegrini, G. (2005). Il viaggio come esperienza geografica e psicologica. In G. Sangiorgi (a cura di). Turista e turismi, contributi psicologici allo sviluppo del settore. *Atti del II Convegno Nazionale A.R.I.P.T.* Cagliari: Cuec., pp. 137–145.

Cummins, R. A. (1998). The second approximation to an international standard for life satisfaction, *Social Indicators Research* 43.
de Rosa, A.S. (1990). Per un approccio multi-metodo allo studio delle Rappresentazioni Sociali, *Rassegna di Psicologia*, VII (3), 101–152.
de Rosa A.S. (2003). Le « reseau d'associations » une technique pour détecter la structure, les contenus, les indices de polarité, de neutralité et de stéréotypie du champ sémantique liés aux Représentations Sociales. In J.C. Abric (Ed). *Méthodes d'étude des représentations Sociales.* (pp. 81–117). Paris: Edition Erés.
Di Franco, G. (1989). Qualità della vita: dai modelli alle ricerche empiriche. In S. Vergati (Ed.), *Dimensioni sociali e territoriali della qualità della vita* (pp. 61–96). Roma: La Goliardica.
Ferrari, M.G., Bocci, E., Bianchi, P., Cavallero, P., & Rombai, L. (2014). Qualità territoriale, ambienti e paesaggi. Età a confronto in alcune aree tosco-laziali. Atti del XIV Congresso del Comitato Scientifico Nazione "Psicologia e Turismo" - I Congresso Nazionale A.R.I.P.T.Fo.R.P. Invecchiamento e turismo. Salute, cultura, intergenerazionalità. (Brescia, 11 ottobre 2014). *Turismo e Psicologia. Rivista Interdisciplinare di Studi e Ricerche e Formazione*, 2, 171–190. Padova: Padova University Press. ISSN: 2240–0443 (www.turismoepsicologia.it)
Giua, M. (2015). Memories for ageing people. Progetto Innovation Label. Ordine Psicologi del Lazio (18 maggio 2015). Roma, Italia (www.ordinepsicologilazio.it)
Havighurst, R. J., Munnichs, J. M., Neugarten, B., & Thomae, H. (1969). *Adjustement to retirement*, Van Goram: Assen.
Knez, I., & Eliasson, I. (2017). Relationships between Personal and Collective Place Identity and Well-Being in Mountain Communities. *Front. Psychol.* 8:79.
Lewin, K. (1946) Action research and minority problems, *Social Issues*, 2, 34–46.
Mead, G.H. (1934). *Mind, Self, Society*. Chicago: Chicago University Press. (Trad. it. Mente, Sé e Società. Firenze: Editrice Universitaria, 1966)
Markus, H. (1977). Self schemata and processing information about the self. *Journal of Personality and Social Psychology*, 35 (2) 63–80.
Moscovici, S. (1961/1976). *La Psychanalyse, son Image et son Public. Étude sur la re-présentation sociale de la psychanalyse*, Paris: Presses Universitaires de France; secon-da edizione (1976). La Psychanalyse, son Image et son Public. Paris: Presses Universi-taires de France
Nenci, A. (2005). Ambienti turistici e benessere. Le possibilità rigenerative dei luoghi [Tourism environments and well-being. The restorative potentialities of places]. In G. Sangiorgi (Ed.), Turista e turismi, contributi psicologici allo sviluppo del settore [Tourist and tourisms, psychological contribution to the development of the sector]. *Proceedings of the II A.R.I.P.T. National Congress* (pp. 31–39). Cagliari, IT: Cuec.
Passafaro, P., Mura, M., Albanese, A., & Bocci, E. (2017) Potentialities and Preferences for Alternative Forms of Sustainable Tourism: The Case of Rural and Intergenerational Tourism. In R. H. Price (ed) *Ecotourism and Sustainable Tourism: Management, Opportunities and Challenges.* Nova Science Publishers, NY. (pp. 29–84). ISBN 978-1-53610-799-9.
Reinert, M. (1993). Les mondes lexicaux et leur logique à travers l'analyse statistique d'un corpus de récits de cauchemars. *Langage & Société*, 66, 5–39.
Schalock, R. (1990). *Quality of life*. Washington, DC: American Association on Mental Retardation.
Schalock, R. L., & Felce, D. (2004). Quality of Life and Subjective well being: conceptual and measurement issues. In Emerson, E. (2004). *The international handbook of applied research in intellectual disabilities*. New York: Wiley.
Serino, C. (1999). Prototipi mediterranei: prodotti e paesi [Mediterranean prototypes: products and countries]. *Proceedings of the VIII National Congress Of The Interdisciplinary Scientific Committee Of "Psychology And Tourism"*. Gorizia, IT, September, 23–26, 1999.
Sherif, M. (1966). *In common predicament: social psychology of group conflict and cooperation.* New York: Houghton Mifflin.
Tajfel, H. (1978). *Differentiation between social groups: studies in the social psychology of intergroup relations*. London: Academic Press.

Tajfel, H. (1981). *Human groups and social categories.* Cambridge Uk: Cambridge University Press.
WHOQOL Group. (1994). WHOQOL Group, The Development of the World Health Organization Quality of Life Assessment Instrument. In J. Orley & W. Kuyken, (Eds.) *Quality of life assessment: International perspectives*, pp. 41–57. Berlin: Springer.

Territories and Landscapes: Place Identity, Quality of Life and Psychological Well-Being in Rural Areas

Maria Gabriella Ferrari, Elena Bocci, Erika Lepisto, Paola Cavallero, and Leonardo Rombai

Abstract Different perspectives describe different characteristics related to the places of daily life: "territories" spatial-geographical areas with material and concrete dimensions, "landscape" environmental areas as perceived by the inhabitants, with cognitive, affective, social and aesthetical meanings. In the environmental psychology the term "place identity" means the aspects of the image of Itself in relationship to the meanings and in partnership values to a physical environment.

In the Central Italy there are historically and culturally recognized geographical areas, of rural-agricultural tradition, rich in natural landscapes and historical-

M. G. Ferrari (✉)
Department of Neurosciences, Psychology, Drug Research and Child Health (NEUROFARBA), University of Florece, Florence, Italy
e-mail: mg.ferrari@unifi.it

Association of Interdisciplinary Research in Psychology of Tourism: Training, Research and Planning (A.R.I.P.T. Fo.R.P.), Milan, Italy
e-mail: mg.ferrari@unifi.it

E. Bocci
Department of Developmental and Social Psychology, Sapienza University of Rome, Rome, Italy

Association of Interdisciplinary Research in Psychology of Tourism: Training, Research and Planning (A.R.I.P.T. Fo.R.P.), Milan, Italy
e-mail: elena.bocci@uniroma1.it

E. Lepisto
Department of developmental and social psychology, Sapienza University of Rome, Rome, Italy
e-mail: erikalepisto91@gmail.com

P. Cavallero
Association of Interdisciplinary Research in Psychology of Tourism: Training, Research and Planning (A.R.I.P.T. Fo.R.P.), Milan, Italy
e-mail: paolacavallero@alice.it

L. Rombai
History, Archaeology, Geography, Fine and Performing Arts (SAGAS), University of Florence, Florence, Italy
e-mail: leonardorombai@gmail.com

A. Bianco et al. (eds.), *Italian Studies on Quality of Life*, Social Indicators Research Series 77, https://doi.org/10.1007/978-3-030-06022-0_19

cultural remembrances, like Lunigiana, Media Valle del Serchio, Crete Senesi and Maremma, these territories are considered traditionally marginal and disadvantaged. The study investigates to understand how "everyday landscapes" and the on-going processes of change are perceived by the inhabitants also in relation with Quality of Life. The results presented showed distinctions between different age groups examined: youth, adults and elderly.

Territory and Landscape

The terms territory and landscape, although applying to the same spatial units, refer to different perspectives and involve complex, multi-meaning concepts.

"Territory" denotes a spatial and geographical area which is subject to management and transformation measures in terms of living environment. In geography, territory refers to a space controlled and altered by the civilizations that lived and live in it and includes the idea of physical or administrative "boundaries" (Sack 1986). As to the specific natural and anthropic elements, territory can be defined as a "circumscribed space with a communitarian dimension" (Banini 2013).

The notion of territorial representation or image is similar to the concept of "landscape", a term used by the European Landscape Convention (2000) to designate parts of territory as perceived by their inhabitants. This also involves the conception of cognitive, affective and aesthetic meanings and importance for the quality of life (Council of Europe 2000).

The Italian territory is pervaded by geographical areas, predominantly rural, that are historically and culturally recognizable. They are composed of municipalities and share similar anthropological, historical and geographical characteristics (Rombai 2001; Regione Toscana 2015).

These territories are still mainly intact: mountainous fields, hilly and flat countryside or coastal and insular areas/regions. However, their physical characteristics and the morphological, hydrographical, climatic conditions related to animal and vegetable patrimony vary significantly. Moreover, historical inheritance of several ancient civilizations is evident in the smaller urban areas with rich civil and religious architectures. They reveal the archaeological and artistic heritages of the long period between ancient and contemporary times.

In the Central Italy, particularly in the central Tyrrhenian area – the ancient Etruscan and later Romanised region – there are landscapes that are rich of historical-cultural remembrances (historical-geografical rural areas). The focus of the present work is on such landscapes: the Lunigiana (high and middle valley of river Magra), Media Valle of river Serchio, Crete Senesi, Maremma of Tuscany (Grossetana) and of Lazio (Viterbese).

In the current society the geographical and natural characteristics, the historical-cultural elements, the urban and productive installations shape the look of the territories affecting the place attachment and, subsequently, the quality of life (Carta et al. 2012) and psychological well-being (Ryff and Keyes 1995; Ruini et al. 2003).

The multi-disciplinary research presupposes that the territory, described by geographers and aesthetically and symbolically appreciated by the inhabitants, may be better understood if studied from a psycho-social perspective in relation to the quality of life of individuals and communities.

It is highlighted the importance of sharing the results of research not only in the academic sphere, but also with stakeholders of the territory, to outline together "possible futures" (Testa 2017).

Background

In "Person-Environment-Behaviour" (PEB) relationships, Ittelson (1973 pag.18) notes that: "man is never encountered independent of the situation through which he acts, nor is the environment ever encountered independent of the encountering individual". To understand PEB relationships means studying people, their place attachment, their future intentions as well as the physical settings in which they live and act.

From a psycho-social point of view, our focus is on quality of life and on psychological well-being in relation to the environment (Bonnes and Secchiaroli 1992; Twigger-Ross and Uzzell 1996) in rural areas by considering the importance of living in suitable environments, fitting needs and expectations (Zani and Cicognani 2000).

Consistent with the "biophilia hypothesis" (Wilson 1984; Kellert and Wilson 1993; Ulrich 1993) the literature provides ample accounts of the positive influence of natural environment on physical health (cfr. Inter alia: Ulrich, 1984; Cooper-Marcus and Barnes 1999; Velarde et al. 2007).

Also from a psychological perspective (Wohlwill 1983; Kaplan and Kaplan 1989; Kaplan 1995; Hartig 2003, 2004; Berto 2005; Lafortezza et al. 2009; Scopelliti et al. 2016; Carrus et al. 2017), contact with nature brings about positive psycho-physical effects. Indeed, as Grinde and Patil (2009 pag. 2335) pointed out, contact with nature seem to reduce stress and improve people's attention and mental state.

The research distinguishes between the satisfaction of living in rural/urban areas (Saporiti 2016) and focuses on the benefits of nature in the cities as an important component of urban inhabitant's attachment (Bonnes et al. 2004) and quality of life (Burgess et al. 1988). But it also highlights some ambivalent attitudes towards nature in the city in terms of "appreciation" and "devaluation" (Bonnes et al. 2011).

General preferences for rural areas seem associated with the cognitive and emotional bond of place identity (Proshansky 1978; Proshansky et al. 1983). By focusing on rural and mountain sites, Knez and Eliasson (2017 pag. 1) the attention is drawn to the fact that: "Definitions of landscape include not only objective natural characteristics (Turner 1989), but also subjective human views, perceptions, identifications and memories (Knez 2006; Knez and Thorsson 2008; Lewicka 2008)". In fact, the results of the study conducted by Knez and Eliasson (2017) in mountain communities have shown that residents have individually and collectively pinpointed their favourite sites in mountains to which they have evolved emotional and cognitive bonds. In this context, the subjects perceive and experience high levels of well-being associated with a cognitive and emotional bond of place-identity.

According to their results: "the stronger the attachment/closeness/belonging (emotional component of place identity) residents felt to favourite personal and collective sites the more well-being they perceived when visiting these places. Similarly, the more remembrance, thinking and mental travel (cognitive component of place identity) residents directed to these sites the more well-being they perceived in these places. In both types of sites well-being was more strongly predicted by emotional than cognitive component of place-identity" (Knez and Eliasson, 2017 pag. 1).

The importance of closeness has been emphasised by Hidalgo and Hernàndez (2001) by discussing the desire to maintain closeness to the object of attachment.

By incorporating closeness into the previous definition of place attachment (Shumaker and Taylor 1983) Hidalgo and Hernàndez (2001 pag. 274) state: "it could take the following form: a positive affective bond between an individual and a specific place, the main characteristic of which is the tendency of the individual to maintain closeness to such a place".

Due to its multi-dimensionality, the place attachment has been synthesized by Scannell and Gifford (2010) in a comprehensive model, including many aspects into three dimensions: "Person–Place-Process" (PPP Framework).

In particular, the psychological process dimension refers to: the emotional component of place attachment (Hidalgo and Hernàndez 2001), the cognitive component – memories, beliefs, meaning, and knowledge – (Proshansky 1978) and actions to maintain closeness to places as indicated by Hidalgo and Hernàndez (2001).

The bond to lived places (i.e. emotional, cognitive and actions aspect) is challenged by the demands of the contemporary society as they affect the perception of the environmental changes.

Currently, many *non places* (Augé, 1992) surround urban areas so that mountain and countryside areas risk to become "new" places of uncertain destiny, if transformation does not respect valuable landscape elements and is carried out without considering sustainability and social sharing.

In these places, people and communities may not develop a sense of attachment due to the environmental transformations as they may negatively affect their historical and cultural settings. Subsequently, the places become less familiar (Mazza and Minozzi 2011) and may led to phenomena of deterioration and of abandonment.

Studying the bond with the territory, Castiglioni (2016) investigates the psycho-social relapse of the type of territorial management.

She highlights the differences (in terms of opinions, practices, but also attachment) among citizens of North-eastern Italian territories: "institutional landscapes" managed by institutions and experts, versus "everyday landscapes" managed by the whole community and continuously subject to transformations.

She finds that "institutional landscapes" produce a detriment to the creation of a sense of personal attachment, due to the fact that citizens are not involved; while the position of people as "insiders" in "everyday landscapes" results in a "sense of belonging", "affective bonds" and "social relations" (strong place attachment), even if there is often little awareness.

Therefore, Castiglioni (2016 pag. 37) proposes that: "an increase of awareness of different sets of values existing in a landscape seems the most appropriate strategy to overcome the opposition between the two landscape ideas and the questions of landscape change, through a wide process of 'landscape literacy', focused to the acquisition of a way to 'look at' the landscape and to act responsibly on it".

Based on research findings mentioned above, the aim of this study is to assess the impact of "everyday landscapes" on place identity, quality of life and psychological well-being for the rural inhabitants of specific areas in Central Italy. These territories are characterized by that type of natural and historical-cultural landscapes that unite natural habitats, outstanding natural beauties, farming and forestry lands with historical and cultural traces (cf. inter alia: Sestini 1963; Sereni 1984).

In the last century, as a consequence of industrialization, these areas have also been experienced different degrees of urbanization which have not always respected the dimensions of landscape and historical-cultural.

Objectives

The research investigates at an exploratory level some rural areas in Central Italy, from hills to mountain and coastal areas in Tuscany and Northern Lazio, in order to understand how "everyday landscapes" and the on-going processes of change are perceived.

The objective is to investigate how the inhabitants of Lunigiana, Media Valle of river Serchio, Crete Senesi and Maremma express their place identity, including its cognitive and emotional components:

- cognitive component: knowledge of the specific places of the territory and their history, local dialect and values attributed to the everyday landscape elements as well as to elements of degradation;
- emotional component: attachment/belonging/closeness.

As Knez and Eliasson (2017) the cognitive and emotional components of place identity are considered in relation to quality of life and psychological well-being about "everyday landscapes".

Historical-Geografical Rural Areas Research Context

In almost all the Italian, and particularly Tuscan and Lazio extra-urban or rural territories, the physical and natural elements are strongly linked to the historical and cultural ones. Traces, identities, material and immaterial memories are the result of

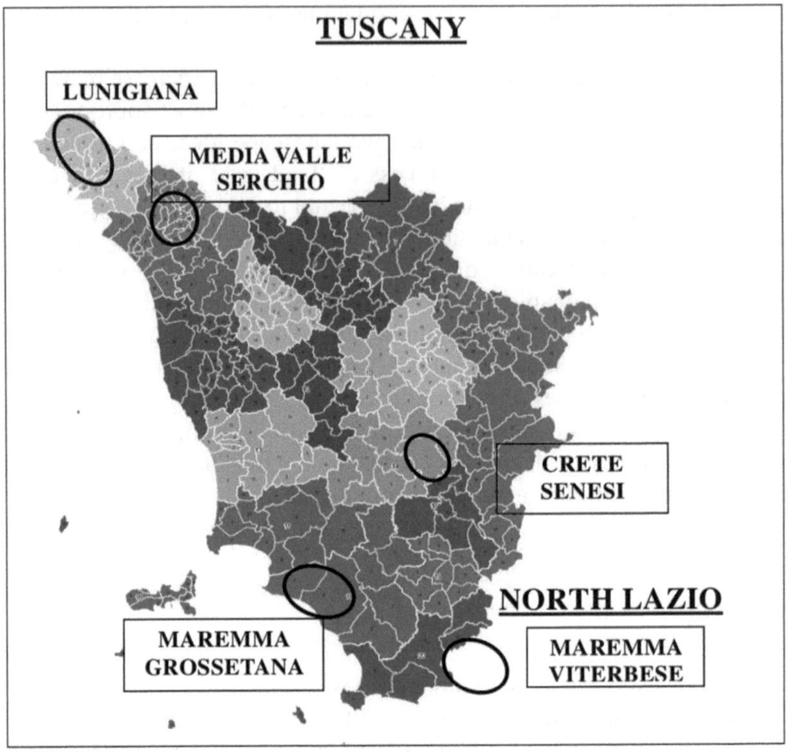

Fig. 1 Tuscany region and North Lazio: historical-geographical areas under study. (Adapted from the Regional Landscape Plan of Tuscany, 2015)

three millennia of human history and the high influence of urban pressure that have shaped environments of unquestionable landscape value (Fig. 1).

These rural areas are high nature-value territories and they preserve the historical heritage of infinite civilizations from prehistory till today. But although they are not immune from the risks and degradation.

LUNIGIANA (LUN): – The northernmost part of Tuscany, a mountainous area in the province of Massa Carrara, on the border between Emilia and Liguria, and extending between the Tuscan-Ligurian Apennines, and the high ridges of the Tuscan-Emilian Appennines and the Apuan Alps, is crossed by the valley of the river Magra, coinciding with the ancient Via Francigena. It includes parts of the Tuscan-Emilian Apennines National Park and of the Regional Natural Park of the Apuan Alps, an area of very high naturalistic interest with sharp peaks, just a few kilometres from the sea. It is also characterized by ancient villages and medieval castles and villas and houses of the eighteenth century. In the lower valley of the river there are some industrialized areas, but no large commercial areas.

MEDIA VALLE of the river Serchio (MVS) – On the border with the Lucchesia–mountain, wooded and hilly area of the province of Lucca, flanked to the south by the city of Lucca and to the north by the Garfagnana, in between the Tuscan-Emilian Apennines and the Apuan Alps. It stretches along the banks of the river Serchio. Downstream there are some recent industrialized areas.

CRETE SENESI (CRETE) – Tuscany's geographical area in the south-east of Siena. It is difficult to point out its exact limits because the administrative boundaries do not coincide with the specific physical-natural features of the clay area. It means that some parts belong to nearby territorial areas. The name "Crete" comes from clay – or argil – component of the area's soil, which gives the landscape its characteristic colours depending on the season. The economy benefits from farming and family farm activities. The landscape is intact and healthy as there are no industrialized or commercial areas.

MAREMMA – The geographical area of Maremma extends for approximately 5000 sq. Km covering southern Tuscany and Northern Lazio, and is divided into Maremma Grossetana and Maremma Laziale, mosaic of environments and colours due to the variety of landscapes.

MAREMMA GROSSETANA (MAR.GR.) – Hilly, flat and coastal area of southern Tuscany overlooking the Tyrrhenian Sea, in the province of Grosseto. It extends from the Gulf of Follonica to the north to the border with the Lazio region. From the coast the southern islands of the Tuscan Archipelago are visible. Ancient villages are present in the inland such as Pitigliano or on the coast like Castiglione della Pescaia. Some industrial and commercial areas are located in the north.

MAREMMA VITERBESE (MAR.VT.) – The northernmost area of Lazio at the borders with Tuscany, in the province of Viterbo. Valentano is located in the Volsini mountain chain, near the Lake Bolsena and about 30 km from the Tyrrhenian Sea. The surrounding natural environment is still intact, with important prehistoric testimonies of the Bronze Age and the small lake of Mezzano. The economy of the area is still predominantly based on agriculture and livestock farming, with an emphasis on ancient agro-food productions. Industries and businesses are poorly developed.

Methodology

Procedure, Tool and Data Analysis

The data collection took place in the period 2015–2016, with an anonymous and self-administered *ad hoc* questionnaire (Ferrari et al. 2014). In each territory, it was asked to consider the historical-geographical area of belonging. The questionnaire is divided into four sections in order to investigate:

A. cognitive component: knowledge of the specific places of the territory and the history, local dialect and value attributed to the everyday landscape elements as well as to the elements of degradation;
B. emotional component: attachment/belongingness/closeness;
C. quality of life and psychological well-being;
D. socio-demographic data.

As to the types of items referring to different territories, the cognitive component was explored: the knowledge and awareness of "everyday landscapes" including multiple choices items (for example: Thinking about your Territory how much do you think you know it? Not at all/slightly/somewhat /much/very much) and single items on a scale from 0 to 10.

For the evaluation of the emotional component, at first the single item method with dichotomous answer was used (Trentin 1991): Do you identify "..." as your geographic territory of belonging? Yes/No with subsequent request to specify the reasons – open question – (for example: Are you able to synthetically motivate your choice of answer, why you feel or do not you feel bound to this territory?).

Later, for psycho-social constructs related to place identity: for place attachment/belongingness a series of 30 items was applied, on a 5-point Likert scale, from "0 = strongly disagree" to "4 = strongly agree".

These items were adapted from two studies. The first evaluated attachment to the neighbourhood (Fornara et al. 2010), through 8 items related to rooting, personal identity and social identity. Some examples of these items are: "This is an ideal territory for me", "I would find it difficult to leave this territory", "I recognize myself in the people of this territory".

Additional 22 items were derived from the model of Raymond et al. (2010), which identifies the connection with the place of belonging in natural and rural contexts. Some examples of these items are: "This is the best territory for the activities I enjoy", "I feel that this territory is a part of me", "The friendships developed through sporting activities in this territory are very important to me".

Moreover, in order to assess the tendency of the individual to maintain closeness with the place of daily life, participants were asked about the intentions of future residence. This was done by using the single item followed by the open question on the motivations: "I would like to spend the rest of my life in this territory: No/In part/Yes. Can you synthetically motivate your choice of answer?"

Answers to open questions have been categorized through semantic categories, following the method of content analysis (Losito 2002).

Descriptive analyses were performed; the subjects were compared by the four territorial areas, and by age group using test chi^2, ANOVA test and post-hoc tests.

Structure and reliability for the two dimensions of place identity: "place attachment" and "belongingness" were tested by item analysis, some exploratory factor analyses (Principal Component Analysis) and Cronbach's alpha test.

Item analysis eliminated some non-discriminant items, and with the principal component analysis and the reliability analyses, for the place-attachment scale a 6-item scale was obtained (KMO index = .854; explained total variance = 55.352% and Cronbach's Alpha reliability = .821).

For the belongingness scale a 13-item scale was obtained (KMO index = .880; explained total variance = 55.858% and Cronbach's Alpha reliability = .783).

From these procedures, a measure for place attachment and one for belongingness were obtained through average scores (with range 0–4).

The Sample

The study sample consists of 366 inhabitants of the four territorial areas and sub-areas (Table 1). Data collection was performed in municipalities in the following areas:

1 – LUNIGIANA (n = 125) – High Valley of river Magra (LUN HVM): Pontremoli, Filattiera (n = 58) and Middle Valley of river Magra (LUN MVM): Aulla – (n = 67),

2 – MEDIA VALLE of the river Serchio (MVS): Borgo a Mozzano (n = 15),

3 – CRETE SENESI: Asciano (n = 86),

Table 1 Research sample (n = 366): inhabitants of historical-geographical rural areas, research context

Variable	Modality	f	%
Gender	M	179	48.9
	F	187	51.1
Age years: M=43.2 ± 21.5			
Age classes	Youth (14–24)	110	30.0
	Adults (25–64)	173	47.3
	Elderly (>65)	83	22.7
Territories	1 – Lunigiana (n=125)		
	High Valley of Magra	58	15.8
	Middle Valley of Magra	67	18.3
	2 – Media Valle of Serchio	15	4.1
	3 – Crete Senesi	86	23.6
	4 – Maremma (n=140)		
	Grossetana	37	10.1
	Viterbese	103	28.1
Place of birth	Native	289	79.0
	Non native	77	21.0
Total		N = 366	100.0

f frequencies; % percentage

4 – MAREMMA (n = 140) – grossetana (MAR.GR.): Grosseto, Castiglione della Pescaia (n = 37) and Maremma viterbese (MAR.VT): Cellere and Valentano (n = 103).

48.9% of the respondents were male and 51.1% female. The age was in between 14 and 88 years, mean 43.2 (sd = 21.5), of which 30.0% young adults, 47.3% adults, 22.7% elderly people.

79.0% of the participants are native of the place, in each territory: Lunigiana 90/125 (72.0%), Media Valle of the Serchio 15/15 (100.0%), Crete 67/86 (77.9%), Maremma 117/140 (83.6%).

Results

Section A. Cognitive Component

A medium-high level of knowledge of the territory is highlighted in the answers provided by the total sample: knowledge of the territory, its history and local dialect, as well as high appreciation of the natural and historical-cultural elements (Table 2). Regarding the responses for the individual territories it is noted that:

Table 2 Cognitive component: knowledge of the specific places of the territory and the history, local dialect and territorial differences (chi^2)

Cognitive component	Total (n=366) N (%)	Lunigiana (n=125) N (%)	Media Valle Serchio (n=15) N (%)	Crete (n=86) N (%)	Maremma (n=140) N (%)	Chi2 (df; p)
Knowledge of Territory						
Very much-Much	171 (46.7)	54 (43.5)	3 (20.0)	36 (42.4)	78 (55.7)	
Somewhat	162 (44.3)	61 (49.2)	10 (66.7)	40 (47.1)	51 (36.4)	
Not at all/slightly	31 (8.5)	9 (7.3)	2 (13.3)	9 (10.6)	11 (7.9)	10.879 (6; .092)
Knowledge of territorial history						
Very Much-Much	83 (22.7)	30 (24.0)	3 (20.0)	19 (22.1)	31 (24.0)	
Somewhat	167 (45.6)	71 (56.8)	5 (33.3)	29 (33.7)	62 (48.1)	
Not at all/slightly	105 (28.7)	24 (19.2)	7 (46.7)	38 (44.2)	36 (27.9)	18.939 (6; .004)
Local Dialect						
Very much-Much	113 (30.9)	29 (23.0)	3 (20,0)	36 (41,9)	45 (34.9)	
Somewhat	87 (23.8)	27 (21.6)	2 (13.3)	21 (24,4)	37 (28.7)	
Not at all/slightly	155 (42.3)	69 (55.2)	10 (66.7)	29 (33.7)	47 (36.4)	17.913 (6; .006)

Table 3 Cognitive component: evaluation in average values of landscape elements (natural and historical–cultural) and territorial differences (ANOVA)

Evaluation elements	Total (n=366)	Lunigiana (n=125)	Media Valle Serchio (n=15)	Crete (n=86)	Maremma (n=140)	
	m (SD)	m (SD)	m (SD)	m (SD)	m (SD)	F(df); p
Natural (range 0–10)	8.7 (1.3)	8.6 (1.2)	7.9 (1.8)	8.8 (1.3)	8.8 (1.0)	F(3.362) = 2.453; p=.063
Historical–Cultural (range 0–10)	8.1 (1.7)	8.1 (1.5)	7.5 (1.4)	7.6 (1.9)	8.5 (1.5)	F(3.353)=5.43; p=.001

m mean; *SD* standard deviation; *F* ANOVA

for the knowledge of the specific places of the territory, the participants claim to know the territory “Very much”, “much” and “somewhat” in Lunigiana 92.7%, in Maremma 92.1%, in Media Valle 86.7%, in Crete 89.5% (p = N.S.);

they affirm to know the history of territory “Very much”, “much” and “somewhat” in Lunigiana 80.8%, in Maremma 72.1%, in Crete 55.8%, in Media Valle 53.3% (p = .004);

about the local dialect they claim to know it: “Very much”, “much” and “somewhat” in Crete 66.3%, Maremma 63.6%, Lunigiana 44.6% and Media Valle Serchio 33.3%. Furthermore in Media Valle 66.7% and in Lunigiana 55.2% they speak it Not at all/slightly (p = .006).

The value attributed to the everyday landscape’s natural and historical/cultural elements and to the elements of degradation was also examined (Table 3).

regarding the evaluation of natural elements on a scale from 0 to 10, Table 3 shows that the levels are very high in all territories, in particular in Maremma (M = 8.8, SD = 1.0), while they are slightly inferior in Crete (M = 8.8, SD = 1.3) and in Lunigiana (M = 8.6, sd = 1.2). The lowest values, albeit always high, have been found in Media Valle Serchio (M = 7.9, SD = 1.8) with no significant difference among the four territories (F(3.362) = 2.453; p = .06).

For the historical/cultural elements the highest values have been found in Maremma (M = 8.5, SD = 1.5) and slightly inferior in Crete (M = 7.6, SD = 1.9) and in Lunigiana (M = 8.1, SD = 1.5). The lowest values, albeit always high, have been found in Media Valle Serchio. (M = 7.5, SD = 1.4). A significant difference among the four territories has been found (F(3.353) = 5.43; p = .001), post-hoc test: Crete/Maremma (p = .001).

By providing the respondents nine categories (on a scale from “0 = no degradation” to “10 = maximum degradation”), i.e. the main ones considered as sources of pollution and environmental degradation, very complex results were obtained as shown in the Graph 1.

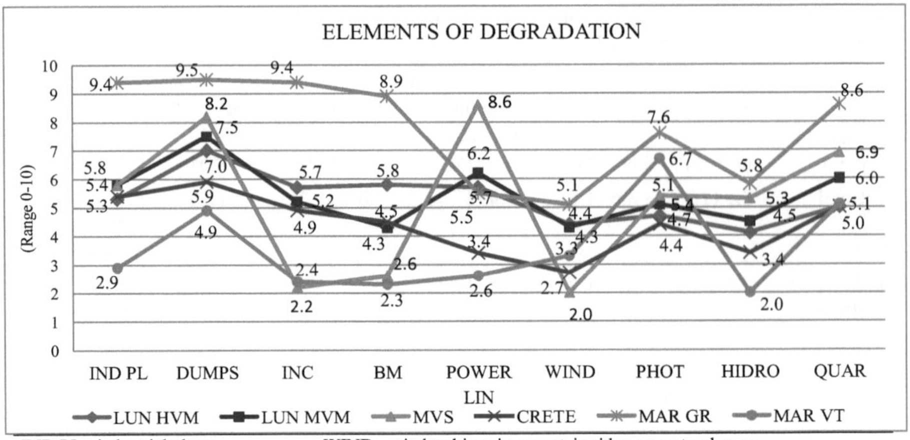

IND PL - industrial plants	WIND - wind turbines in mountain ridges or natural areas
DUMPS – dumps	PHOT - photovoltaic panels in agricultural lands or natural areas
INC - incinerators	HYDRO - hydroelectric stations on rivers
BM - biomass power stations	QUAR - quarries of mineral resources or other materials
POWER LIN - Power lines	

Graph 1 Perception of the elements of landscape degradation. (Lunigiana High an Middle Valley Magra; LUN HVM and LUN MVM); Media valle Serchio MVS; Crete Senesi: CRETE; Maremma grossetana: MAR GR; Maremma Viterbese: MAR VT)

In this graph the territorial subdivision among territorial areas has been maintained: Lungiana: high and middle valley of Magra river and Maremma Grossetana and Maremma Viterbese to explore the experience of the specific elements of degradation, derived by different industrial plants in the sub-areas.

Respondents are most concerned about the factors already present in their area and the inhabitants of the Maremma Grossetana are those who worry the most.

Moreover, elements of degradation are extracted from the open question: "Do you believe that other elements of environmental or sanitary risks may increase in your territory? If yes, can you specify which?" Some answers have pointed out further elements of environmental worry: land abandonment, hydro-geological instability, land consumption, pollution, overbuilding, coastal erosionn and sea pollution, increased use of herbicides and pesticides.

Section B – Emotional Component

The emotional component has been assessed through two different methodologies: the single item method with dichotomous answer (Table 4) and the Likert scale (Table 5).

Table 4 Emotional component: specific place, sense of belonging and territorial differences (chi^2)

Emotional component	Total (n=366) N (%)	Lunigiana (n=125) N (%)	Media Valle Serchio (n=15) N (%)	Crete (n=86) N (%)	Maremma (n=140) N (%)	Chi2 (df; p)
Sense of belonging						
Yes	338 (92.3)	118 (94.4)	14 (93.3)	72 (83.7)	134 (95.7)	
No	28 (7.65)	7 (5.6)	1 (6.7)	14 (16.3)	6 (4.3)	12.071 (3; .007)
Specific place						
Yes	322 (87.9)	113 (90.4)	13 (100)	71 (82.6)	125 (89.9)	
No	41 (11.2)	12 (9.6)	-	15 (17.4)	14 (10.1)	5.465 (3; .141)

Table 5 Emotional component: place attachment and belongingness in average values and territorial differences. (ANOVA)

Emotional component	Total (n = 366) m(SD)	Lunigiana (n=125) m(SD)	Media Valle Serchio (n = 15) m(SD)	Crete (n = 86) m(SD)	Maremma (n = 140) m(SD)	F (df); p
Place attachment (range 0–4)	2.9 (.87)	2.7 (.82)	2.7 (.85)	2.7 (1.04)	3.2 (.71)	F(3.365) = 8.113;p <.000
Belongingness (range 0–4)	2.6 (.72)	2.5 (.67)	2.5 (.96)	2.5 (.79)	2.9 (.65)	F(3.365) = 8.704;p <.000

m mean, *SD* standard deviation, *F* ANOVA

According to the answers of the single items the respondents perceive the territory in which they live as a place of belonging in the 92.3% of cases. The largest percentage is recorded in Maremma 95.7%, followed by Lunigiana 94.4%, Media Valle 93.3% and the Crete 83.7% (p=.007).

Moreover, for the sense of belonging to a specific place, the majority of people (87.9%) expresses a feeling of belonging. In particular: Media Valle 100%, Lunigiana 90.4%, Maremma 89.9%, Crete 82.6%. (p = N.S.).

The motivations of belonging refer to concepts like: "place of birth and childhood", "origins, generational roots", "I live, choose to live there", "well-being, I am fine", "beauty, nature charm, uncontaminated landscapes", "tranquillity and healthiness", "natural", "attachment bond", "belongingness, it is my land", "memories and affections, place of childhood and adolescence", "family ties", "social relationships, valid social context", "rich in history, traditions and culture".

Those who do not express a sense of belonging (7.65%) give reasons such as: "it is not my place of origin", "disagree with environmental management policies", "land of poverty, suffering and migrants".

Through the Likert Scale the following results for the constructs of place attachment and belongingness were obtained (Table 5):

Table 6 Emotional component: closeness operationalized as intentions of future residence: "In this area I would like to spend the rest of my life" and territorial differences (chi^2)

Closeness: "Intentions of future residence"	Total (n = 366) N (%)	Lunigiana (n = 125) N (%)	Media Valle Serchio (n = 15) N (%)	Crete (n = 86) N (%)	Maremma (n = 140) N (%)	Chi2 (df; p)
Yes	166 (45.6)	67 (54.5)	10 (66.7)	26 (30.2)	63 (45.5)	
In Part	157 (43.1)	41 (33.3)	5 (33.3)	41 (47.7)	70 (50.0)	
No	41 (11.2)	15 (11.2)	-	19 (22.1)	7 (5.0)	28.676 (6; .000)

Note: not all subjects answer to all questions

for place attachment (from 0 = extremely low to 4 = extremely high) the highest values have been found in Maremma (M = 3.2, SD = .71), in Crete (M = 2.7, SD = 1.04), in Media Valle (M = 2.7, SD = .85) and in Lunigiana (M = 2.7, SD = .82); ($F_{(3.365)} = 8.113$; $p < .000$) post-hoc test: Maremma/Lunigiana ($p < .000$) Maremma/Crete (p = .003);

for belongingness (from 0 = extremely low to 4 = extremely high) the results are: Maremma (M = 2.9, SD = .65), Lunigiana (M = 2.5, SD = .67), Media Valle (M = 2.5, SD = .96) and Crete (M = 2.5, SD = .79); ($F_{(3.365)} = 8.704$; $p < .000$) post-hoc test: Maremma/Lunigiana (p = .001) Maremma/Crete ($p < .000$).

The closeness was assessed as "intentions of future residence" in the specific territory (Table 6). We found that: 45.6% is willing to stay, while 43.1% intends to remain only "in part" and the remaining 11.3% wants to leave (Chi^2: $p < .000$).

The details of the three response choices showed that people wanting to stay correspond to the following percentages: Media Valle 66.7%, Lunigiana 54.5%, Maremma 45.5% and Crete 30.2%. The answer "In part" was recorded respectively: in Maremma 50.0% and in Crete 47.7% and both in Lunigiana and Media Valle 33.3% (Chi^2: $p < .000$).

In relation to the closeness as intention of future residence, the relation between age and closeness was further investigated. By verifying the answer by age, as regards future intentions of residence, the majority of the elderly (53.0%) intends to remain, followed by adults (48.3%) and then young people (35.8%). As to the "in part" answers, the percentages are: adults 48.8%, elderly 44.6% and finally young people 33.0%. It is also noted that young people are rather evenly distributed along the three response options and that they do not take for granted a future departure from the place of origin.

It suggests that young people who do not foresee a future residence in the area, are willing to go away not because they dislike where they live, but because they feel the need to experience other places and other opportunities. This is supported by the high percentage of young people who report their sense of belonging (88.2%),their medium-high level of attachment (M = 2.56, sd = .95) belongingness (M = 2.36, sd = .72), and the value they give the natural (M = 8.37, sd = 1.35) and cultural-historical elements (M = 7.42, sd = 1.86).

The motivations expressed by those who wish to reside in the territory are consistent with their stated sense of belonging; the motivations for wanting "in part" to stay reveal a conflict, particularly in young people, between living in a loved and valued place, looking for new jobs and relational opportunities or wanting to travel and make new experiences. Finally, the motivations reported by the few subjects who do not intend to stay refer to: lack of job opportunities and relational difficulties in the social community.

Section C. Quality of Life and Psychological Well-being

As to the quality of life the results are "Very much", "much" and "somewhat" Maremma 98.6%, Lunigiana 92.0%, Media Valle 86.7%, Crete 84.9% ($p < .000$).

For the psychological well-being "Very much", "much" and "somewhat" Maremma 98.6%, Lunigiana 94.3%, Media Valle 93.3%, Crete 87.2% ($p < .001$) (Table 7).

Consistent with the findings of recent studies (Knez and Eliasson 2017) the results of the present study suggest that the cognitive and emotional components of place identity play an active role in the quality of life and psychological well-being.

In fact, in this section the results were coherent with the those previously presented in sections A and B.

Table 7 Quality of life, psychological well-being and territorial differences (chi^2)

	Total (n = 366) 1	Lunigiana (n = 125)	Media Valle Serchio (n = 15)	Crete (n = 86)	Maremma (n = 140)	
	N (%)	N (%)	N (%)	N (%)	N (%)	Chi2 (df; p)
Quality of life						
Very much-Much	250 (68.3)	90 (72.6)	9 (60.0)	43 (50.0)	108 (78.3)	
Somewhat	86 (23.5)	24 (19.4)	4 (26.7)	30 (34.9)	28 (20.3)	
Not at all/slightly	27 (7.4)	10 (8.1)	2 (13.3)	13 (15.1)	2 (1.4)	27.131 (6; .000)
Psychological well-being						
Very much-Much	257 (70.2)	96 (77.4)	9 (60.0)	43 (50.0)	109 (79.0)	
Somewhat	85 (23.2)	21 (16.9)	5 (33.3)	32 (37.2)	27 (19.6)	
Not at all/slightly	21 (5.7)	7 (5.6)	1 (8.7)	11 (12.8)	2 (1.4)	30.096 (6; .000)

Note: not all subjects answered to all questions

Considering the differences already highlighted between Maremma and Lunigiana, in both territories elevated values have been found regarding knowledge of the territory and the history together with belongingness. This is consistent with the high values registered for quality of life and psychological well-being.

The same coherence has been noted for the territories of Media Valle Serchio and Crete, presenting less elevated levels of quality of life/psychological well-being and less elevated levels in both the cognitive and emotional components of place identity. However, on the whole a general appreciation for "everyday landscapes" was found.

Finally, the quality of life and psychological well-being associated with the cognitive and emotional components of place identity were assessed.

In fact, in the total sample ($n = 366$) positive correlations are highlighted between: attachment and psychological well-being ($rho = .534$; $p < .01$), attachment and quality of life ($rho = .407$; $p < .01$), belongingness and psychological well-being ($rho = ,551$; $p < .01$); belongingness and quality of life ($rho = .460$; $p < .01$).

Interestingly, the inhabitants of Maremma have the highest scores in place identity, quality of life and psychological well-being, but they, especially the inhabitants from Maremma Grossetana, are also the most concerned about elements of degradation.

In other territories the concern is more associated with present elements or new industrial installations, but it is generally expressed with smaller intensity.

This emphasises the importance of sharing this kind of research findings not only in the academic environment but also directly with stakeholders of territory as it may help to increase awareness of territories and landscapes and the collaboration of outlining "possible futures" (Testa 2017).

Conclusions

The results of the research show that in the examined rural areas the inhabitants mainly associated psychological well-being and a good quality of life with motivations related to the pleasant environment that is suitable for their needs.

These data draw attention to often marginal and disadvantaged realities where the inhabitants still perceive a strong attachment as a psychological dimension that is correlated with psychological well-being and quality of life.

Following Saporiti (2016) from Report COOP 2016, based on studies ISTAT, in relation to the environments of the province (that often corresponds with the rural areas) in which the inhabitants perceive relational and social psychological well-being (Saporiti 2016): Italians living in small municipalities are on average more satisfied than city people, i.e. who lives in urban centres up to 2.000 inhabitants feels more satisfied than who lives in big cities. Thus, it seems that territories that combine natural and cultural elements, derived from history and tradition and aspects of modern life, have more resources than urban areas to increase their inhabitants' psychological well-being, through a good integration between natural elements and community contexts.

In details, Maremma and Lunigiana slightly more than Crete and Media Valle.

Rural areas are comfortable both for adults and elderly people, who find in their "everyday landscapes" suitable dimensions for their material and psycho-social needs. This is also the case for young people who, even though they may decide to leave, still regard it as a valid and pleasant place to come back to if they wish.

These territories, also subject to depopulation – as pointed out by ISTAT – are mostly abandoned because of the lack of job opportunities rather than for discomfort toward the physical or psycho-social "everyday landscapes".

These contributions can explain the reactions of the inhabitants of other similar rural areas of Central Italy, recently devastated by earthquakes (2016–2017). In an interview, the Mayor of Norcia (Perugia), Nicola Alemanno, in line with the respondents of the present research, said with determination: "...Here we are born, here we have built our future, no one will move from here", in the hope that it will be possible to rebuild the village and that citizens can reconstruct community life, without being forced to emigrate (Cecchi 2016).

It is essential that the involvement of the local population in environmental reconstruction, change and transformation does not increase the risk of disrupting the "everyday landscapes" and transform then in "new" places of uncertain destiny.

Thanks for the data collection: Dr. Paola Bianchi in Lunigiana and Dr. Emanuela Stoppolini in the Crete Senesi.

References

Augé, M. (1992). Non-Lieux. *Introduction à une anthropologie de la surmodernité*. Paris: Seuil.

Banini, T. (2013). *Identità territoriali. Questioni, metodi, esperienze a confronto*. Milano: Franco Angeli.

Berto, R. (2005). Exposure to restorative environments helps restore attentional capacity. *Journal of Environmental Psychology*, 25, 249–259.

Bonnes, M., Carrus, G., Bonaiuto, M., Fornara, F. & Passafaro, P. (2004). Inhabitant's environmental perceptions in the city of Rome within the framework of Urban Biosphere Reserves of the UNESCO Programme on Man and Biosphere. *Annals of the New York Academy of Sciences*, 1023, 175–186.

Bonnes, M., Passafaro, P. & Carrus, G. (2011). The ambivalence of attitudes toward urban green areas: between pro-environmental worldviews and daily residential experience. *Environment and Behavior*, 43, 207–232.

Bonnes, M. & Secchiaroli, G. (1992). *Psicologia ambientale. Introduzione alla psicologia sociale e ambientale*. Roma: Carocci.

Burgess, J. Harrison, C.M. & Limb, M. (1988). People, parks and the urban green: a study of popular meanings and values for open spaces in the city. *Urban studies*, 25, 455–473.

Carrus, G., Scopelliti, M., Panno, A., Lafortezza, R., Colangelo, G., Pirchio, S., Ferrini, F., Salbitano, F., Agrimi, M., Portoghesi, L., Semenzato, P. & Sanesi, G. (2017). A Different Way to Stay in Touch with "Urban Nature": The Perceived Restorative Qualities of Botanical Gardens. *Frontiers in Psychology*, 8:914 (2017). doi:https://doi.org/10.3389/fpsyg.2017.00914

Carta, M.G., Aguglia, E., Caraci, F., Dell'Osso, L., Di Sciascio, G., Drago, F., Del Giudice, E., Faravelli, C., Hardoy, M.C., Lecca, E., Moro, M.F., Calò, S., Casacchia, M., Angermeyer, M. & Balestrieri, M. (2012). Quality of life and Urban/Rural Living: Preliminary Results of a

Community Survey in Italy. *Clinical Practice & Epidemiology in Mental Health*, 8, 169–174. doi: https://doi.org/10.2174/1745017901208010169.
Castiglioni, B. (2016). "Institutional" vs "everyday" landscape as conflicting concepts in opinions and practices. Reflections and perspectives from a case study in Northeastern Italy. *Journal of Research and Didactics in Geography* 1. 5., 37–46. doi: https://doi.org/10.4458/6964-03.
Cooper-Marcus, C. & Barnes, M. (1999). *Healing Gardens: Therapeutic Benefits and Design Recommendations.* New York: John Wiley & Sons.
Ferrari, M.G., Bocci, E., Bianchi, P., Cavallero, P., Mazza, R. & Rombai, L. (2014). Qualità territoriale. ambienti e paesaggi. Età a confronto in alcune aree tosco-laziali. *Turismo e Psicologia.* 7.2, 171–190
Fornara, F., Bonaiuto, M. & Bonnes, M. (2010). *Indicatori di Qualità Urbana Residenziale Percepita (IQURP). Manuale d'uso di scale psicometriche per scopi di ricerca e applicativi.* Milano: Franco Angeli.
Grinde, B. & Patil. G.G. (2009). Biophilia: does visual contact with the nature impact on health and well-being? *Int. J. Environ. Res. Public Health* 2009. 6, 2332–2343.
Hartig, T. (2003). Tracking restoration in natural and urban field settings, *Journal of Environmental psychology*, 23(2), 109–23.
Hartig, T. (2004). Restorative environments. In C. Spielberger, (Ed.). *Encyclopedia of applied psychology* (vol, 3, pp.273–278). San Diego, CA: Academic Press.
Hidalgo, M.C. & Hernàndez, B. (2001). Place Attachment: conceptual and empirical questions. *Journal of Environmental Psychology,* 21, 273–281.
Ittelson, W.H. (1973). *Environment and cognition.* New York: Seminar Press.
Kaplan, S. (1995). The restorative benefits of nature: towards an integrative framework. *Journal of environmental psychology*, 15(3), 169–82.
Kaplan, R. & Kaplan, S. (1989). *The experience of nature: a psychological perspective.* New York: Cambridge University Press.
Kellert, S.R. & Wilson, E.O. (1993). *The biophilia hypothesis.* Washington, D.C.: Island Press.
Knez, I. (2006). Autobiographical memories for places. *Memory,* 14, 359–377.
Knez, I. & Eliasson, I. (2017). Relationships between personal and collective place identity and well-being in mountain communities. *Front. Psychol.* 8:79. doi: https://doi.org/10.3389/fpsyg.2017.00079.
Knez, I. & Thorsson, S. (2008). Thermal, emotional and perceptual evaluations of a park: cross-cultural, and environmental attitude comparisons. *Build. Environ.* 43(2008), 1483–1490.
Lafortezza, R., Carrus, G. Sanesi, G. & Davies, C. (2009). Benefits and well-being perceived by people visiting green spaces in periods of heat stress. *Urban Forestry & Urban Greening*, 8, 97–108.
Lewicka, M. (2008). Place attachment, place identity, and place memory: restoring forgotten city past. *Journal of Environmental.Psychology.* 28, 209–231.
Losito, G. (2002). *L'analisi del contenuto nella ricerca sociale.* Milano: Franco Angeli.
Mazza R. & Minozzi S. (2011). *Psico(pato)logia del Paesaggio. Disagio psicologico e degrado ambientale.* Bologna: Erreciedizioni.
Proshansky. H. M. (1978). The city and self-identity. *Environment and Behavior,* 10, 147–170.
Proshansky, H. M., Fabian, A.K. & Kaminoff, R. (1983). Place identity: physical world socialization of the self. *Journal of Environmental Psychology*, 3(1), 57–83.
Raymond, C.M., Brown, G. & Weber, D. (2010). The measurement of place attachment: Personal, Community and Environmental Connections. *Journal of Environmental Psychology*, 30(4), 422–434.
Rombai, L. (2001). La geografia storica. In D. Ruocco et Al. (Eds). *Cento anni di geografia in Italia.* pp 42–152. Novara: Istituto Geografico De Agostini.
Ruini, C., Ottolini, F., Rafanelli, C., Ryff, C. & Fava, G.A. (2003). La validazione italiana delle Psychological Well-being Scales (PWB). Italian validation of Psychological Well-being Scales (PWB). *Rivista di Psichiatria*, 38, 3, 117–130.
Ryff, C.D. & Keyes, C.L. (1995). The structure of psychological well-being revisited. *Journal of Personality and Social Psychology*, 1995, 69 (4), 719–727.

Sack, R.D. (1986). *Human Territoriality: Its Theory and History*. Cambridge: Cambridge University Press.
Scannell, L. & Gifford, R. (2010). Defining place attachment: A tripartite organizing framework. *Journal of Environmental Psychology,* 30, 1–10.
Scopelliti, M., Carrus, G., Adinolfi, C., Suarez, G., Colangelo, G., Lafortezza, R., Panno, A. & Sanesi, G. (2016). Staying in touch with nature and well-being in different income groups: The experience of urban parks in Bogotá. *Landscape and urban planning,* 148, 139–148.
Sereni, E. (1984). *Storia del paesaggio agrario italiano*. Bari: Laterza.
Sestini, A. (1963). *Il paesaggio*. Milano: Touring Club Italiano.
Shumaker, S.A. & Taylor, R.B. (1983). Toward a clarification of people-place relationships: a model of attachment to place. In N. R. Feimer & E. S. Geller (Eds.). *Environmental Psychology. Directions and perspectives*. New York: Praeger.
Turner, M. G. (1989). Landscape ecology: the effect of pattern on process. *Annu. Rev. Ecol. Syst.* 20, 171–197.
Trentin, R. (1991). *Gli atteggiamenti sociali. Teoria e ricerca.* Torino: Bollati Boringhieri.
Twigger-Ross, C. L. & Uzzell, D. L. (1996). Place and identity processes. *Journal of Environmental Psychology*, 16, 205–220.
Ulrich, R.S. (1984). View through a window may influence recovery from surgery. *Science*, 224, 420–421.
Ulrich, R. S. (1993). Biophilia, biophobia, and natural landscapes. In S.R. Kellert & E.O. Wilson (Eds.). *The biophilia hypothesis*. Washington, D.C.: Island Press.
Velarde, M.D., Fry, G. & Tveit, M. (2007). Health effects of viewing landscapes – Landscape types in environmental psychology. *Urban Forestry & Urban Greening*, 6, 199–212.
Wilson, E. O. (1984). *Biophilia: The Human Bond with other species.* Cambridge, MA: Harvard University Press.
Wohlwill, J. F. (1983). The concept of nature: A psychologist's view. *Human Behavior & Environment: Advances in Theory and Research*, 6, 5–37.
Zani, B. & Cicognani, E. (2000). *Psicologia della salute.* Bologna: Il Mulino.

SITOGRAPHY

Cecchi, S. (2016). Terremoto, la rivolta degli sfollati. "Ecco le tende, restiamo a Norcia" Le istituzioni cedono: arrivano le strutture, in attesa dei container. *Quotidiano.net*. https://www.quotidiano.net/cronaca/terremoto-30-ottobre-norcia-1.2642525. Accessed 1 November 2016.
Council of Europe (2000). European Landscape Convention. Florence. 20.X.2000. *European Treaty Series* – No. 176. https://rm.coe.int/1680080621. Accessed 20 October 2000.
Regione Toscana (2015). Piano di indirizzo territoriale con valenza di Piano Paesaggistico. Cartografia identificativa degli ambiti http://www.regione.toscana.it/documents/10180/12604310/cartografia_identificativa.pdf/89e8ace0-ad95-4c92-bbb1-3ef0f4626cbc.
Russo A. (a cura di) "*Rapporto Coop 2016* Consumi e distribuzione. Assetti, dinamiche, previsioni" COOP. https://italiani.coop/rapporto-coop-2016-ecco-ledizione-aggiornata/. Accessed 11 November 2016.
Saporiti, R. (2016). "Gli italiani più felici abitano in provincia. Sembrerebbe di sì". *Il Sole24ore.*http://www.infodata.ilsole24ore.com/2016/11/11/gli-italiani-piu-felici-abitano-in-provincia/. Accessed 11 November 2016.
Testa, R. (2017). "Qualità della vita: il futuro che ci costruiamo". *L'Indro.* L'approfondimento quotidiano indipendentemente. http://www.lindro.it/qualita-della-vita-il-futuro-che-ci-costruiamo. Accessed 1 June 2017.

Part III
Economy, Welfare and Quality of Life

Economic Growth, Quality of Life, Life Styles and Sustainability: Correlations and New Variables to Be Considered as Indicators in Recent Literature

Manuela Ciani Scarnicci, Antonella Laino, Maria Francesca Belcaro, and Chiara Vita

Abstract Lifestyle affects the quality of life and the economic growth traditionally measured in terms of GDP, Gross Domestic Product. In the first part of the paper we highlight the reasons for GDP is not an indicator of well-being, defined by the Commission of the European Observatory on Health as '*an emotional, mental, physical, social and spiritual state which enables people to reach and maintain their personal potential in society*'.

In the second part, it is emphasized as this definition points out the link between well-being of the subject and the progress of society in which he lives. It is no longer sufficient to assess growth only on the basis of the produced wealth.

Already Pigou, studied the relationship between wealth and well-being, overcoming the variables considered by the marginalist analysis, investigating social costs and benefits arising from the fulfillment of subsequent needs to the primary ones.

Introduction

GDP Limits as an Indicator of a Country's Growth

It is now widely believed that the success, or failure, of a country depends on the rate of growth and economic development; high growth rates represent improvements of the economic state, the productivity growth and, in an indirect way, the flow of foreign investment. It is therefore not difficult to understand why GDP, a country's gross domestic product indicator, has for many years been a priority indicator of

M. C. Scarnicci (✉) · A. Laino
Universita' e-Campus, Como, Italy
e-mail: manuela.cianiscarnicci@uniecampus.it; antonella.laino@uniecampus.it

M. F. Belcaro · C. Vita
Laboratorio Qumap-PIN, UNIFI, Prato, Italy
e-mail: chiara.vita@pin.unifi.it; mfbelcaro@gmail.com

A. Bianco et al. (eds.), *Italian Studies on Quality of Life*, Social Indicators Research Series 77, https://doi.org/10.1007/978-3-030-06022-0_20

wealth, especially among neoliberals, who have made it the main instrument for assessing economic policies (Nafziger 2006).

The true strength of GDP as an indicator of wealth has always been its simplicity of calculation: it is rather simple, by means of national accounting elements, to calculate the value of goods and services produced in a given year in a country, including the balance of transactions with foreign economies.

Nevertheless, for many years, GDP has marked considerable limits on the actual indication of the growth and development of society as an advancement of its well-being: not always have better values of the indicator been accompanied by an improvement in living standards. First of all, not all social and territorial areas enjoy the same degree of GDP growth, which does not allow to highlight the geographical and social distribution of wealth and therefore does not analyze the socio-spatial distribution of growth. Moreover: we could detect increases in GDP due to natural events, such as floods, earthquakes, which stimulate new investment for reconstruction, far from being considered events that increase growth and/or development (Sen et al. 2010).

The weakness of GDP as a key indicator of a country's growth has started to emerge from the beginning of the 1970s: it is noted that GDP does not reflect the value of the gray economy, i.e. the total of non-recorded cash transactions which occur to escape taxation and, as in some countries the weight of this area of the economy almost reaches 50% of GDP, completely wipes out the indicability. It is also shown that GDP does not consider non-market-based economic activities, such as the domestic production of households, which is, above all, for the developing countries a key element of the economy. Lastly, the calculation of GDP considers the depreciation of capital, but only in its sense of productive capital, such as facilities, without paying any attention to a broader concept of capital, which may include natural capital, forests, natural resources, biodiversity, human capital, education, health, and social capital. The difficulty of accommodating the measures of these forms of capital lies in the complexity of their measurement, despite their importance (Cheli 2000).

The Relationship Between Quality of Life, Well-Being and Income

GDP and GNP (Gross National Product), another indicator of wealth and growth in a country, have not been designed to reflect the well-being of a given society, yet this is the goal pursued by modern societies, who have also experienced significant increases in GDP at the cost of worsening the quality of life and experiencing radical change in lifestyles. Already Pigou, in "the Economics of Walfare" (1920) founder of the modern welfare economy, acknowledges that an increase in national incomes is not always an improvement in well-being.

The relationship between happiness and available income according to various studies (Clark et al. 2008), exists and is positive, as individual well-being is positively correlated to income, but in a limited way; and the correlation is stronger in the lower income brackets. In this respect, the concept of relative income in relation to the social group to which it belongs is relevant (Ferrer-i-Carbonell 2005). This conclusion is associated to a more general result introduced in 1974 under the name of Easterlin's paradox, (Easterlin 1974), also referred to as the paradox of happiness, which destabilized the widespread growth assessment approach measured on the basis of GDP or GNP, stimulating the search for alternative targets and indicators. The paradox leads to the conclusion that throughout life, people's happiness depends very little on changes in income and wealth. According to Easterlin, when income increases, human happiness rises up to a certain value, but then begins to decrease, following the trend of a reversed U.

Almost all the hypotheses explain the paradox and point to the need to include not only consumer goods but also relational goods in the wealth analysis, such as the affective situation and participation in social life. According to many, the economic analysis should also consider the environmental heritage that reverberates most of the negative externalities of human activity not counted in the logic of the market.

For many years now, the concept of quality of life is inseparably linked to sustainability, and vice versa. The concept of quality of life is a concept of great evidence and topicality, especially if it is related to the one of sustainability of life and sustainable development of society (Van de Kerk and Manuel 2008).

The World Health Organization provides its own definition of quality of life, which implies the perception individuals have of their position in the cultural context and the system of values accepted and shared by the society they belong to, and also in relation to the goals, the expectations and the interests they establish. The definition highlights the subjective dimension of the quality of life, considering that the individual can determine the quality of his life by referring to his own judgment. In this regard, we see a growing number of authors interpreting the phrase 'quality of life', considering the use of development potential, adaptation of the individual's expectations to the social environment, possibilities of self-development, the characteristics of the organization of social life (Dolan and Metcalfe 2012).

The stimulus to look for the measure of the development of a community in a man-centered (I prefer individual-centered) vision, and not the income, stems from Amartya Sen's studies and intuitions. He considered the concept of need as strongly related to that of capacity and functions, in terms of resources, rather than what pleases the human being in terms of GDP. An individual's well-being is linked to the quality of life he leads, and life is a 'collection' of functions, even very different from one another, ranging from the primary need for healthy eating, good health, to more complex results such as the sense of dignity, and active participation in social life. The quality of life, therefore, is shaped by individual preferences and experiences. According to Sen, the quality of life depends, for everyone, on the freedom it enjoys, the economic opportunities that come out of it, social opportunities, guarantees and social security. The basis of the quality of life is the consideration of the opportunity for the individual to use the assets held for pursuing a dignified existence. So, goods are just a tool through which the individual allows his life to 'work', to reach a definite quality of life and well-being. The ability to use a product in a fruitful way is even more important than owning it.

The concept of well-being involves two distinct approaches that, despite the many attempts of reconciliation, remain in contradiction.

The first approach is what refers to the theory of welfare, with reference to the conditions that must be met for people to live a good life, embracing fundamental human rights, considered universal. In one of the most widespread versions of this approach, Sen (1999) argues that satisfaction of these needs helps society create opportunities such as the flexibility in human beings, helpful for overcoming hunger, oppression, and exploitation.

The second approach, defined as subjective well-being, is defined as a multidimensional evaluation of one's life, including both cognitive and emotional reactions (Pavot and Diener 2003). Thus, through the indicators of subjective well-being, the level of well-being of autonomous individuals is measured.

Subjective well-being refers to the ability to function optimally, which depends on physical health, the interest in the surrounding environment, the motivation to achieve the goals: an essential attribute of the concept of well-being is the sense of power of emancipation (Gough and McGregor 2007). Stiglitz's subjective well-being (Stiglitz et al. 2009) argues that it covers various aspects such as cognitive assessment of one's life, happiness, satisfaction, positive emotions such as joy and pride, but also negative ones such as pain and anxiety, and each of these must be measured separately to evaluate the well-being of individuals.

Sen's studies have amplified the interest in identifying alternative growth indicators with the aim of measuring the progress of long-term development in terms of prosperity and well-being of the population. Discussion on the concept of well-being is very complex and links the concept of social relations, confidence and participation rather than consumption, focusing on the creation and exchange of social value through activating cultural relations rather than focusing on the economic value of a transaction.

In 2009, the Fitoussi Commission sends a strong message in this regard: less attention should be paid to the development of indicators that measure economic performance, placing the focus on measuring the quality of life and the well-being of individuals, including rational and prudent management of natural and cultural resources, especially if not renewable. In this regard, the Commission emphasized how the concept of well-being consists of multi-dimensional aspects, thus recommending measuring life levels in addition to income, consumption and material resources, and including assessing non-material needs such as health, education, personal, political and civil activities, social relations and environmental conditions.

One of the most important studies on quality of life is that conducted by H. Cantril (1965) who investigated the reality of 13 countries including the USA. A scale that is still current has been used to assess the quality of life.

When we talk about measuring well-being in research literature, we can therefore distinguish three measurement categories (Diener and Suh 1997):

- Economic welfare
- Social well-being
- Subjective well-being

Economic welfare refers to measurements carried out through GDP, which, as mentioned at the beginning of this study/paper, does not however appear exhaustive as an exclusive measure of well-being. By overcoming the mere consideration of monetary aspects, and by assessing the negative environmental effects of unmanaged growth, we refer to a wider concept of well-being by trying to build indicators in which activities that do not create well-being are removed, and introducing activities that instead increase it, such as leisure, even though they are difficult to measure.

The Indicators

An example in this sense is the MEW (Measure of Economic Welfare) created by Nordhaus and Tobin in 1972 (Nordhaus and Tobin 1972) which increases the social value of GDP by adding an estimate of the value of free time and unpaid work, and reduces this value by considering the damage caused by production and consumption. MEW is a first attempt to change GDP to achieve a better measure of progress that realistically affects a country. Non-directly productive utility activities are not counted, while monetization of leisure activities and home work are included, which can improve well-being (McGillivray and Clark 2006).

Nordhaus and Tobin start from the assumption that GDP is a measure of production, while economic welfare depends on consumption; for the calculation of a welfare indicator it is necessary to separate the consumption from the investment and the intermediate costs, excluding public expenditure, as it is already considered within the investments (Cheli 2000).

Samuelson and Nordhaus in 1983 published a study that sets out the trends of GNP and MEW in the US between 1929 and 1980 (Samuelson and Nordhaus 1983): the trend shows that after an initial prevalence of net welfare based on GNP, from the forties onwards there has been a surplus of the GNP value on the MEW, with a constantly opening scissor since the sixties.

One of the main criticisms raised at MEW is for not taking into consideration environmental degradation in a specific and significant way, although this legitimate criticism is opposed by the fact that health damage resulting from degradation and pollution is almost entirely offset by incomes from non-monetary transactions (Masetti and Merola 2006). In addition, according to detractors, the indicator is not sensitive to changes due to inequalities, and overestimates leisure, considering it to both the employed and the unemployed.

In 1989 Daly and Cobb (1994), produce an alternative measure, based on the sustainable development theory, that the ISEW (Index of Sustainable Economic Welfare) where consumer spending considers the distribution of income, and the cost of environmental pollution. The index seeks to subtract the wealth value from urbanization costs, the cost of automobile accidents, air and noise pollution, wanting to deduct the value of all activities that undermine the sustainability of natural resources such as depletion of non-renewable resources and long-term environmental damage. The aim is to find an alternative to GDP, inspired by the MEW, integrated by a careful assessment of the environmental and social aspects of well-being. Rather than sum up all the expenses, such as GDP, consumption is correct considering the distribution of income, depreciation of natural resources, environmental degradation, while enhancing leisure time and home based work. The assessment of sustainable economic welfare is carried out by starting from weighing individual consumption against an index of income distribution. To this a value assessment of services rendered by durable consumer goods and unpaid domestic work, from that part of non-defensive public spending, is added. Thus negative aspects of growth are being considered and assessed because of the worsening of quality such as pollution, loss of productivity of agricultural land, income needed to offset future generations for the reduction of non-renewable energy resources and long-term environmental costs.

According to Asheim (2000) this welfare measurement methodology refers to three concepts: sustainable income, welfare equivalent income and net social benefit. Sustainable income is defined as Hicks' income definition (Hicks 1939[1]): for this purpose, the calculation of the ISEW deduces from the value of production, measured by GDP, the depreciation of natural capital, of capital and defensive expenditures.[2]

The concept of implicit income, in this type of measurement, however, turns out to be still wider than that identified by Hicks. In fact, the equivalent income welfare refers to the definition of well-being identified by Fisher (1906), which Daly and Cobb have further expanded by including natural and human capital. Knowing that the process of economic growth implies the existence of many activities that negatively affect well-being, the authors interpret the psychic income net of these activities. It follows that ISEW deducts from personal consumption the costs of substitution, purchase and maintenance of durable goods; subsequently, integrations and deductions are made, the purpose of which is to compute, within the index, negative or positive externalities associated with consumption. Net social profit, on the other hand, expresses a measure of the effectiveness of some policy choices. It

[1]It is recalled that according to Hicks (1939) '*the purpose of calculating income in practical life is to provide individuals with an indication of the quantity they can consume without depleting ... and this quantity coincides with the value of individual consumption plus the increase of the monetary value of consumption expectations*'.

[2]Recall that the defensive expenses are all expenses incurred to prevent or repair damage caused by the production or consumption, but useless in terms of the welfare production: therefore, the enhancement of negative externalities.

consists of an extensive version of the cost/benefit analysis that, instead of using monetary values expressed by GDP, uses welfare equivalent income and sustainable income. So, net social profit is defined as the difference between the value that ISEW assumes as a result of the adoption of a given policy and the value of the index in the absence of it. ISEW, considering jointly the income dimension, the environmental dimension and the social dimension, can be defined as an indicator of sustainable development, whose purpose (Lawn 2003) is to express a quantitative measure of social well-being within a territory, in a given period, while contemplating the effects of past and present activities (Rinaldi and Zelli 2014). The basic idea is that the relationship between individual consumption and well-being is not necessarily proportional, especially for people with different income sources: in fact, an increase in a unit of consumption produces different levels of well-being for individuals with different incomes.

Despite the inspiration that MEW's calculation has represented for the composition of the ISEW, the two indicators show significant differences, precisely for the introduction of environmental degradation into the latter. Moreover, ISEW does not consider leisure as excessively subjective and questions its assessment. The ISEW ultimately has a structure similar to the MEW but it differs for the fundamental role assigned to inequality in assessing well-being and attention to the environment. It has the great advantage of being able to compare with GDP, and returns a synthetic and aggregate value, but unlike GDP, it takes account, albeit indirectly, of the income distribution.

The ISEW is conceptually criticized for its inter-temporal interpretation as a sustainability index. According to Neumayer (2000), the indicator cannot be interpreted simultaneously as an indicator of well-being and sustainability because the two concepts are distinct and sometimes antithesis: just think of the numerous cases where consumer choices that provide significant perceptible well-being today may not be sustainable on a prospective basis. In addition, the concept of sustainability to which the index refers is weak substitutability: in fact, being an aggregate index, it assumes the perfect substitutability of the different types of capital.

An alternative to the ISEW is the GPI (Genuine Progress Indicator) developed by the Redefining Progress Association,[3] which considers both the economic dimension and the social dimension (Talberth et al. 2007). It is based on the private consumption data used to determine GDP, but also considers the distribution of income, the value of domestic work, the value of volunteering, the costs of crime and that of pollution. The GPI can be divided into two components: the present measure of economic prosperity and the measure of sustainable economic development. It attempts to rectify GDP so that it can provide a good estimate of economic welfare, which also ponders environmental and social aspects. To achieve this result, the defensive expenditure is deducted from GDP, but the items that contribute to the improvement of well-being are increased, although not included

[3]Redefining Progress is the nation's leading public policy think tank dedicated to smart economics. It finds solutions that ensure a sustainable and equitable world for future generations.

in national accounts, such as volunteering or housework, care for children and the elderly by relatives. Critics' greatest concern is the fact that it confuses social and environmental challenges, that it is not prospectively structured and requires a large amount of information. For Italy, this indicator was only once calculated with the name of RIBES (Ricostruzione dell'Indice di Benessere Economico e Sostenibile), with reference to the period 1960–1990. Until the 1980s both indicators grew, while from the 1980s the GPI tended to stop growing unlike GDP: this means that despite continued economic growth, the welfare of Italian citizens had stopped following the same trend.

Social well-being (or social phase) historically begins in the sixties, with the movement of social indicators which originate in the US and spread rapidly in all developed countries (Carlucci 2005). It is based on the socio-economic dimension defined on the basis of quantitative indicators with the main objective of showing the degree of satisfaction of aggregated needs in groups.

One of the most important proposals in this area is the Human Development Index (HDI) used in the United Nations Development Program's global human development relations. For the calculation of this index we use the data relative to the average life expectancy, literacy, level of education and standard of living measured by GDP. This information helps determine the country's level of development and the impact of economic policies on quality of life. The purpose of the index is to compare the relative level of human development of populations/communities in the world. For the calculation of the index, the geometric mean of three indices indicating life expectancy at birth, average education years, to highlight access to knowledge, the measurement of gross national income per capita, calculated in terms of purchase power, is used to show the lifestyle.[4] This index was created in 1990 by the Pakistani Mahbub ul Haq, economist and international development Theorist, (Haq 1995) according to which human development is a process of expanding people's choices and expanding personal choices through the expansion of human capacity and operations. It has been used by the UN since 1993 to assess the quality of life of member countries. In 2012 the country with the highest level of this index was Norway, followed by Australia, USA and the Netherlands. (Ciani Scarnicci 2012).

This index increases awareness of social problems with the information it can provide, and can be used to mobilize support for specific projects and interventions to combat the poverty of less developed countries. The information potential of the index in question is much higher than GDP: In fact, the results of studies using HDI can encourage governments to incorporate non-economic goals into their policies. Critics concern the lack of inclusion of human rights development, or indicators of freedom, as well as the lack of attention to the poverty line.

[4]For more in-depth information on the value of the index please refer to the 'Summary – Human Development Report 2011 – Sustainability and Equity: a Better Future for All – http://hdr.undp.org

Different results have been achieved with the calculation of the Happy Planet index, developed in 2006 by the New Economics Foundation to measure the level of well-being in different countries. In this case, the experience of subjective well-being was considered as well as the perception of the individual on his own level of happiness and the expectation of life.

Another recent research report on measuring subjective well-being was announced by the UN in 2012 by the "World Happiness Report 2012". The inspiration for the creation of the World Happiness Report came from Bhutan, which, according to the levels of GDP it expresses, is one of the poorest countries in the world with a pro capita revenue of $ 670 per year (Della Casa 2008). Since 2008, the country starts referring to GNH (Gross National Happiness), which officially replaces GDP as the basis for public policy decisions. The basic idea is that the development of human society can only be achieved if material growth is associated with spiritual growth: for this reason, the pillars of the indicator are economy, but also culture, environment and good governance. The possibility of replicating the system based on the calculation of the indicator in countries other than Bhutan, which do not have a strong identity, still leaves many perplexities in international organizations (OECD 2008).

Conclusions

ESW (equitable and sustainable well-being) is an indicator that is born with the aim of measuring the progress of a society not only from the economic point of view, but also socially and environmentally. Its elaboration comes from a joint project of CNEL (National Council of Economics and Labour) and ISTAT (National Institute of Statistics), and it is part of the international debate on overcoming GDP.

ESW incorporates a concept of multidimensional well-being, and describes, through the identification of 12 measures of well-being, the aspects that contribute to determining the quality of life. One of the strengths of ESW is the attention to the different dimensions of well-being, allowing from time to time the use of the different aspects of well-being investigated to gather information on the progress of society and the aspects on which to invest in the future (Maggino 2015).

With the 2017 DEF (Economy and Finance Document), Italy is the first country in the EU and in the G7 to include in addition to GDP not only economic planning, but also indicators of equitable and sustainable well-being. On an experimental basis, it will be introduced considering past evolution and the prospects of four quality of life indicators: average income available, inequality index, non-participation rate at work, CO_2 emissions.

References

Asheim, G.B. (2000). Green National Accounting: Why and How?. *Environment and Development Economics*, (1), 25 48.

Cantril, H. (1965). *The Pattern of Human Concern*. New Brunswick, Rutgers University Press.

Carlucci, F. (2005). *La misurazione della condizione umana*. Roma, Università La Sapienza.

Cheli, B. (2000). Sulla misura del benessere economico: i paradossi del PIL e le possibili correzioni in chiave etica e sostenibile, con uno spunto per l'analisi della povertà. *Rivista Italiana di Economia, Demografia e Statistica*, LIV (1).

Ciani Scarnicci, M. (2012). *Il PIL un problema di valutazione*. Milano, FrancoAngeli.

Clark, A., Fritjers, P., Shields, M. (2008). Relative Income, Happiness and Utility: an Explanation for the Easterlin Paradox and Others Puzzles. *Journal of Economic Literature*, 46 (1), 95–144.

Daly, H.E., & Cobb, J.B. (1994). *For the Common Good: Redirecting the Economy Toward Community, The Environment and a Sustainable Future*. Boston, Beacon Press.

Della Casa, G. (2008). *L'ecologia profonda. Lineamenti per una nuova visione del mondo*. Firenze, Macro Edizioni.

Diener, E., & Suh, E. (1997). Measuring Quality of Life: Economic, Social. And Subjective Indicators. *Social Indicators Research*, 40 (1), 189–216.

Dolan, P., & Metcalfe, R. (2012). Measuring Subjective Wellbeing: Recommendations on Measures for Use by National Governments. *Journal of Social Policy*, 41 (2), 409–427.

Easterlin, R. (1974). *Does economic growth improve human lot? Some empirical evidence, Nation and Households in economic growth: Essays in honor of Moses Abromowitz* (edited by P.A. Davis e M.W. Reder). New York e London, Academic Press.

Ferrer-i-Carbonell, A. (2005). Income and Well-being: an empirical Analysis of the Comparison Income Effect. *Journal of Public Economics*, 89, 997–1019.

Fisher, I. (1906). *The Nature of Capital and Income*. London, The Macmillan Company.

Gough, I., & McGregor, J.A. (2007). *Wellbeing in developing countries: from theories to research*. Cambridge, Cambridge University Press.

Haq, M. (1995). *Reflections on Human Development*. New York, Oxford University Press.

Hicks, J.R. (1939). *Value and Capital: An Inquiry into Some Fundamental Principles of Economic Theory*. Oxford, Oxford Clarendon Press.

Lawn, P.A. (2003). A Theoretical Foundation to Support the ISEW, GPI and Other Related Indexes. *Ecological Economics*, 44 (1), 105–118.

Maggino, F. (2015). *A New Research Agenda for Improvements in Quality of Life*. New York, Springer.

Masetti, E., & Merola, M. (2006). *Gli indicatori della qualità della vita e dello sviluppo umano sostenibile*. Pavia, Fondazione Lombardia per l'ambiente.

McGillivray, M., & Clark, M. (2006). *Understanding Human Well-Being*. Tokyo, United Nation University Press.

Nafziger, E.W. (2006). *Economic Development*. Cambridge, Cambridge University Press.

Neumayer, E. (2000). On the Methodology of ISEW, GPI and Related Measures: Some Constructive comments and some doubt on the 'threshold' hypothesis. *Ecological Economics*, 34(3), 347–361.

Nordhaus, W.D., & Tobin, J. (1972). *Is Growth Obsolete? Economic Growth. Fiftieth anniversary colloquium V, National Bureau of Economic Research*. New York, Columbia University Press.

OECD (2008) Measuring the Progress of Societies. OECD.org. Accessed 15 Jan2017.

Pavot, W., & Diener, E. (2003). *Well-being (Including life satisfaction)*. Encyclopedia of Psychological Assessment, (2), 1097–1101. Thousand Oaks, CA: Sage.

Rinaldi, A., & Zelli, R. (2014). *Misurare il benessere. La sfida degli indicatori alternativi al PIL*. Roma, Donzelli editore.

Samuelson, P.A., & Nordhaus, W.D. (1983). *Economia*. Bologna, Zanichelli.

Sen, A. (1999). *Development as Freedom*. New York, Anchor Books.

Sen, A.K., Fitoussi, J.P., Stiglitz, J.E. (2010). *La misura sbagliata delle nostre vite. Perché il PIL non basta più per valutare benessere e progresso sociale*. Milano, Rizzoli Etas.

Stiglitz, J.E., Sen, A., Fitoussi, J.P. (2009). The Measurement of Economic Performance and Social Progress Revisited. http://www.ofce.science-po.fr. Accessed 25 Jan 2017.

Talberth, D.J., Cobb, C., Slattery, N. (2007). The Genuine Progress Indicator 2006: A Tool for Sustainable Development. http://www.rprogress.org. Accessed 25 Jan 2017.

Van de Kerk, G., & Manuel, A.R. (2008). A comprehensive index for a sustainable society: The SSI- the Sustainable Society Index. *Ecological Economics*, 66 (2–3), 228–242.

World Happiness Report 2012, http://worldhappiness.report/ed/2012. Accessed 15 Jan 2017

European Welfare States: Does Decentralization Affect Poverty?

Alessandra Coli and Barbara Pacini

Abstract The shifting of welfare systems to the local level may have positive or negative consequences. On the one hand, it may be argued that local governments better tailor welfare policies to the specific needs of population, given their direct knowledge of territory; on the other hand, especially in the presence of weak supervision by the central government, decentralization may cause inequalities and territorial fragmentation. The main objective of the paper is to explore the relationship between welfare state typologies – with different degrees of decentralization – and the level of monetary poverty and material deprivation of citizens. Using data from official statistics, we model individual binary outcomes (living or not under the poverty line, being or not able to make ends meet) as a function of both family-level and country-level characteristics. The empirical analysis is run on a selection of European countries for the year 2013.

Introduction

The decentralization of responsibilities to increasingly lower levels of government may have positive or negative consequences. On the one hand, decentralization could produce welfare policies better tailored to the population's specific needs; on the other hand, especially in the presence of weak supervision by the central government, it may lead to negative implications like territorial fragmentation and inequalities (Redriguez-Pose and Ezcurra 2009; Andreotti et al. 2012).

According to some scholars, effectiveness of decentralization depends on the national welfare framework and especially on the form of the welfare state. For example, Sellers and Lidstrom (2007) argue that a strong territorial decentralization

A. Coli (✉)
Dipartimento di Economia e Management, Università di Pisa, Pisa, Italy
e-mail: alessandra.coli1@unipi.it

B. Pacini
Dipartimento di Scienze Politiche, Università di Pisa, Pisa, Italy
e-mail: barbara.pacini@unipi.it

A. Bianco et al. (eds.), *Italian Studies on Quality of Life*, Social Indicators Research Series 77, https://doi.org/10.1007/978-3-030-06022-0_21

is essential for a public welfare state built around universalist egalitarian ends, since it allows for ensuring equal provision regardless of the place.

This study explores the relationship between welfare states typologies – having different degrees of decentralization – and poverty. We consider several aspects of welfare systems such as the amount of resources assigned to social protection, the rules for accessing benefits (whether means-tested or not), the origin of social protection funding (if public or private), the different mix of benefits supplied (in cash or in kind benefits) and, finally, their level of decentralization. To this end, we estimate pooled logistic regressions for a sample of 127,324 households selected in 14 European countries. Data are taken from Eurostat and Oecd databases. The empirical analysis aims to assess whether decentralization is a significant predictor of poverty.

The paper is organized as follows. Section "European official statistics on social protection" describes European official statistics on social protection. Section "Variables and indicators" describes the variables and indicators used in the empirical analysis, section "Methodology and results" sets out the methodology adopted and presents main results. Finally, section "Final considerations" provides commentary on the results in terms of their strengths and weaknesses.

European Official Statistics on Social Protection

Eurostat and Oecd supply internationally harmonized statistics on social protection receipts and expenditures through two thematic databases: the Esspros (European system of integrated social protection statistics) and the Socx (Social expenditure) databases.

Esspros is an accounting framework developed in the late 1970s by Eurostat and the EU member states to allow international comparison among administrative national data on social protection (Eurostat 2011). Here, social protection is defined as encompassing "all interventions from public or private bodies directed to relieve households and individuals of the burden of a defined set of risks and needs, provided that there is neither a simultaneous reciprocal nor an individual arrangement involved" (Eurostat 2011, p. 9). The categories of risks and needs covered are eight, namely: sickness/health care, disability, old age, survivors, family/children, unemployment, housing, social exclusion not elsewhere classified. Esspros is composed of a core system and of modules. The core system records the accounting of social protection schemes distinguishing receipts (origin of financing) from expenditures (uses of financing). Modules contain supplementary statistical information on particular aspects of social protection, namely on pension beneficiaries and on net social benefits. Receipts are analysed according to the nature of the payment (social contributions, general government contributions, transfers from other schemes and other receipts) but also according to the paying sector (e.g. whether from central or local government). On the expenditure side, social benefits are analysed by risk or need covered and by type (if in cash or in kind, if means-tested or not).

In the 1990s, Oecd developed the Socx database for monitoring trends in aggregate social expenditure and analysing changes in its composition, across Oecd countries. Oecd defines social expenditures as "the provision by public and private institutions of benefits to, and financial contributions targeted at, households and individuals in order to provide support during circumstances which adversely affect their welfare, provided that the provision of the benefits and financial contributions constitutes neither a direct payment for a particular good or service nor an individual contract or transfer" (Adema et al. 2011, p. 90). Oecd distinguishes nine social different policy areas, which only approximately correspond to the risks/needs specified by Esspros: old age, survivors, incapacity-related benefits, health, family, active labour market programmes, unemployment, housing, and other social policy areas. Like Esspros, Socx database analyses social benefits by function and by type. Furthermore, it allows one to separate public from private benefits. Social benefits are classified as public when general government (central, state/local governments, social security funds) controls the relevant financial flows.

Also, National Accounts (NAs) disseminate statistics on social protection accounting. According to the ESA 2010 definition "Social benefits are transfers to households, in cash or in kind, intended to relieve them from the financial burden of a number of risk or needs, made through collectively organized schemes, or outside such schemes by government units and NPISHs; they include payments from general government to producers which individually benefit households and which are made in the context of social risks or needs" (Eurostat 2013a, par. 4.83). The following are risks or needs covered: sickness, invalidity/disability, occupational accident or disease, old age, survivors, maternity, family, promotion of employment, unemployment, housing, education, general neediness (Eurostat 2013a, par. 4.84). It is worth noting that NAs include education within the boundaries of social protection, which, at the opposite, is excluded both by Esspros and by Socx. With respect to the other data sources, NAs supply estimates of social benefits at sub-national level, more precisely by Nuts 2 regions (Eurostat 2013b). This data is currently published by Eurostat, within the Households regional accounts.

National statistical offices disseminate also micro statistics on the supply and use of social protection services. However, these statistics seldom permit sound comparisons among countries. Eusilc (EU Statistics on Income and Living conditions, Eurostat 2016) represents an exception, providing internationally comparable details on cash social benefits received by households and individuals. Although Eusilc definition of social benefits is based on Esspros concepts, some differences are present. In fact, Eusilc social benefits include education and cover current transfers only; furthermore, they do not include in kind benefits with the only exception of housing benefits.

The above described data sources allow us to obtain a complete and detailed picture of social protection supply and demand at the country level (Coli et al. 2016).

Welfare systems can be compared by looking at several aspects suggested in literature (Esping-Andersen 1990; Ferrera et al. 2012; Powel and Boyne 2001; Titmuss 1974): the functional dimension, which accounts for changes in the composition of risks and needs covered; the allocation dimension, which looks at the rules for accessing benefits (e.g. if benefits are means-tested or not); the profile of the productive unit delivering services (public, private and third sector); the different mix of economic transactions performed (benefits in cash, benefits in kind or tax breaks with social purposes).

Unfortunately, accurate, relevant and comparable statistics are lacking when focusing on sub-national areas. According to our analysis, the distribution of cash benefits by region (Nuts 2) from NAs represents the only official data currently disseminated on social protection expenditure at the local level. Eusilc individual data permit to estimate cash benefits (plus housing in kind benefits) at sub-national level, but only for large geographical areas.

Finally, it is worth reminding that data sources on social protection receipts and expenditure are not fully homogeneous, because of differences in the boundaries of the social domain (i.e. the distinction between social spending and non-social spending) and in the breakdown of social expenditure among functions (Coli et al. 2016; Coli and Valentini 2017).

Variables and Indicators

We define binary outcome variables which allow us to separate poor from non-poor households and a set of predictors concerning country welfare systems. Furthermore, we select/compute a set of variables and indicators to control for household social and demographic characteristics as well as country economic well-being.

We use both individual and country variables. Given the lack of data for some countries, we limit our analysis to a set of countries, namely Austria (AT), Belgium (BE), Germany (DE), Denmark (DK), Spain (ES), Finland (FI), France (FR), Ireland (IE), Italy (IT), Netherlands (NL), Norway (NO), Portugal (PT), Sweden (SE), and United Kingdom (UK). We end with a cross-section data set, including 127,324 households for the year 2013.

Table 1 shows a synthetic description of variables and indicators, also specifying the data source from which data are taken.

Nowadays, the multidimensional nature of well-being is a worldwide recognized concept, both in academic studies (e.g. Anand and Sen 1997; Stiglitz et al. 2010; Whelan et al. 2014; Aaberge and Brandolini 2015; Betti et al. 2015) and in official statistics (Eurostat 2017; Oecd 2017; Istat 2017). Well-being encompasses several aspects of life (topics or dimensions) such as the availability of economic resources, the level of education attained, the health status, the quality of interpersonal relations and the overall level of satisfaction about life. We consider a subset of well-being indicators, focussing on those aspects more probably affected by social policies.

Table 1 Variables and indicators description

Name	Description	Categories	Data source
HCR	Monetary poverty	0 = above poverty threshold	Eusilc
		1 = under poverty threshold	
DEPRIVATION	Being or not able to make ends meet	0 = with some difficulties, relatively easily, easily, quite easily	Eusilc
		1 = with great difficulties, with difficulties	
KIND TOT	Share of in kind benefits over total benefits	Percentage values	Esspros
MEANS TOT	Share of means-tested benefits over total benefits	Percentage values	Esspros
PRIVATE TOT	Share of private social benefits over total social benefits, 2011	Percentage values	Soxc
SOC EXP	Social expenditure as a percentage of GDP	Percentage values	Soxc
DECENTR	Decentralization measure based on the legal system of the country	5-point scale from the most federalist and decentralized countries (score 5) to the most unitary and centralized ones (1)	Ljiphart 1999
LOCAL EXP	Share of general government expenditure for social protection paid by lower levels of government	Percentage values	Esspros
CV BEN NUTS2	Variation coefficient of per capita social benefits across regions (NUTS 2)- 2011	Percentage values	Eurostat, NAs
HSIZE	Numbers of members	Number	Eusilc
FAMTYPE	Type of household	1 = one person household	Eusilc
		2 = households without dependent children	
		3 = single parent with dependent children	
		4 = households with dependent children	
		5 = other households	
NDEGREE	Number of members with tertiary education	Number	Eusilc
NLOW	Number of members with up to lower secondary education	Number	Eusilc
NFEM	Number of female members	Number	Eusilc
NWORKERS	Numbers of members with a job	Number	Eusilc
NUNEMP	Numbers of unemployed members	Number	Eusilc
NOLD	Number of members aged 75 or more	Number	Eusilc

(continued)

Table 1 (continued)

Name	Description	Categories	Data source
NRETIRED	Number of retired members	Number	Eusilc
NKIDS	Number of members aged less than 16	Number	Eusilc
BENEFITS	Benefits received (old age and survivors' benefits excluded) as a quota of households' average disposable income	Number	Eusilc
GDP PPP	GDP per inhabitant	PPP (Purchasing Power Parity	Eurostat, NAs

In particular, we consider two outcome variables, the first (HCR) focuses on monetary poverty, whereas the latter (DEPRIVATION) considers the household inability to make ends meet. The first variable identifies as poor, those households whose equivalised disposable income is below the at-risk-of-poverty threshold (HCR = 1). Following official statistics, the threshold is set at 60% of the national median equivalised disposable income. The second outcome variable identifies as poor (DEPRIVATION = 1) those households that report difficulty to make ends meet. This last indicator is included among the deprivation measures published by Eurostat (Eurostat 2017). Thought a significant stream of literature encourages the development of composite indicators of well-being/poverty (see Alkire et al. 2015 for a review of main methodologies), we prefer to consider separated indicators. This approach allows us to avoid confounding due to the weighting procedure and to assess clearly if and to what extent welfare systems may affect each indicator.

To characterize different social protection systems across countries, we propose the following set of indicators: share of social benefits in kind over total benefits (KIND TOT), share of means-tested benefits over total benefits (MEANS TOT); share of private social benefits over total social benefits (PRIVATE TOT), social expenditure as a percentage of GDP (SOC EXP).

For what concerns decentralization, we identify several indicators. The DECENTR indicator, taken from (Lijphart 1999), classifies countries according to the form of the state (whether federalist or unitary) and to the level of delegation of power from central to local governments. A classification of democracies is proposed which ranges from the most federalist and decentralized countries (score 5.0) to the most unitary and centralized ones (1.0). This indicator still represents one of the most influential typology of modern democracies, although this classification has been criticized by many scholars on conceptual, empirical and normative grounds (Sellers and Lidstrom 2007). Lijphart's indicator accounts for the level of decentralization in general, whereas our purpose is to measure the territorial decentralization of welfare policies specifically; furthermore, it limits to consider constitutional provisions, whereas it is also necessary to consider their implementation as performed by decentralised entities (Addis et al. 2016).

To overcome these limits, we propose two supplementary indicators. The first (LOCAL EXP), defined as the share of social protection expenditures funded by sub-national government, can be viewed as a proxy of the level of autonomy of local governments in delivering social protection; a larger proportion of expenditures funded by lower government levels indicates that fiscal impact is shifted away from central government (Schneider 2003). The second indicator (CV BENEFITS NUT2) measures the territorial heterogeneity of social benefits received by households. This indicator is computed as the coefficient of variation of per capita social benefits across Nut 2 regions. Higher levels may imply either a higher territorial heterogeneity of the risks or needs to be covered, or a different behaviour of local governments in terms of resources to be devoted to social protection.

Finally, we control for those household social and demographic characteristics which could affect outcome variables. Particularly, the following variables are selected: size of household (HSIZE), Family social-demographic type (FAMTYPE), number of members with tertiary education (NDEGREE), number of members with up to lower secondary education (NLOW), number of female members (NFEM), numbers of members with a job (NWORKERS), number of unemployed members (NUNEMP), number of retired members (NRETIRED), number of old-age members (NOLD), number of kids (NKIDS). Furthermore, for each household, we compute the amount of benefits received (excluding pensions) as a percentage of household average disposable income of the country (BENEFITS). Finally, we use GDP per inhabitant in power purchased parities (GDP PPP), as a proxy of the value of each country economy.

Table 2 shows country variables values for the year 2013, including the head count ratio and the share of households suffering of deprivation. This comparison points out important differences among country welfare systems. Greater values of institutional decentralization, not necessarily agrees with higher levels local government expenditure, nor with the territorial heterogeneity of social protection benefits. In the following section, we investigate the relationship between these different measures of decentralization and the risk of being poor or experiencing difficulties to make ends meet, controlling for both welfare states characteristics and households typologies.

Methodology and Results

The objective of our analysis is to contribute to a better understanding of the potential effects of decentralization on monetary poverty as well as on the inability of households to make ends meet. To this end, we model individual binary outcomes (HCR and DEPRIVATION variables) as a function of both family-level and country-level characteristics.

There is a natural hierarchy within the data: there are observations at the family level nested within the country level. This multilevel structure affects model

Table 2 Country variables values for the year 2013

COUNTRY	HCR	DEPRIVATION	KIND TOT	MEANS TOT	PRIVATE TOT
AT	15.78	14.55	30.22	8.35	6.80
BE	17.18	21.98	31.81	5.16	6.50
DE	20.33	10.40	37.60	12.09	11.10
DK	16.19	12.22	40.07	35.91	14.50
ES	18.87	36.75	30.52	14.45	1.90
FI	16.62	7.55	38.35	5.34	4.10
FR	14.02	19.86	36.33	11.51	10.30
IE	15.57	34.61	37.28	31.47	7.90
IT	19.25	39.94	24.61	5.69	7.50
NL	11.99	16.59	35.36	13.44	24.10
NO	14.24	7.34	41.46	4.23	9.00
PT	18.27	46.08	26.50	8.37	7.20
SE	18.97	6.88	45.55	2.66	10.50
UK	17.15	19.68	38.33	13.64	21.50
COUNTRY	SOC EXP	GDP PPP	DECENTR	LOCAL EXP CV	BEN NUTS2
AT	0.30	35,000	4.50	22.31	7.16
BE	0.30	32,000	3.20	11.91	9.24
DE	0.30	33,200	5.00	27.31	8.33
DK	0.32	33,700	2.00	32.14	4.15
ES	0.25	24,300	3.00	39.35	16.52
FI	0.31	30,200	2.00	31.15	3.12
FR	0.35	28,900	1.30	8.78	7.55
IE	0.20	35,300	1.00	1.73	0.10
IT	0.29	26,200	1.50	19.64	13.55
NL	0.30	35,500	3.00	13.22	7.16
NO	0.23	49,300	2.00	24.66	5.49
PT	0.27	20,600	1.00	1.28	17.08
SE	0.29	33,300	2.00	44.28	4.27
UK	0.27	29,000	1.00	5.78	8.99

specification and estimation. Possible strategies in quantitative analyses of multi-country data sets include the following: pooling the data for all countries (and using cluster- robust standard errors), using separate models for each country, country fixed effects models, or multilevel models (also known as random effects models or hierarchical models). Multilevel models appear to be the natural choice when one is interested in country-level predictors or in the variance component structure, investigating to what extent unobserved country factors affect population units (families). Our data set contains thousands of observation at the individual level, but the number of countries is small. Recently, Bryan and Jenkins (2016) argued that the small number of countries in most multi-country data sets severely constrains the ability of multilevel regression models to provide robust conclusions about the effects of country-level characteristics on outcomes (see also Austin 2010). Based on this literature, we opted to estimate a pooled logistic regression model (as a generalized linear model with link function logit) using the whole sample and computing cluster robust standard errors to account for the multilevel structure of data.[1]

Table 3 shows our results. Columns (1) and (2) refer to the pooled logistic model for the monetary poverty as dependent variable, while columns (3) and (4) contain results when deprivation is used as outcome variable. Significant positive coefficients indicate that corresponding variables increase the probability of poverty. Conversely, significant negative signs mean that predictors reduce the risk of poverty. In case of categorical variables, the coefficient sign indicates whether the risk increases or decreases compared to a reference category.

The level of institutional decentralization seems to increase the probability of monetary poverty but, at the opposite, it seems to decrease the probability of having difficulties to make ends meet. Higher shares of social protection expenditure held by local governments seem to reduce the probability of incurring in both the kinds of poverty whereas the level of territorial heterogeneity in the distribution of social benefits does not seem to be a significant predictor.

Higher shares of means tested benefits seem to diminish the probability of monetary poverty and increase that of experiencing deprivation. Symmetrically, the presence of kind benefits seems to increase the probability of monetary poverty and reduce households' difficulty to make ends meet. These apparently contradictory results are due to the different nature of well-being aspects measured by the two outcome variables. Social protection systems mainly based on cash benefits (i.e. with lower levels of in kind benefits) affect household disposable income and therefore monetary poverty. Conversely, systems with higher shares of in kind benefits make probably easier to make ends meet since people do not have to pay for some services like health services. In line with this last evidence, we find that cash benefits reduce the probability of monetary poverty but increase the possibility of deprivation. However, the level of country expenditure for social protection significantly reduces both monetary poverty and deprivation whereas the origin of social protection expenditure (whether public or private) is not a significant predictor of poverty. Single parent with dependent children or One-person families are the more vulnerable groups. In particular, the first group has the highest probability of experiencing difficulties to make ends meet whereas the probability of incurring in monetary poverty is not significantly different for the two typologies of family. The probability of being a poor household increases with the size of the household, the presence of members with a low level of education, the presence of female members (but only for predicting deprivation) and the number of unemployed members. At the opposite, it decreases with the number of members with tertiary education, the number of members aged 75 or more, the number of

[1]It is worth noting that we obtained consistent results applying a multilevel (random intercept) logistic regression. Due to space constraints we decided not to show them in the paper, however they may be required to the authors.

Table 3 Logit model with standard errors and cluster adjusted standard errors

Dependent variable:				
	HCR		DEPRIVATION	
	Coefficient	Std. Error	Coefficient	Std Error
DECENTR	0.176^{***}	(0.057)	-0.065^{*}	(0.035)
LOCAL EXP	-0.015^{**}	(0.007)	-0.019^{***}	(0.007)
CV BEN NUTS2	−0.010	(0.023)	0.050	(0.030)
SOC EXP	-3.233^{**}	(1.623)	-3.577^{*}	(1.961)
GDP PPP	-0.00005^{***}	(0.00001)	−0.00003	(0.00002)
KIND TOT	0.051^{**}	(0.024)	-0.053^{***}	(0.011)
MEANS TOT	-0.026^{***}	(0.009)	0.022^{**}	(0.011)
PRIVATE TOT	−0.011	(0.026)	−0.013	(0.009)
HSIZE	0.390^{***}	(0.047)	0.136^{***}	(0.035)
NDEGREE	-0.586^{***}	(0.059)	-0.511^{***}	(0.051)
NLOW	0.210^{***}	(0.053)	0.233^{***}	(0.069)
FAMTYPE2	-0.670^{***}	(0.155)	-0.389^{***}	(0.088)
FAMTYPE3	−0.126	(0.115)	0.372^{***}	(0.067)
FAMTYPE4	-0.565^{***}	(0.146)	-0.279^{***}	(0.079)
FAMTYPE5	-0.906^{***}	(0.319)	-0.632^{***}	(0.202)
NFEM	0.035	(0.032)	0.102^{***}	(0.020)
NOLD	-0.214^{**}	(0.090)	-0.174^{***}	(0.067)
NKIDS	−0.051	(0.054)	−0.009	(0.031)
NWORKERS	-1.420^{***}	(0.100)	-0.546^{***}	(0.040)
NUNEMP	0.424^{***}	(0.086)	0.589^{***}	(0.059)
NRETIRED	-0.999^{***}	(0.162)	-0.578_{***}	(0.065)
BENEFITS	-1.446^{***}	(0.350)	0.690^{***}	(0.195)
Constant	0.432	(0.952)	2.546^{*}	(1.300)
Observations	127,324		126,981	
Log likelihood	43,007.030		51,720.610	
Akaike Inf. Crit.	86,060.070		103,487.200	

Note: $^{*}p < 0.1$; $^{**}p < 0.05$; $^{***}p < 0.01$.

members with a job and the number of retired. The number of kids does not result to be a predictor of the risk of poverty. In particular, we find that the probability of being poor increases with the number of elderly people as far as we do not control for the number of family members with tertiary education and that the number of dependent children ends to be a predictor of poverty, once considered the number of workers of the family.

Finally, it is worth noting that the size of the country economy is a significant predictor of the risk of poverty: in line with intuition, higher levels of per inhabitant GDP reduces the probability of poverty.

Final Considerations

This work deals with the relationship between welfare state typologies and poverty. We report the results of a pooled logistic regression analysis for a sample of 127,324 households sampled in 14 European countries. Two different outcome variables are defined, namely monetary poverty and a measure of deprivation.

According to our results, institutional decentralization is a risk factor for monetary poverty while it represents a factor of protection against deprivation. Such seemingly contradictory outcome is due to the different nature of well-being aspects measured by the two outcome variables. Social protection systems mainly based on cash benefits affect household disposable income and therefore monetary poverty. Conversely, systems with higher shares of in kind benefits make probably easier to make ends meet since people need not pay for some services directly provided by general government, like health services.

Furthermore, there is evidence that a higher involvement of local governments in the funding of social protection expenditure is associated to lower levels of both monetary poverty and deprivation.

As a direction for future work, we plan to extend the analysis to identify supplementary indicators of decentralization, consider multiple outcomes covering multiple poverty dimensions and use panel data to investigate the dynamic of welfare states evolution. Moreover we are going to devote particular attention to the effects of the recent economic crisis on vulnerable individuals and families, to support specifically-targeted social policies.

Acknowledgements This work was developed under the framework of the University of Pisa research project PRA 2016-35 PO.WE.R (POlicy, WElfare and financial Resources: the impact of crisis on territories). We thank Eurostat for making Eusilc micro data available. The responsibility for all conclusions drawn from the data lies entirely with the authors.

References

Aaberge, R.,& Brandolini, A. (2015). Multidimensional poverty and inequality. In B. Atkinson and F. Bourguignon (Eds.), *Handbook of Income Distribution*, vol. 2A. Amsterdam: Elsevier.

Addis, P., Coli, A., Pacini, B. (2016). Welfare State and Local Government: the Impact of Decentralization on Well-being, 34th IARIW General Conference, Dres- den, Germany, August 21–27 2016.

Adema, W., Fron, P., Ladaique, M. (2011). Is the European Welfare State Really More Expensive? Indicators on Social Spending, 1980–2012; and a Manual to the Oecd Social Expenditure Database (Socx). *Oecd Social, Employment and Migration Working Papers*, No. 124. https://www.oecd- ilibrary.org/content/paper/5kg2d2d4pbf0-en. Accessed 20 September 2017.

Anand, S., Sen, A. (1997). Concepts or Human Development and Poverty! A Multi- dimensional Perspective. *United Nations Development Programme, Poverty and human development: Human development papers* pp. 1–20.

Alkire, S., Foster, J. E., Seth, S., Roche, J. M., Santos, M. E.(2015). *Multidimen- sional poverty measurement and analysis*. Oxford University Press.

Andreotti A., Mingione, E. Polizzi, E. (2012). Local welfare systems: A Challenge For Social Cohesion, *Urban studies*, 49(9),1925–1940.
Austin, P. C. (2010). Estimating Multilevel Logistic Regression Models When the Number of Clusters is Low: A Comparison of Different Statistical Software Procedures, *International Journal of Biostatistics*, 6 (1), doi: https://doi.org/10.2202/1557- 4679.1195.
Betti, G., Gagliardi, F., Lemmi, A., Verma, V. (2015). Comparative measures of multidimensional deprivationin the European Union, *Empirical Economics*, 49(3) 1071–1100.
Bryan, M. L., Jenkins, S. P. (2016). Multilevel Modelling of Country Effects: A Cautionary Tale, *European Sociological Review*, 32 (1) 3–22. doi: https://doi.org/10.1093/esr/jcv059.
Coli A., Micheletti, E., Pacini, B. (2016). European welfare state in times of crisis according to macroeconomic official statistics. In *Proceeding of the 48th scientific meeting of the Italian Statistical Society*.
Coli, A., Valentini, A. (2017). Mapping Social Protection Statistics. In A. Coli, B, Pacini, E. Stradella (Eds), *Policies, Welfare and Financial Resources, the Impact of the Crisis on Territories*. Pisa: Pisa University Press.
Esping-Andersen, G. (1990). *The three worlds of welfare capitalism*. Polity Press.
Eurostat (2011). *The European System of European System of Integrated Social Protection Statistics*.Eurostat.
Eurostat (2013a).*European System of Accounts (ESA 2010)*. Eurostat.
Eurostat (2013b). *NUTS Nomenclature of Territorial Units for Statistic, by regional level*. Eurostat.
Eurostat (2016). *EU, cross-sectional, version Jan 05 2016*. Eurostat.
Eurostat (2017). Material deprivation statistics – early results. *Statistics explained*. Eurostat. http:ec.europa.eueurostatstatistics-explainedA˙ ccessed 20 September 2017.
Ferrera, M., Fargion, V., Jessoula, M. (2012). *Alle radici del Welfare all'italiana Origini e futuro di un modello sociale squilibrato*. Saggi e ricerche, collana storica della Banca d'Italia. Marsilio.
ISTAT. Benessere e sostenibilita' database (2017). www.istat.it/it/benessere-e-sostenibilita'. Accessed 21 September 2017.
Lijphart A. (1999). *Patterns of Democracy. Government Forms and Performance in Thirty-Six Countries*. New Haven/London.
OECD. Better life index database (2017). www.oecdbetterlifeindex.org. Accessed 21 September 2017.
Powel, M., & Boyne, G. (2001). The spatial strategy of equality and the spatial division of welfare. *Social policy and administration*, 33 (2).
Rodriguez-Pose, A.,& Ezcurra, R. (2009). Does decentralization matter for regional disparities? A cross-country analysis. *Journal of Economic Geography*, Oxford University Press.
Schneider, A. (2003). Decentralization: Conceptualization and Measurement. *Studies in Comparative International Development* 38(3) 32–56.
Sellers, J. M., Lidstrom, A. (2007). Decentralization, Local Government and the Welfare State. *Governance*,24(2) 609–632. Wiley Online Library.
Stiglitz, J., Sen, A. Fitoussi (2010). *Report by the Commission on the Measurement of Economic Performance and Social Progress*. The Commission. http://ec.europa.eu/eurostat/documents/118025/118123/Fitoussi+Commission+report. Accessed 21 September 2017.
Titmuss, R. (1974). *Social policy, An introduction*. Allen&Unwin.
Whelan, C. T., Nolan, B., Maitre, B.(2014). Multidimensional poverty measurement in Europe: An application of the adjusted headcount approach. *Journal of European Social Policy*. 24(2), 183–197. UK, SAGE Publications.

Decent Work Principles and Job Quality Criteria to Improve Sustainable and Equitable Well-Being

Paola Conigliaro

Abstract The principles of Decent Work inspire today the struggle against poverty and the promotion of an equitable, inclusive and sustainable development. The aim to provide a job for all and the commitment to improve working conditions for every worker are mutually supporting aspects of a virtuous action. Well-being at work and well-being in the whole society are interrelated.

A political and economic system based on decent work principles must guarantee social protection to those that cannot work. It also has to preserve leisure, private life, and lifelong learning of worker and non-workers.

Relationships between working conditions and subjective well-being lie on multiple levels. This article aims to highlight the multidimensionality of the quality of work. It also provides a brief description of the data on actual working conditions, which allows comparing the plausible conditions with the targets assumed under international agreements.

Introduction

Work has a central role in the determination of quality of life although relationships between individuals and their job change according to different conditions and contexts. For many people, paid work is a guarantee of livelihood, an opportunity to be autonomous, to affirm their own role, identity and dignity. For some (especially women), it is the sole way to emancipate themselves from seclusion and abuse (Nussbaum 2011), as long as work relationships do not replicate analogous forms of subjection.

P. Conigliaro (✉)
Sapienza University of Rome, Rome, Italy

Italian National Institute of Statistics, Rome, Italy
e-mail: paola.conigliaro@istat.it

A. Bianco et al. (eds.), *Italian Studies on Quality of Life*, Social Indicators Research Series 77, https://doi.org/10.1007/978-3-030-06022-0_22

Work supports inclusion of more vulnerable people, such as those suffering from mental illness, but it may also represent a threat to the mental health of workers in stressful working conditions (WHO 2010).

The Declaration of Philadelphia (ILO 1944) affirms that workers have the right to pursue, through work, "their spiritual development" as well as "their material well-being" because they are able to "make their greatest contribution to the common wellbeing" (Art.3, b). Work allows self- realization. During World War II at its height, the Declaration proclaimed its particular principle of "War against want".

The Declaration is the document which states the aims and purpose of the International Labour Organisation, the tripartite agency founded in 1919 as part of the Versailles Treaty at the end of World War I. The mission of the ILO is to support peace and social justice, promoting the development and adoption of a fair set of roles in the work system. On 10th December 1948, in a social and historical context shaped by the post-war climate and debate, the United Nations adopted the Universal Declaration of Human Rights (UDHR), whose Article 23 ratified the universal right to work.

Other fundamental acts have reiterated the importance of work in terms of equity and social peace. The concepts of human development and sustainability nowadays subsume these values. This is the framework of the *Decent Work* principles.

Decent work concerns universal rights, job quality, and subjective well-being in relation to work.

All domains intersect with the normative asset.

Universal rights are consubstantial with the nature of human beings, without any other specific qualification. So, the right to work impacts on those that can work (labour force), as much as on those that cannot.

The job quality domain concerns all those aspects that define the actual experience of work, e.g. contracts, earnings, working time, work-life balance, career, work intensity, health and safety, human relations.

The domain of subjective well-being in relation to work concerns the relationships of people (workers and non-workers) with work. It is influenced by macro and micro social conditions.

Furthermore, organisational and workers' well-being may have great effect even on customers' and users' rights and safety.

The article is a multi-facetted description of several approaches and definitions of what work should encompass in order to enable human development and sustainability for all. It also presents diverse sets of indicators adopted by major international institutions, which refer to particular knowledge needs. The article aims to highlight common assumptions or peculiarities between different domains in order to meditate on the capability of influencing labour and human conditions, adopting a conjoint strategy. It also provides a brief description on actual working conditions to compare global trends on labour conditions with targets assumed as a consequence of international agreements.

The Right of Decent Work for All

The principles of decent work inspire today the struggle against poverty and the promotion of an equitable, inclusive and sustainable development.

The eradication of slavery and juvenile labour are the absolute priorities. Nonetheless, freedom of choice, equitable salary, safety and salubriousness, respect and the absence of discrimination are necessary conditions in the aim of decent work for all. A political and economic system based on decent work principles must guarantee social protection to those that cannot work (e.g. sick workers, invalids, elderly, unemployed). It also preserves time for leisure, rest, private life and lifelong learning of workers.

The UDHR affirms that everyone has the right to work to free choice of employment, just and favourable working conditions, protection against unemployment, equal pay for equal work without discrimination, remuneration ensuring an existence worthy of human dignity, supplemented, if necessary, by other means of social protection, and to form and to join trade unions for the protection of their interests. Article 24 also promotes the right to rest and leisure, to ensure with reasonable limitation of working hours and periodic paid holidays.

The UN International Covenant on Economic, Social and Cultural Rights (1976) consolidated these principles, and settled that States Parties have to submit reports on the measures adopted and the progress made in achieving the observance of the rights (art.16, p.1).

The ILO promulgated in 1999 the Decent Work Agenda, which rests on four pillars: rights at work; employment creation; social protection; social dialogue and tripartism. Providing the agreed definition of the concept of decent work, the ILO also defined (ILOL 2013) the operative tools to measure it at national and international level; it identified ten substantive dimensions and a set of 90 indicators, including indicators revealing information on the legal frameworks for decent work.

Decent work principles assumed a significant role in the definition of Sustainable Development Goals (SDGs 2015). Even if there is the specific Goal 8, "Decent Work and Economic Growth",[1] ILO's Director-General, Guy Ryder, affirms that decent work is not just a goal; it is, in fact, a driver of sustainable development. Within the SDGs indicators set, there are indeed many indicators connected with the decent work dimension (Table 1). Nevertheless, some goals or targets that could be connected with decent work principles are not associated to specific indicators, so that it is not possible to assess the impact of the statements and their capability of intercession on real life conditions. This is, for instance, the case of lifelong learning, which is quoted in the title of Goal 4, but is not measured by any indicator. Although it is not included in the ILO indicators set, it is a strategic topic in an ever-changing labour system.

[1] In full "Promote sustained, inclusive and sustainable economic growth, full and productive employment and decent work for all".

Table 1 ILO decent work principles compared with indicator in SDGs

ILO Decent Work	Sustainable development goals indicators
Pillars (i–iv) and Dimensions (1-10)	C = Indicators where ILO is custodian I = Indicators where ILO is involved
(ii) Employment creation	Informal employment 8.3.1 – **C**
(1) Employment opportunities	Unemployment rate, by sex, age and persons with disabilities 8.5.2 – **C**
(6) Stability and security of work	Proportion of youth (aged 15–24) not in education, employment or training 8.6.1 – **C**
	8.b.1 Existence of a developed and operationalized national strategy for youth employment, as a distinct strategy or as part of a national employment strategy
(i) Employment opportunities	Proportion and number of children aged 5–17 engaged in child labour, by sex and age 8.7.1 – **C**
(3) Decent working time	Frequency rates of fatal and non-fatal occupational injuries, by sex and migrant status 8.8.1 – **C**
(4) Combining work, family and personal life	
(5) Work that should be abolished	
(8) Safe work environment	
(2) Adequate earnings and productive work	Average hourly earnings of employees, by sex, occupation, age and persons with disabilities 8.5.1 – **C**
(7) Equal opportunity and treatment in employment	Proportion of women in managerial position 5.5.2 – **C**
(iii) Social protection	Proportion of population covered by social protection 1.3.1 – C
(9) Social security	Equity: Labour share of GDP, comprising wages and social protection transfers 10.4.1 – **C**
	Education, health and social protection 1.a.2 government expenditure on essential services – **I**
(iv) Social dialogue and tripartism	Level of national compliance of labour rights (freedom of association and collective bargaining) 8.8.2 – **C**
(10) Social dialogue, employers' and workers' representation	Fundamental freedoms: 16.10.1 killing, kidnapping, enforced disappearance, arbitrary detention and torture of trade unionists and human rights advocates – **I**

Lifelong learning is indeed a very important issue in terms of social sustainability. It is part of the first key principle of the European Pillar of Social Rights (EC 2017). In fact, Europe 2020 fixed as a benchmark an average of at least 15% participating in learning.

The European Pillar draws on the European Social Charter of 1961, the Revised European Social Charter of 1996, the 1989 Community Charter of the Fundamental Social Rights of Workers and the European Code of Social Security of the Council of Europe. It builds upon 20 key principles, structured around three categories: equal opportunities and access to the labour market, fair working conditions, social protection and inclusion. For each principle, the Pillar describes the Union acquis, and how Member States and the social partners could effectively implement it.

The Pillar emphasizes, in particular, those aspects connected with European conditions, nonetheless, it can also represent a model for other regional or national politics. It takes into consideration the need for flexibility to match market pressure; nevertheless, it reaffirms that flexibility cannot justify precariousness. Fair working conditions and access to social protection must be granted to all workers, in standard or non-standard contracts, including various forms of self-employment. Wages have to provide a decent standard of living; this is necessary to prevent in-work poverty. There is no tolerance for any form of discrimination. Adopting the holistic human rights-based approach, the Pillar affirms the key principle of inclusion of people with disabilities in the labour market and in society. Eurostat publishes on its website[2] the social scoreboard of indicators related to the Pillar. There are 36 indicators of which 14 indicators relate to decent work, and five indicators focus on social security. These indicators do not measure some principles which are peculiar to the Pillar, such as social inclusion.

The Quality of Working Conditions

The United Nations Economic Commission for Europe (UNECE) established a statistical framework to measure the quality of employment, collecting information at social macro, meso and micro level. The 2015 edition is just the latest revision on this topic, arranged for the UNECE by the Expert Group on Measuring Quality of Employment of the Conference of European Statisticians (CES). The framework consists on seven dimensions, twelve sub dimensions (Table 2) and almost 70 indicators.

The handbook aims to provide a coherent structure for measuring a multidimensional concept defined as quality of employment. "The statistical framework defines quality of employment from the point of view of the employed person. It refers to the entirety of aspects of employment that may affect the well-being of employed persons" (UNECE 2015, p.6).

The job quality analysis, on its part, takes place at social micro level. It concerns safety and health at work and prevention of risks, including organisational well-being. *Job quality*, as well as *decent work* and *quality of employment*, is a multidimensional concept.

[2]http://ec.europa.eu/eurostat/web/european-pillar-of-social-rights/indicators/social-scoreboard-indicators

Table 2 Quality of employment dimensions – UNECE framework (2015)

Dimension	Sub-dimension
1. Safety and ethics of employment	(a) Safety at work
	(b) Child labour and forced labour
	(c) Fair treatment in employment
2. Income and benefits from employment	(a) Income from employment
	(b) Non-wage pecuniary benefits
3. Working time and work-life balance	(a) Working hours
	(b) Working time arrangements
	(c) Work-life balance
4. Security of employment and social protection	(a) Security of employment
	(b) Social protection
5. Social dialogue	
6. Skills development and training	
7. Employment-related relationships and work motivation	(a) Employment- related relationships
	(b) Work motivation

Eurofound[3] outlined a conceptual framework, which relies on seven objective dimensions and 21 sub-dimensions (Table 3). Most of these indicators, or their components, have an evident relationship with decent work indicators. Eurofound measures work intensity particularly in terms of the availability of time to perform a task, and the capability to manage it.

Studies and policies for the prevention of occupational risks have been mainly directed at the physical environment and the effects on physical health. However, there is a raising awareness of other aspects which influence psychosocial conditions at work. They concern autonomy and control, social relationships, availability of necessary support and work-life balance.

The European Agency for Safety and Health at Work (EU-OSHA), in the same way as Eurofound, conducts surveys and analyses data concerning occupational safety and health at a national level. Its mission is to promote knowledge about risks at work, implement instruments of risk prevention and encourage the improvement of working conditions. It also provides assessment tools for enterprises and organisations, developing a specialized branch on, work-related stress and psychosocial risks at work (EU-OSHA – Eurofound 2014).

Psychosocial risks relate to job design, and concern the potentiality of particular organisational working conditions and contexts, to cause physical or psychological damage (Cox and Griffiths 1995). Poor work design and poor social context of work, for example, may result in work-related stress, burnout or depression.

[3]European Foundation for the Improvement of Living and Working Conditions is a tripartite European Union Agency, whose role is to provide knowledge to assist in the development of better social, employment and work-related policies

Table 3 Dimensions and Sub-dimensions of job quality – Eurofound 2012

Dimension	Sub-dimension
Physical environment	Posture-related (ergonomic)
	Ambient (vibration, noise, temperature)
	Biological and chemical
Work intensity	Quantitative demands
	Pace determinants and interdependency
	Emotional demands
Working time quality	Duration
	Atypical working time
	Working time arrangements
	Flexibility
Social environment	Adverse social behaviour
	Social support
	Management quality
Skills and discretion	Cognitive dimension
	Decision latitude
	Organisational participation
	Training
Prospects	Employment status
	Career prospects
	Job security
	Downsizing
Earnings	

Workers' illnesses, especially those connected with stressful conditions, may have severe consequences on performance and even on the safety and health of clients, users and further stakeholders.

The concept of job quality evolves towards the broader concept of working life quality that embraces a wider range of life aspects connected with labour status and working conditions (Gallie et al. 2012). Macroeconomic and social dynamics, as well as technological changes, lead to the extension of the reference horizon.

The Organisation for Economic Co-operation and Development (OECD) defined the framework for measuring and assessing job quality (Cazes et al. 2015), considering three objective and measurable dimensions: earning quality labour, market security, and quality of the working environment. The framework outlines a simplified description of the concept of working life quality, to allow comparison between countries, and in longitudinal terms. The aim is to consider the multidimensionality of the concept of job quality, including it into the wider OECD well-being framework.

Subjective Well-Being in European Statistics and Its Relationships with Labour Status

The VI European Working Conditions Survey (Eurofound 2016) dedicates a part of its questionnaire to the subjective well-being of workers. It applied the World Health Organization's Well-Being Index (WHO-5), which assesses: 'positive mood' (good spirits and relaxation), 'vitality' (being active and waking up fresh and rested) as well as 'general interest' (being interested in things). The index score ranges from 0 to 100. The average subjective well-being score of workers in Europe is over 65.

The European Statistics Office (Eurostat 2015) dedicated a specific analysis to the relationship between labour status and subjective well-being of workers and non-workers, within the framework of Life Conditions studies. It processed data from the European Union Statistics on Income and Living Conditions, which adopted in 2013 an ad-hoc module on subjective well-being.

To assess subjective well-being, it identified the three dimensions recognized by literature as the most significant: cognitive, affective and eudaimonic (OECD 2013).

In cognitive terms, individuals value their level of satisfaction. This evaluation involves comparison with past conditions, ambitions and performance of other people that they consider themselves more similar or closer to (Michalos 1985 and ff.). On the emotional side, subjects show their affects, which may be positive (trust, joy, happiness) or negative (worry, fear). Eudaimonia corresponds to a sense of purpose, and regards self-realization. It appears as a satisfactory integration with the surrounding world (Huppert et al. 2009).

The relationship between working conditions and subjective well-being should be particularly connected with the eudaimonic dimension.

A micro data analysis of the Italian dataset from Eu-SILC survey (Conigliaro 2018), revealed that the three dimensions of subjective well-being (i.e. life satisfaction, meaning of life and a composite dimension of emotional status) are related with labour conditions. Comparing the level of each dimension of well-being with labour status, the emotional status shows a more evident variation according to labour status. Meaning of life, which is considered in the survey a measure of eudaimonia, is very high for most of the respondents. It seems less influenced by labour conditions, even if it is depleted among unemployed males.

The analysis at the individual level reveals how being involved in a specific labour condition may be associated to a particular level or to a particular dimension of subjective well-being. For example, meaning of life for women is lower in the unemployed, but differences are less evident when compared to that of men.

Paid jobs allow workers to become independent, full and valued actors in society. The workplace is itself an important site of socialization. Sharing a common work experience feeds trust in a community and forges a relevant part of social identity (Dubar 2000).

For these reasons, unemployment may have effects that go beyond the economic disease, affecting psychological well-being and social behaviour (WHO 2010).

The salutary effects of work depend, however, on its nature and conditions. Instability of relationships and isolation may produce insecurity, alienation, high levels of competitiveness, less solidarity, and the acceptance of poorer working conditions. These circumstances increase the risks of mental stress at work, even in standard employment.

Economic and Labour Market Conditions

Before introducing further aspects of the relationship between work and subjective well-being, we need to draw a sketch of the general situation in which this relationship develops. We take here, as implicit, the relevance of some contextual conditions like demographic trends, climate change, depletion of natural resources, micro and widespread conflicts, globalization, financialisation and technological innovation. They are unanimously acknowledged as strongly influencing the structure and dynamics of work.

With regard to the work system, data on economic performance (ILO 2017a) describe an economic context unable to improve quality or quantity of employment. Even economic growth does not guarantee, per-se, decent jobs and income equality (social justice). "This is (...) the paradox that the extraordinary advances in the productive capacity of the global economy now provide the material means to eliminate poverty and meet human needs as never before, but are singularly failing to do so." (ILO 2015, p. 2).

SDG 1 aims to eradicate poverty, but data (Box 1) registers a dramatic persistence of poor-quality employment. Especially in emerging and developing countries, vulnerable work is synonymous with extreme poverty. In developing countries, workers cannot usually count on social transfers because there are no strong social security systems. On the other hand, many mature systems of protection are faced with challenges of economic sustainability.

Box 1: Worst Working Conditions in the World

There are still 152 million child workers and 40.3 million victims of forced labour all over the world; in a year, 2.78 million workers' deaths were work related (ILO 2018).

Half of the workers are in countries that have not yet ratified the Freedom of Association and Protection of the Right to Organise Convention (1948). Only 45 percent of workers have a singular form of social protection, while multiple social protection measures are available for less than 30 percent of the world's population (ILO 2015, 2017b, 2018).

In 2016, nearly half of the workers in Southern Asia and nearly two-thirds in sub-Saharan Africa lived in moderate or extreme poverty (less than

(continued)

Box 1 (continued)

US$3.10 per day in purchasing power terms). The reduction in working poverty was slowing, "endangering the prospects for eradicating poverty as set out in the Sustainable Development Goals." (ILO 2017a, p.2).

It is expected that differences between developed, emerging and developing countries will not diminish, maintaining inequality between countries unacceptable. A high level of inequality also endures within countries between different social groups. Discrimination concerns mainly gender, disability, ethnicity and somatic traits, and religion. Although gender inequality is more severe in many developing countries, it also persists in developed countries; differences concern vulnerability at work, more serious forms of occupational segregation, wage differential and rigid gender roles. "Women continue to be over-represented in both non-standard forms of work and unpaid family labour." (ILO 2015, p.5).

A persistent high level of long-term unemployment affects many countries, including Europe.

Employment growth remains weak and without substantial improvement in quality (Box 2).

The rate of workers in vulnerable employment,[4] marked by precariousness and limited access to contributory social protection schemes, continues to decrease, but at a reduced rate. Temporary and part-time employment (particularly the latter) frequently offer lower wages, poorer prospects for career advancement and less access to social security than full-time permanent contracts. Countries across the EU-28 that have high levels of both involuntary part-time and temporary employment are typically associated with higher rates of in-work poverty.

Box 2: Unemployment, Vulnerable Work, Estrangement

The total number of unemployed is expected to remain stable in 2018, above 192 million (5.5% of the active population). In 2019, the global unemployment rate is expected to remain essentially unchanged, whereas the number of unemployed is projected to grow by 1.3 million (ILO 2018).

Unemployment rate was 5.7% in 2016 (12.8% for 15–24 year-olds and 6.2% for females). In developed countries, unemployment is expected to fall

(continued)

[4]ILO defines workers in vulnerable employment as the sum of own-account workers and contributing family workers. They are less likely to have formal work arrangements, and are therefore more likely to lack decent working conditions, adequate social security and 'voice' through effective representation by trade unions and similar organizations. Vulnerable employment is often characterized by inadequate earnings, low productivity and difficult working conditions that undermine workers' fundamental rights.

Box 2 (continued)

both in level (a reduction of 670,000 people) and in rate (6.2% in 2017 compared to 6.3% in 2016). Within Western, Northern and Southern Europe, the unemployment rate is projected to reach 9.1% in 2017, down by 0.2 percentage points in respect to values anticipated for 2016. Progress towards returning to pre-crisis level of 7.4% (in 2008) is slowing down (ILO 2017a).

Workers in vulnerable employment remain at 1.4 billion in 2017. They represent 42% of total workers, 50% in emerging countries, and even 80% in developing countries. Projections draw an improvement in vulnerable workers of 11 million annually. This will happen particularly in Southern Asia and sub-Saharan Africa. In EU-28, part-time employment amounts to 20.5%. Non-voluntary part-time is higher in those countries where the part-time portion is smaller, and it has risen faster in recent years, e.g. Italy and Spain, a 4% increase (ILO 2017a).

The VI European Working Condition Survey registered very few advancements in job quality over the last 10 years in Europe. Structural inequality continued to result as the most significant. Despite an improvement in the working time quality index, "one worker in five (22%) works in their free time to meet work demands at least several times a month" (Eurofound 2016, p.8), within a generally positive social environment, "around 16% of workers – more women than men – report exposure to adverse social behaviour" (ibidem). All the considered part-time workers score a lower level of job quality (59) compared to full-time workers (66). Job insecurity perception remains at the same level as in 2010.

In the EU-28, young NEETs (Not in Education, Employment or Training) amount to 12% of the 14–24 years-old population in 2015 (Eurofound 2016b).

Data confirm that European countries are facing a profound crisis in the world of work despite clearly better working conditions and more advanced and universalistic social protection.

The Meaning of Work, and Its Future Perspectives

To achieve the goal of decent work for all, the entire complex set of rules and recommendations defined at international level has to be translated into practical applications which impact on workers' lives and personal well-being.

The referring pattern of decent work is the "standard" job, which corresponds to a stable job, lasting for the whole working life, a professional or technically specialized competence and an educational and training coherent course.

If we assume a global vision, we have instead to recognize the absolute prevalence of "non- standard" working conditions. In the pursuit of decent work for all, it is necessary to take account of these constraints.

Companies, stressed by market pressure, require more flexibility by workers. This often means short-term contracts or adaptation to spatial and functional changes. Workers always have to be available and efficient; frequently, they are not sufficiently updated, informed and consulted. These circumstances increase physical and psychological risks. Ever-changing sets or jobs deplete relationships with colleagues and undermine social support in the work context.

There is a portion of workers, especially in developed and emerging countries, that are completely monopolized by work because the boundaries between private life and work collapse. They follow a pattern of total and absolute readiness; the 24/7 model (Crary 2013).

Many forms of self-employment conceal a subordination, pillaged of every elementary right, or a form of precarious work without rules and social protection. Most people, especially young people, have little opportunity of choosing the job they get.

In the context of fragmented functions, and highly specialised training, competence becomes rapidly obsolete. Professional identity becomes weaker because working paths lose their clearness, further compromising connections with colleagues. These conditions affect the solidity and serenity of workers (Gallino 2011).

Furthermore, due to high unemployment rates and precarious job security, younger generations do not see many opportunities of stable income and professional development. The majority of them may consider work not central in their life projects, but as part of a hostile system in which they cannot self-identify.

These signals are now a cause of concern. However, this problem can be observed from another angle. Sociological and philosophical studies demonstrate that work has not always been considered consubstantial with human essence. In a broad interpretation of Max Weber's theory, many scholars associate the positive value of labour to the Protestant ethic. Indeed, Francesco Totaro (1998) identified the first evidence of a new work ethic in St. Paul's writings. However, the author situated the concrete change of labour physiognomy in modern times. Work in modernity became decisive, both in terms of the concept of action and the concept of being.

This reflection leads to conclude that work has not always had an ethical value, therefore, it may assume a completely different meaning in the future. Humankind has the faculty to imagine it as more tailored to the essence of human capabilities, and to act in order to realize this vision. Within this framework of principles, conditions and constraints, it is compelling to reflect on the meaning of work and the role of work, in satisfying human needs. The question of the value of work, according to different age cohorts, geographical areas, and social, political, cultural and economic conditions is therefore fundamental. The ILO meeting "The Future of Work We Want: a Global Dialogue" (Geneva, April 2017) focused attention on the work wanted, imagined, and desired, rather than forecast, assuming that our vision can influence work, economy, policy and justice.

We can register, in fact, a wide agreement on the general principles of decent work, and considerable disputes in defining problems, answers and solutions. Some perspectives may consider a condition or a trend mainly as an opportunity, others as a threat.

In the ILO debate, represented the main different visions which are commonly found in all current discussions on the future perspective of work. They concern the threats and potential associated with some phenomena, such as technological innovation or globalisation, whose centrality is undisputed.

Technological innovation and automation increase productivity level. They have the potential to release humankind from hard work, allowing them to invest time and energy into richer pursuits. Nevertheless, we register a significant dissonance between technological and human development; an inexplicable proportion of people in the world still work to survive.

The oligopoly of a few huge companies on the global market makes any regulation within the labour system ineffective; companies control the market and set out the rules. Some experts consider small and medium companies, which represent the backbone of the local economy, strategic in promoting more widespread wealth and supporting local development. Others sustain that, in a system composed of small companies and independent workers, it is more difficult to assure the quality of working conditions.

There are also other issues underlying completely different visions of the future. One of these regards the future of education. The role of education is widely recognized, but what kind of education? Training oriented to fit the labour market offers highly specialized profiles. It provides a strong identification with a role or a profession, high levels of competence and better performance, but it is threatened by precariousness. For this reason, to address the challenges of an ever-changing world of work, education focused on the person is considered more effective when it makes the individual capable of facing many different problems with an open mind.

Other reflections go a step beyond the frontiers, challenging concepts regarding the meaning of work or the future of the standard model.

These are just few examples of a wider panorama of perspectives. Unfortunately, it is not possible to find evidence in any of them that the actual trends will lead to the achievement of global social justice. The current situation may result in many different scenarios that could coexist as a consequence of extremely segmented and unequal labour markets. In a sustainable perspective, the existence of such a level of inequality is unacceptable.

Final Considerations

The contribution of labour to human development is commonly recognized, provided that work relationships take place respecting human dignity.

External and internal determinants influence working conditions and opportunities, with a huge impact on individual expectancy. Social and employment policies, economic context and organisational rules concern job quality, social relationships at work and subjective well-being.

As figures demonstrate, current external conditions greatly threaten internal determinants, bringing one to consider work for all, and dignity at work, as fungible factors. But it is not effective to assume the existence of a trade-off between these two elements of decent work.

The aim to provide jobs for all and the commitment to improve working conditions for every worker are indeed mutually supporting aspects of a virtuous action. A systemic vision, capable of putting into relation macro levels (political, ethical, and cultural) and micro levels (organisational), is crucial to defining more effective actions in line with ethical objectives.

Each indicator set, briefly presented in this paper, enriches the knowledge of such an articulated phenomenon, highlighting some elements of it. However, this wealth of information can work to the detriment of the interpretative capacity and the definition of clear objectives and effective policies. For these reasons, it is necessary to acquire a common awareness of the different approach to the concept, paying attention to an unambiguous use of terminology and definitions.

References

Cazes, S., Hijzen, A., Saint-Martin, A. (2015). Measuring and Assessing Job Quality – The OECD Job Quality Framework. OECD Social, Employment and Migration Working Papers No. 174. Paris: OECD Publishing. doi:https://doi.org/10.1787/5jrp02kjw1mr-en

Conigliaro, P. (2018). Labour Status and Subjective Well-being. A Micro-level Analysis and a Multidimensional Approach to Well-being. *Working Paper Series. PhD course in Applied Social Sciences. 4 (2018).* Department of Social Sciences and Economics. Sapienza University of Rome

Cox, T., & Griffiths, A. (1995). The nature and measurement of work-related stress: Theory and practice. In Wilson, J. R. and Corlett, N. (Ed.), *Evaluation of human work*, 3rd ed. London: CRS Press.

Crary, J. (2013) *24/7. Late Capitalism and the Ends of Sleep*. London: Verso Editions

Dubar, C. (2000). *La socialisation. Construction des identités sociales et professionnelles*. Paris: Armand Colin Editeur. 3e édition.

Eurofound. (2012). *Trends in job quality in Europe*. Luxembourg: Publication Office of the European Union. doi:https://doi.org/10.2806/3516

Eurofound. (2016). *VI European Working Condition Survey – Overview report*. Luxembourg: Publication Office of the European Union. doi: https://doi.org/10.2806/25823

Eurofound. (2016b). *Exploring the diversity of NEETs*. Luxembourg: Publication Office of the European Union. doi:https://doi.org/10.2806/62307

EU-OSHA – Eurofound. (2014). *Psychosocial risks in Europe Prevalence and strategies for prevention*. Luxembourg: Publication Office of the European Union. doi: https://doi.org/10.2806/70971

European Commission. (2017). *European Pillar of Social Rights*. Brussel: European Commission. doi:https://doi.org/10.2792/95934

Eurostat. (2015). *Quality of life, fact and views*. Luxembourg: Publication Office of the European Union. doi:https://doi.org/10.2785/59737

Gallie, D., Gosetti, G, La Rosa, M. (2012). *Qualità del lavoro e della vita lavorativa*. Sociologia del lavoro 127. Milano: Franco Angeli

Gallino, L. (2011). Il lavoro oggi: merce o valore. In Gosetti, G. (Ed.). *Lavoro e lavori. Strumenti per comprendere il cambiamento*, 17–28. Milano: Franco Angeli

Huppert, F. A., Marks, N., Clark, A., Siegrist, J., Stutzer, A., Vitterso, J., Wahrendorf, M. (2009). Measuring Well-being Across Europe: Description of the ESS Well-being Module and Preliminary Findings. *Social Indicators Research, 91,* 301–315

ILO. (1944). *Declaration of Philadelphia*. Geneva: International Labour Office

ILO. (2013). *Decent work indicators. Guidelines for producers and users of statistical and legal framework indicators*. Geneva: International Labour Office. ISBN: 9789221280187; 9789221280194 (web pdf)

ILO. (2015). *Future of work centenary initiative report*. Geneva: International Labour Office. ISBN 9789221289982 (web pdf)

ILO. (2017a). *World Employment Social Outlook Trends 2017*. Geneva: International Labour Office. ISBN 9789221288824 (web pdf)

ILO. (2017b). World Social Protection Report 2017–19. Universal social protection to achieve the Sustainable Development Goals. Geneva: International Labour Office. ISBN 978–92–2-130016-8 (web pdf)

ILO. (2018). *World Employment Social Outlook Trends 2018*. Geneva: International Labour Office. ISBN 9789221315360 (web pdf)

Michalos, A. C. (1985). Multiple Discrepancy Theory. *Social Indicator Research, 16,* 347–413

Nussbaum, M. C. (2011). *Creating Capabilities. The Human Development Approach*. Cambridge (Mass): The Belknap Press of Harvard University Press

OECD. (2013). *Guidelines on Measuring Subjective Well-being*. Paris: OECD Publishing. doi:https://doi.org/10.1787/9789264191655-en

Totaro, F. (1998). *Non di solo lavoro – Ontologia della persona ed etica del lavoro nel passaggio di civiltà*. Roma: Vita e pensiero

UN Office of the High Commissioner for Human Rights. (1976) *International Covenant on Economic, Social and Cultural Rights*. UN-OHCHR

WHO. (2010). *Mental health and well-being at the workplace – protection and inclusion in challenging times*. Copenhagen: WHO Regional Office for Europe. ISBN 9789289002059

Patient Satisfaction and Uncertainty in Illness in Oncology: Which Are the Relevant Aspects When Planning a Qualitatively Adequate Assistance?

Maria Daniela Giammanco and Lara Gitto

Abstract This study, aimed at assessing oncology patient satisfaction, was carried out at four operating units of the ARNAS Garibaldi of Catania. The analysis involved 300 cancer patients.

The patients responded to a questionnaire designed to collect epidemiological and socio-demographic data. The questionnaire included the Mishel Uncertainty in Illness Scale (MUIS), as well as a tool measuring patient satisfaction with, respectively, the service received, the medical and nursing staff, the access, the waiting time and the comfort.

An ordered logit model was estimated. The results suggest that Uncertainty in Illness and its components (Ambiguity, Inconsistency Complexity and Unpredictability), patient participation and other service-related aspects, impact on patient satisfaction.

The findings confirm the need for a greater involvement of the patient as part of a Customer Satisfaction Management model.

The same model can be applied in different settings to strengthen patients' empowerment process and their ability to manage the disease.

Introduction

Any approach to care for chronic and long term diseases should address patients' needs and requirements (Miles 2009), especially when patients are suffering from chronic illnesses (Miles and Asbridge 2014). In this perspective, social policy

M. D. Giammanco (✉)
Dipartimento di Scienze Politiche e Sociali, Università di Catania, Catania, Italy
e-mail: mdgiamma@unict.it

L. Gitto (✉)
CEIS EEHTA (Economic Evaluation & Health Technology Assessment), Università di Roma "Tor Vergata", Rome, Italy
e-mail: Gitto@CEIS.uniroma2.it

A. Bianco et al. (eds.), *Italian Studies on Quality of Life*, Social Indicators Research Series 77, https://doi.org/10.1007/978-3-030-06022-0_23

makers should develop programs aimed at improving patient satisfaction as well as their health conditions (Bottomley 2002).

The assessment of patients' personal experiences and expectations in healthcare are crucial factors for planning a qualitatively adequate assistance. Their perspectives may help to draw guidelines and protocols aimed at improving assistance and support: the latter, together with accountability and innovation, are a priority in all cancer-related services (Husson et al. 2011).

Patient satisfaction is of major importance in the implementation of the *Customer Satisfaction Management model* by the *European Primer on Customer Satisfaction Management* (EUPAN 2017): it requires the involvement of citizens/users in programming, producing and assessing a service. Successful organizations use customers' expectations as the starting point: managing satisfaction has to do with services and/or products, but also with the ultimate satisfaction of the citizen/customer (EUPAN 2017).

Several factors appear to cause the gap between expectations and the actual experience of the service. The latter is highly influenced by interaction with sources other than the service provider itself (e.g. family, colleagues, media, etc.) and by statements heard from staff members or read on leaflets or other publicity material. Even external factors such as the appearance of the buildings may create expectations on the patients (Huisman et al. 2012).

Many of these factors are considered in the present analysis, which was carried out on a sample of patients at four oncology units of a public hospital in Sicily, Southern Italy. In Sicily, the number of cancer patients increased in the 3-year period 2009–2011: the average annual number of ordinary admissions for tumor diseases was 42,171, of which 55.9% were male patients and 44.1% female (Ministero della Salute 2007).

The aim of this paper is to analyse oncology patient satisfaction with the services received.

The study is organized as follows: the next section illustrates the framework of analysis, reporting the relevant literature dealing with patient satisfaction and uncertainty in the oncology setting. Then, the tools employed to collect the relevant information, some statistics about the observed sample and the econometric model are presented. The discussion of the results, together with some comments, conclude this contribution.

Background

Health services researchers, healthcare providers and regulators have acknowledged that patient satisfaction, together with clinical results, economic measures and Health Related Quality of Life (HRQoL), is a constituent part of healthcare quality (Lin and Kelly 1995; Heidegger et al. 2006).

Patient satisfaction has been considered a key patient-focused outcome to assess and enhance (Gesell and Gregory 2004) as it is the result of the interpersonal process of care stemming from the patient's general opinion on the quality of care (Donabedian 1988).

In the case of oncology patients, who often face prolonged care and become highly dependent on the health care system, satisfaction becomes a facet of general life satisfaction (Locker and Dunt 1978; Blanchard et al. 1990; Gupta et al. 2014).

It has been stressed how oncology patient satisfaction is determined by several factors such as accessibility of care and clinical environment; technical aspects of care; patients' education and the information provided by medical personnel (Sitzia and Wood 1998).

The importance of the information received in determining patient satisfaction is embedded in the questionnaires typically used to assess it (Sandoval et al. 2006; Brédart et al. 2005; Kleeberg et al. 2005), as patients consider both physicians and nurses as a relevant source of information (Oberst 1984; Tishelman 1994; Hutchison et al. 1991) likely to reduce uncertainty (Mishel 1999). Moreover, information improves patients' satisfaction in relation to perceived trust and responsiveness from providers (Mowen et al. 1993).

Tightly linked to the impact of the interpersonal aspects of care and the information received on oncology patient satisfaction is the perceived Uncertainty in Illness.

Uncertainty has been defined as "*the inability to determine the meaning of illness-related events*", characterized by the subjective interpretation made by the patient about illness-related events (Mishel 1981). Uncertainty may be divided into four different dimensions: Ambiguity, Inconsistency, Complexity and Unpredictability. In particular, Ambiguity relates to the vagueness of the state of illness; Inconsistency concerns contradictory information received; Complexity relates to the cues about the treatment; Unpredictability accounts for the difficulty of connecting the treatment to the health outcome (Mishel 1997).

Uncertainty is a determinant of stress for people suffering from life-threatening illness and their caregivers, such as parents and relatives (Santacroce 2003). It might negatively affect their HRQoL, promoting the onset of anxiety and depression (Taylor et al. 1991; Carleton et al. 2012) and lowering the compliance to medical treatments (Brouwers and Sorrentino 1993; Bailey Jr. et al. 2009).

Data and Methods

According to the National Cancer Plan, in Italy the health assistance for cancer patients is provided by hospitals (Ministero della Salute 2014). The present study was carried out at four operating units of a public hospital, the ARNAS Garibaldi, located in Catania. The units were: the Reception of the Oncology Centre, the Day Hospital Division, the Medical Oncology Division and the Weekly Surgery Division.

The analysis involved 300 consecutive cancer patients. Between February and April 2016 they responded to a questionnaire designed to collect epidemiological and socio-demographic data. The duration of the survey was, on average, 30–35 min.

The questionnaire consisted of several parts aimed at assessing the various dimensions of the patient's disease experience, related to the oncological hospital service. It included internationally validated scales, such as the European Organization for Research and Treatment of Cancer in Patient Satisfaction with Care Measure (EORTC IN-PATSAT32) and the Mishel Uncertainty in Illness Scale (MUIS).

The EORTC IN-PATSAT32 (Brédart et al. 2005) is a 32-item questionnaire assessing patients' appraisal of hospital doctors and nurses, as well as specific aspects of the care organization and services. It contains 11 multi-item and 3 single-item scales. The scales assess technical competence, information provided and interpersonal skills of both physicians and nurses. The questionnaire also evaluates interpersonal skills and information provided by other hospital staff, waiting time, access, exchange of information, comfort and overall satisfaction with care.

In line with the questionnaire items, an additional question was introduced to capture the patient's experience of her/his involvement in all the medical choices impacting her/his own health.

The MUIS assesses the uncertainty associated with the course and the treatment of the disease and it has often been used for oncology patients (Mishel 1981; Mishel et al. 1984; LaPushin 2009; Parker et al. 2013; Hagen et al. 2015).

The first part of the empirical analysis concerned a statistical problem related to the correlation among subscales of the same questionnaire, that may arise in such a context. When jointly analyzing two variables from the same source (e.g. two items of the MUIS questionnaire), the variation among two variables may be spurious due to the causal effect of a third variable impacting on the other two. For example, a positive correlation between patient satisfaction and Inconsistency (the dimension related to the soundness of information given to the patients), which implies that the more contradictory the information, the higher the patient satisfaction, may be due to the circumstance that Inconsistency is correlated with other dimensions, such as Complexity, which concerns the cues about the treatment. Complexity, in turn, is correlated with patient satisfaction (0.292). Therefore, the positive link between Inconsistency and patient satisfaction may derive from the positive and stronger correlation with Complexity.

This issue is addressed with partial correlations. For each MUIS dimension, the partial correlations estimate the relationships between such dimension and the dependent variable, while controlling for each of the other three MUIS subscales (Bailey Jr. et al. 2009).

The formula for partial correlations is:

$$r_{\mathrm{xy.z}} = \frac{r_{\mathrm{XY}} - r_{\mathrm{XZ}} r_{\mathrm{ZY}}}{\sqrt{1 - r_{\mathrm{XZ}}^2} \cdot \sqrt{1 - r_{\mathrm{ZY}}^2}}$$

Hence, partial correlations, in this context, help to select which dimensions within a validated scale should be selected as regressors and which sign of correlation is to be expected.

In the econometric estimations, the MUIS subscales with significant partial correlations were considered as regressors of an ordered logit regression, whose dependent variable was the satisfaction for the service and the assistance received (item 27 of the EORTC IN-PATSAT32).

In the ordered logit model, the dependent variable Y is a linear function of another latent variable, Y*, continuous and not measured. This latent variable Y* has different thresholds: the probability to observe a given outcome corresponds to the probability that the estimated linear function, plus random error, is within the range of the cut-points estimated for the outcome.

The continuous latent variable is equal to:

$$Y^*{}_{\mathrm{i}} = \sum_{k=1}^{K} \beta_k X_{\mathrm{ki}} + \varepsilon_i$$

The βs are the coefficients to be estimated; x_{1i}, x_{2i}, ..., are the regressors employed; ε_i is the error term, assumed to be logistically distributed. The coefficients βs are estimated together with the cut-points that allow to calculate the probability that Y will take on a particular value (Wooldridge 2010).

The choice of the ordered logit model was motivated by the fact that patients' assessment was expressed on an ordered scale from 1 to 5, where 1 corresponds to the lowest assessment and 5 to a service of excellent quality. The score was then standardized on a 0–100 scale, so that the final values for the dependent variable were 25, 50, 75, 100 (no one rated the service so poorly as to have a final score of 0) (Brédart et al. 2005).

Results

Some descriptive statistics related to the observed sample of 300 oncology patients are reported in Table 1.

Patients were, on average, 59 years old; almost 55% were female and most of them (81.3%) were married. More than 54% of the patients presented other co-morbidities. Most of them had a primary education. On average, individuals had known their diagnosis for 14 months.

As specified in Table 1, patients attributed average scores of 53.43 and 50.50, on a 0–100 scale, to their overall satisfaction and feeling of participation. They rated the physicians' skills at 58.52 and the nurses' interpersonal skills at 65.17. Organizational aspects such as waiting times, access and comfort received the scores of 47.32, 47.74 and 52.93, respectively.

Table 1 Descriptive statistics

Variable	Mean	Std. Dev.	Min	Max
Age	59.16	11.35	28	86
Gender (female = 1; male = 0)	0.545	0.499	0	1
Married (yes = 1; no = 0)	0.813	0.391	0	1
Education level (from 1 = primary to 4 = post graduate)	1.647	0.711	1	4
Time from diagnosis (months)	14.384	18.753	1	180
Comorbidity factors (yes = 1, no = 0)	0.544	0.498	0	1
General satisfaction	3.134	0.784	1	5
Participation	3.023	0.976	0	5
General assessment of physicians' skills	58.519	19.937	0	100
Assessment of nurses' interpersonal skills	65.161	22.859	0	100
Waiting times	47.324	19.461	0	100
Access	47.742	17.170	0	100
Comfort	52.926	19.585	0	100
MUIS Ambiguity	34.711	6.886	12	56
MUIS Inconsistency	24.436	3.950	7	35
MUIS Complexity	15.252	2.819	7	26
Better health comparing to last year (yes = 1, no = 0)	0.117	0.322	0	1

Table 2 Pearson's correlations

	EORTC 27	Ambiguity	Inconsistency	Complexity	Unpredictability
EORTC 27	1				
Ambiguity	0.199***	1			
Inconsistency	0.052	0.710***	1		
Complexity	0.292***	0.333***	0.336***	1	
Unpredictability	−0.090	0.164***	0.217***	−0.064	1

*90% significant; **95% significant; ***99% significant

As far as Uncertainty scales were concerned, Ambiguity scored 34.71 (on a 12–56 range); Inconsistency 24.44 (on a 7–35 range); Complexity 15.25 (on a 7–26 range). On average, patients reported a worsening in their health conditions in comparison to the previous year: only 11.7% affirmed their health status had improved.

Bivariate Pearson's correlations were first used to examine the pairwise correlation between each two MUIS dimensions and then to determine whether the associations of these dimensions with demographic variables and other symptom measures differed in magnitude or direction.

Table 2 shows the Pearson's correlations the pairwise correlations between each couple of the MUIS dimensions, and each MUIS dimension and the EORTC IN-PATSAT32 item no. 27.

When partial correlations are considered, it is possible to observe a high level of significance between patient satisfaction and Ambiguity, Complexity and

Table 3 Partial correlation analysis

MUIS dimensions	Control variables	Correlation with EORTC 27
MUIS-Ambiguity	Inconsistency-Complexity-Unpredictability	0.202** (0.000)
MUIS-Inconsistency	Ambiguity-Complexity-Unpredictability	−0.160** (0.006)
MUIS-Complexity	Ambiguity-Inconsistency-Unpredictability	0.256** (0.000)
MUIS-Unpredictability	Ambiguity-Inconsistency-Complexity	−0.273 (0.212)

*90% significant; **95% significant; ***99% significant

Table 4 Variables employed in the econometric analysis

Control variables	Age (and squared age), sex(f = 1; m = 0), marital status (1 = married, 0 = not married), education level (from 1 to 4), other pathologies (1 = yes, 0 = no)
Health related variables	Health state assessment (1 = improved with respect to the previous year, 0 = not improved).
MUIS (Uncertainty assessment)	Total scores of the MUIS dimensions: Ambiguity, Inconsistency, Complexity, Unpredictability.
EORTC: assessment of the service received, physicians and nurses assessment	Overall satisfaction (**dependent variable**), participation and involvement. Physicians' global skills, nurses interpersonal skills, comfort, access, waiting time.

Inconsistency. The latter is inversely correlated with the dependent variable. The dimension of Unpredictability is not significant.

Table 3 reports the results of partial correlations.

Table 4 reports all the variables included in the econometric estimation.

Finally, the results of the ordered logit estimations can be seen in Table 5.

Overall, the estimates are significant.

Among the variables selected as controls, age presents a non-linear relation with patient satisfaction: hence, the younger the patient the worse her/his assessment of the service This is in line with the existing literature on patient satisfaction (Henley and Davis 1967; Hall and Dornan 1990; Williams 1994).

Education level is positively and significantly related with patient satisfaction: this result contradicts some findings implying that the less educated patients are the more satisfied (Hall and Dornan 1990). Being a woman and married is negatively related to patient satisfaction, though these relations are not statistically significant.

A positive and significant relationship can be observed between the dependent variable and the reporting of a better health compared to the previous year, in line with the existing evidence showing that oncology patients tend to have a variety of unmet needs, which increase as the disease advances (Bitar et al. 2004).

Results also show a positive correlation between the dependent variable and the appreciation of the physicians' global skills and the nurses' interpersonal skills.

With regards to the impact of the organizational aspects of care on patient satisfaction, the coefficients have the expected signs, *i.e.* negative for waiting time

Table 5 Ordered logit estimations

Variable	Coefficient	Standard Err.
Age	−0.203**	0.100
Age2	0.002**	0.001
Education level	0.561***	0.216
Sex(1 = female; 0 = male)	−0.213	0.343
Married (1 = yes; 0 = not)	−0.364	0.342
MUIS: Ambiguity	0.071**	0.032
MUIS: Inconsistency	−0.090*	0.053
MUIS: Complexity	0.007	0.069
Physicians' global skills	0.024**	0.011
Nurses' interpersonal skills	0.038***	0.011
Patient's feeling of participation	1.130***	0.267
Access	0.046**	0.022
Waiting time	−0.008	0.016
Comfort	0.020	0.013
Health betterment	0.954**	0.469

Log pseudolikelihood = −185.199; Pseudo R2 = 0.414; Wald chi2(15) = 180.69
90% significant; **95% significant; ***99% significant

and positive for comfort. Only access is significant and positively correlated (the easier the access to the medical centre, the higher the satisfaction). These results are in line with those contributions stressing the importance of the hospital environment on patient satisfaction (Siddiqui et al. 2005; Lis et al. 2009).

The variable capturing the feeling of participation is strongly significant and has the highest positive coefficient: hence, the more the patient feels he/she has shared decisions with the medical staff, the more he/she is satisfied (Lis et al. 2009).

When considering the results related to the impact of diverse facets of Uncertainty in Illness on patient satisfaction, Ambiguity shows a positive and significant relationship with patient satisfaction, while the dimension of Inconsistency is negatively correlated, though weakly significant. Finally, the MUIS dimension of Complexity is not significantly correlated.

Discussion

The present research is part of the literature that considers patient satisfaction as a measure of the quality of the health care delivered, to be monitored and examined in order to improve providers' performance.

The econometric analysis has outlined the relevance, for oncology patient satisfaction, of subjective factors, diverse aspects of Uncertainty in Illness, specific facets of self assessed HRQoL, the appraisal of professional and interpersonal competences of the personnel and organizational factors.

The results of the regression analysis, with respect to the control variables, mainly confirm the findings of the existent literature.

Moreover, patients seem to give importance to physicians' global skills, i.e. their medical judgment or experience and their interpersonal skills, rather than focusing on technical aspects alone (Lis et al. 2009).

The variable related to nurses' interpersonal skills are significant and positively correlated with patient satisfaction. Nurses have a pivotal role in supplying "*the feeling of concern, regard and respect one human being may have for another*" (Mayer 2007; Mack et al. 2009).

With respect to the Uncertainty related dimensions, the direct and significant correlation of Ambiguity and the inverse and weakly significant correlation of Inconsistency with patient satisfaction are consistent with the aspects of Uncertainty in Illness that these dimensions of the MUIS aim to capture. Ambiguity concerns the patients' perceived inability to control and govern those aspects of their health conditions that are affected by the evolution of cancer, together with the intrinsic uncertainty associated to its treatment. Inconsistency, on the other hand, relies on objective factors, such as the quality of the information received.

The result that the first dimension is positively related to the judgment given to the assistance received may signify that the more challenging and uncertain the illness state *per se*, the greater the extent to which patients need to rely on the hospital and, consequently, the higher their assessment of the service received. On the other hand, the negative sign of Inconsistency suggests that patients require high quality information to be satisfied.

Conclusions

The present contribution has highlighted some determinants of oncology patient satisfaction concerning the assistance received.

The analysis focused on 300 outpatients of four oncology wards at the ARNAS Garibaldi of Catania (Italy). An *ad hoc* questionnaire was built, asking for socio-demographic and epidemiological information and including the EORTC IN-PATSAT 32 and the MUIS.

The suggestions to be drawn from this contribution is that people actively engaged in oncology care should seek as much as possible to embrace the patient's perspective. Involving the patient in the treatment should be a priority, in order to obtain a bilateral understanding of the illness experience and to reduce the Uncertainty in Illness. In this way, medical decisions would respect patients' values and expectations (Epstein et al. 2005).

The analysis could be deepened by considering other socio-economic variables, in order to detect those factors which contribute to the worsening/bettering of the patient's health status. Communication approaches of the diverse professional figures could also be studied, in order to implement strategies specifically tailored for each professional role, to better respond to the patient's queries and doubts emerging during the different stages of the treatment and the progression of the disease.

Acknowledgments The authors would like to thank Giorgio Giulio Santonocito, General Director, Anna Rita Mattaliano, Health Director and Anna Colombo, Head of the Clinical Risk Management Unit of the ARNAS Garibaldi of Catania, for allowing them to carry out the research.

They also thank Maria Avanzato and Chiara Gerratana for having conducted the interviews and collected the data. Usual caveats apply.

References

Bailey Jr., D.E., Landerman, L., Barroso, J., Bixby, P., Mishel, M.H., Muir, A.J., et al. (2009). Uncertainty, Symptoms and Quality of Life in Persons with Chronic Hepatitis C Undergoing Watchful Waiting. *Psychosomatics* 50, 138–146.

Bitar, R., Bezjak, A., Mah, K., Loblaw, D.A., Gotowiec, A.P., Devins, G.M. (2004). Does tumor status influence cancer patients' satisfaction with the doctor-patient interaction? *Supportive care in cancer* 12, 34–40.

Blanchard, C.G., Labreque, M.S., Ruckdeschel, J., Blamchard, E.D (1990). Physician behaviors, patient perceptions, and patient characteristics as predictors of satisfaction of hospitalized adult cancer patients. *Cancer* 65, 186–192.

Bottomley, A. (2002). The cancer patient and quality of life. *Oncologist* 7, 120–125.

Brédart, A., Bottomley, A., Blazeby, J.M., Conroy, T., Coens, C., D'Haese, S.,et al. (2005). An international prospective study of the EORTC cancer in-patient satisfaction with care measure (EORTC IN-PATSAT32). *European Journal of Cancer Care* 41, 2120–2131.

Brouwers, M.C. & Sorrentino, R.M. (1993). Uncertainty orientation and protection motivation theory: The role of individual differences in health compliance. *Journal of Personality and Social Psychology* 65, 102–112.

Carleton, R.N., Mulvogue, M.K., Thibodeau, M.A., McCabe, R.E., Antony, M.M., Asmundson, G.J. (2012). Increasingly certain about uncertainty: Intolerance of uncertainty across anxiety and depression. *Journal of Anxiety Disorders* 26, 468–479.

Donabedian, A. (1988). The quality of care: how can it be assessed? *Journal of the American Medical Association* 260, 1743–1748.

Epstein, R.M., Franks, P., Fiscella, K., Shields, C.G., Meldrum, S.C., Kravitz, R.L., et al. (2005) Measuring patient-centered communication in patient–physician consultations: theoretical and practical issues. *Social Science and Medicine* 61, 1516–1528.

EUPAN. http://www.eupan.eu/. Last accessed: 15 May 2017.

Gesell, S. B., & Gregory, N. (2004). Identifying priority actions for improving patient satisfaction with outpatient cancer care. *Journal of Nursing Care Quality* 19, 226–233.

Gupta, D., Rodeghier, M., Lis, C.G. (2014). Patient satisfaction with service quality as a predictor of survival outcomes in breast cancer. *Supportive Care in Cancer* 22, 129–134.

Hagen, K.B,. Aas, T., Lode, K., Gjerde, J., Lien, E., Kvaløy, J.T., et al. (2015). Illness uncertainty in breast cancer patients: validation of the 5-item short form of the Mishel Uncertainty in Illness Scale. *European Journal of Oncology Nursing* 19, 113–119.

Hall, J.A. & Dornan, M.C. (1990). Patient sociodemographic characteristics as predictors of satisfaction with medical care. *Social Science and Medicine* 30, 811–818.

Henley, B. & Davis, M.S. (1967). Satisfaction and dissatisfaction: a study of the chronically ill aged patients. *Journal of Health and Social Behavior* 8, 65–84.

Heidegger, T., Saal, D., Nuebling, M. (2006). Patient satisfaction with anaesthesia care: what is patient satisfaction, how should it be measured, and what is the evidence for assuring high patient satisfaction? *Best Practice & Research Clinical Anaesthesiology* 20, 331–346.

Huisman, E.R.C.M., Morales, E., van Hoof, J., Kort, H.S.M. (2012). Healing environment: A review of the impact of physical environmental factors on users, *Building and Environment* 58, 70–80.

Husson, O., Mols, F., van de Poll-Franse, L.V. (2011). The relation between information provision and health-related quality of life, anxiety and depression among cancer survivors: a systematic review. *Annals of Oncology* 22, 761–772.

Hutchison, G., Addington-Hall, J., Bower, M., Austen, M., Coombes, C. (1991). Evaluation de la satisfaction des patients quant aux soins dispensés par une équipe pluri-disciplinaire en oncologie. *European Journal of Cancer Care* 1, 16–20.

Kleeberg, U.R., Tews, J.T., Ruprecht, T. et al. (2005). Patient satisfaction and quality of life in cancer outpatients: results of the PASQOC study. *Supportive Care in Cancer* 13, 303–310.

Lapushin, T. (2009). *Theory of uncertainty in illness in patients with cancer of unknown primary origin: Structure providers as antecedents of uncertainty in a population of cancer patients with an unknown primary diagnosis*. Texas Medical Center Dissertations. Paper AAI1467649. Available at: http://digitalcommons.library.tmc.edu/dissertations/AAI1467649.

Lin, B. & Kelly, E. (1995). Methodological issues in patient satisfaction surveys. *International Journal of Health Care Quality Assurance* 8, 32–37.

Lis, C.G., Rodeghier, M., Gupta, D. (2009). Distribution and determinants of patient satisfaction in oncology: A review of the literature. *Patient Preference and Adherence* 3, 287–304.

Locker, D. & Dunt, D. (1978). Theoretical and methodological issues in soc10logical studies of consumer satisfaction with medical care. *Social Science and Medicine* 12, 283–292.

Mack, J.W., Block, S.D., Nilsson, M., Wright, A., Trice, E., Friedlander, R., et al. (2009). Measuring therapeutic alliance between oncologists and patients with advanced cancer: The Human Connection Scale. *Cancer* 115, 3302–3311.

Mayer, D.K. (2007). Oncology nurses' versus cancer patients' perceptions of nursery caring behaviours: A replication study. *Oncology Nursing Forum* 11, 46–50.

Miles, A. (2009). On a Medicine of the Whole Person: away from scientistic reductionism and towards the embrace of the complex in clinical practice. *Journal of Evaluation in Clinical Practice* 15, 941–949.

Miles, A. & Asbridge, J.E. (2014). Clarifying the concepts, epistemology and lexicon of person-centeredness: an essential pre-requisite for the effective operationalization of PCH within modern healthcare systems. *European Journal of Person Centered Healthcare* 2, 1–15.

Ministero della Salute – Dipartimento della programmazione e dell'ordinamento del Servizio sanitario nazionale, Direzione generale della programmazione sanitaria. (2007). *POAT Salute 2007–2013. Linea di attività trasversale 1.Supporto allo svolgimento delle diverse fasi che accompagnano il ciclo della programmazione LT1_SIC_03 Impatto della patologia oncologica ed analisi delle prestazioni e della mobilità in Sicilia*. Available at: http://www.salute.gov.it/portale/temi/documenti/investimenti/73.pdf.

Ministero della Salute (2014). *Documento tecnico di indirizzo per ridurre il burden del cancro - Anni 2014–2016*. Available at: http://www.salute.gov.it/imgs/C_17_pubblicazioni_2324_allegato.pdf

Mishel, M.H. (1981). The measurement of uncertainty in illness. *Nursing Research* 30, 258–263.

Mishel, M.H. (1997). *Uncertainty in illness scales manual*. Unpublished manual. Chapel Hill, NC: University of North Carolina.

Mishel, M.H. (1999). Uncertainty in chronic illness. *Annual Review of Nursing Research* 17, 269–294.

Mishel, M.H., Hostetter, T., King, B., Graham, V. (1984). Predictors of psychosocial adjustment in patients newly diagnosed with gynecological cancer. *Cancer Nursing* 7, 291–300.

Mowen, J.C., Licata, J.W., McPhail, J. (1993). Waiting in the emergency room: How to improve patient satisfaction. *Journal of Health Care Marketing* 13, 26–33.

Oberst, M.T. (1984). Patients' perceptions of care. *Cancer* 53, 2366–2373.

Parker, P.A., Alba, F., Fellman, B., Urbauer, D.L., Li, Y., Karam, J.A., et al (2013). Illness uncertainty and quality of life of patients with small renal tumors undergoing watchful waiting: a 2-year prospective study. *European Urology* 63, 1122–1127.

Sandoval, G.A., Brown, A.D., Sullivan, T., Green, E. (2006). Factors that influence cancer patients' overall perceptions of the quality of care. *International Journal for Quality in Health Care* 18, 266–274.

Santacroce, S.J. (2003). Parental uncertainty and posttraumatic stress in serious childhood illness. *Journal of Nursing Scholarship* 35, 45–51.

Siddiqui, Z.K., Zuccarelli, R., Durkin, N., Wu, A.W., Brotman, D.J. (2005). Changes in patient satisfaction related to hospital renovation: experience with a new clinical building. *Journal of Hospital Medicine* 10, 165–171.

Sitzia, J. & Wood, N. (1998). Patient satisfaction with cancer chemotherapy nursing: a review of the literature. *International Journal of Nursing Studies* 35, 1–12.

Taylor, S.E., Helgeson, V.S., Reed, G.M., Skokan, L.A. (1991). Self-generated feelings of control and adjustment to physical illness. *Journal of Social Issues* 47, 91–109.

Tishelman, C. (1994). Cancer patients' hopes and expectations of nursing practice in Stockholm. *Scandinavian Journal of Caring Sciences* 8, 213–222.

Williams, B. (1994). Patient satisfaction: a valid concept? *Social Sciences and Medicine* 38, 509–516.

Wooldridge, J. (2010). *Econometric Analysis of Cross Section and Panel Data* (2nd ed.). Cambridge: MIT Press.

The Environmental, Economic and Social Sustainability of Energy Sources

Gaetano Borrelli

Abstract The sustainability of energy sources mainly derives from decarbonisation activities. The European Union was the first to move in this direction by defining long-term goals through the communication of a *Roadmap for moving to a competitive low-carbon economy in 2050*, which indicates the strategic path that member states will have to follow to achieve a reduction of atmospheric CO_2 emissions of at least 80% by that year compared to 1990 levels, and medium-term objectives like those identified in the 20-20-20 package. This package envisages a breakdown of European targets by country, e.g. setting for Italy a mandatory renewable energy consumption target of 17% by the end of the decade.

The main purpose of the article is to emphasize the importance of an economic and social approach in order to implement European Union Guideline for decarbonisation.

Introduction

European policies are a clear example of how international and national choices have significant impact even on a regional or local scale. In this regard, in fact, in 2012 the Ministry of Economic Development established a so-called burden sharing decree that broke down the 17% target by region with electricity and thermal quotas, thus excluding consumption in the transport sector and imports from third countries and taking into account the different local realities.

What is certainly of interest to the local decision-makers and offers – indeed, requires – operational margins of action is the analysis, monitoring and government of local energy consumption. Here too, it should be stressed that consumption choices – i.e., investments in energy efficiency – are influenced and governed by policies elaborated at higher levels, yet local policies can play a decisive role. First

G. Borrelli (✉)
ENEA (Italian National Agency for Energy, New Technologies and Sustainable Economic Development), Rome, Italy
e-mail: gaetano.borrelli@enea.it

A. Bianco et al. (eds.), *Italian Studies on Quality of Life*, Social Indicators Research Series 77, https://doi.org/10.1007/978-3-030-06022-0_24

of all, a responsible and knowledgeable local decision-maker should be aware of the weight and relevance of reducing energy consumption and consequent global pollution. In other words, everyone is required to do their part. Normally, however, the local decision-maker is bound to, often exclusively focused on, the perceived problems of utmost urgency of his/her community, namely economic growth and territorial development. These issues can obviously be framed both as harmonised with the rational management of consumption and the local region and as opposed to it, not just for energy. Think, for example, of the hydrogeological damage caused to the local landscape due to its indiscriminate use.

The Energy System

The expression *energy system* indicates that which produces, transforms, transports and distributes energy in a region. The system in question is actually composed of a number of complex systems, the full description of which would distract us from the objective of clearly and linearly defining what kind of awareness is required for a local decision-maker who is sensitive to this issue in managing the local area.

An energy system is logically frameable as a budget, representing a circuit of energy supply and demand. Basically, an energy system supplies energy (producing it, importing it, using stored supplies and transforming it) on the one hand and consuming it on the other. This is an issue that must be considered by every local decision-maker: every human community is bound to a region and consumes energy. Its members can be seen as manufacturers – the businesses – or families according to conventions and classifications that relate to both the actual management of energy production, transformation and distribution and to regulatory control and statistical monitoring of the associated flows. A local area can in fact be the site of power generation and transformation plants and even host a segment of the primary supply system on its lands. The latter, however, is managed and regulated at a national and international level.

An energy system is conceptually rather difficult to define in a simple manner due to the intrinsic extensive nature and complexity of the subject. However, it is possible and essential to communicate the awareness of the weight that every member of the community has (especially decision-makers) in determining its optimal operation. Consider, for example, the energy consumption of families: widespread awareness of the cost of energy both economically and environmentally could significantly reduce the demand, improving the dynamics of the system in its entirety. For example, a reasonable reduction in domestic energy consumption from the perspective of an energy/environmental budget can result in a reduction in imports for certain types of sources (e.g., reduction of electricity demand = reduction of gas imports) and atmospheric emissions of greenhouse gases (due to the reduced workload of thermoelectric power plants). The previous case is obviously a pure approximation of the operating mechanism of an energy system but serves to give an idea of how indispensable it is for every member of the community to understand his/her role and weight in determining environmentally and economically viable choices.

Social Acceptance of Key Technologies in the Area

The local decision-maker moving towards a low-carbon society, besides needing to deal with technical and economic feasibility or regulatory issues related to new technologies (such as geographic boundaries, intermittent and discontinuous nature of renewable sources, efficiency, economic convenience, legislation), is increasingly faced with an additional obstacle that often prevents the implementation of energy technology projects employing renewable sources in the local region: the barriers related to social acceptance. The term social acceptance is here defined as *the conscious acquisition of a change that transforms one's local area, determined by the introduction of a new technology/policy/project.* In this case, acceptance is linked to the way people perceive and interpret energy interventions and plants located in an area. The key question that becomes important to a local administration engaged in promoting the diffusion of renewable or alternative energy sources in its own territory is therefore not if or how much national renewable energy sources (RES)-oriented energy policies are desirable, but rather *whether* and *how* individual *energy projects at the local level* can be socially desirable.

What are the social obstacles that can hinder the spread of energy technologies in the area? There are several reasons that can hinder the social desirability of introducing RES technology. Apart from their new nature, the reasons behind protests are often due to the same issues as those faced by more conventional energy plants. None of these explanations claims to be exhaustive, depending on the case one or the other will be more dominant, and it is possible that more than one can be present in the same situation. Here is a summary.

The Nimby Syndrome The Nimby ("Not In My Back Yard") hypothesis is based on the assumption that the motivation of the protest is linked exclusively to the local reasoning that the population would be in favour of the construction of such facilities provided they are not located in their own area. It should be noted, however, that several scholars believe that this syndrome explains opposition in vast geographical areas and not in limited territories like those in Italy. The authors themselves argue in summary that it is wrong to apply Nimby to all conflicts as often there are other more subtle factors like mistrust in institutions and experts (Borrelli and Guzzo 2011).

The Lack of Transparency and Information Providing the public with technical and scientific information on renewable energies plays a crucial role in determining their favourability or otherwise. Without information there is no awareness, and the conscious acceptance of a change in one's local area caused by the introduction of green technology is also conditioned by the level of information possessed by the public.

The Perception of Risk In protests against RES plants the term *risk* is often used. As with conventional energy plants, there is a fear of adverse effects on biodiversity, health and quality of life determined by wind farms, biomass or geothermal plants, composting plants. Even where the risk associated with some RES plants may seem socially amplified it should not be underestimated and its perception depends on a number of processes and factors of different nature: cultural, communicative, moral values (Borrelli and Sartori 1990).

The Fair Distribution of Risks and Benefits From an analysis of the arguments raised by protesters, it emerges how the social impact of the project is, in some cases, the main source of concern for residents and stakeholders, thereby jeopardising the economic and social desirability of the project. In the specific case of a RES plant a question to be asked in the design phase is: *who loses and who gains from its construction?* The possible repercussions of a wind farm or a biomass plant on strategic sectors such as tourism or agriculture may have a significant impact on the perceptions of the local community. The fear of losing a real or potential source of income for a tourist or agricultural operator or a local shop could prevail over the more distant fear of global warming or dependence on fossil fuels in one's country.

The Decision-Making Process What the latest environmental conflicts have taught us is that in our societies managing technological and industrial risks in general requires the *involvement* of the public. From successful experiences in other countries where the phenomenon of environmental conflict is not new (such as France, the United States or Great Britain) a number of participatory tools have been tested to prevent or avoid such situations, trying in various ways to involve stakeholders during the development of projects that fall within their region and not waiting until the end. Applicable laws in the regions of Tuscany (Law 46/2013) and Emilia Romagna (3/2010) go in this direction.

The Perception of the Local Area One of the distinctive features of renewable plants compared with those for fossil fuels is the increased visual impact on the landscape. Of course this is linked to the generative capacity of the plant, but the visibility aspect also depends on the fact that – while for fossil fuels or nuclear power the extraction is carried out under the earth's surface or is invisible to the public – in the case of RES the supply of raw material takes place on the surface, with a greater impact on landscape and the environment and with greater proximity to places of residence. Various research has highlighted the importance of this dimension in several cases of protest. The dominance of an *idyllic* view of the landscape among tourists, returning immigrants and vacation homeowners is one of these.

Infiltration by Organised Crime The interest and attention of Mafia organisations in energy projects involving RES plants is not a new phenomenon in Italy, which in light of recent Ecomafia reports[1] cannot be ignored. This phenomenon explains

[1]http://www.legambiente.it/contenuti/dossier/rapporto-ecomafia, considered the primary source on this subject.

social resistance that can mobilise local residents and committees against a plant or an energy project, especially in high-Mafia areas, notwithstanding the general benefits to the level of CO_2 in the atmosphere. In these cases it is important for the decision-maker to immediately eliminate any misunderstandings that can perpetuate the perception on a social level of an infiltration of organised crime in certain proposed projects. Efforts should be made to go beyond the basic regulations that in light of recent developments give public entities or other similar bodies (private providers of public services) the right to request anti-Mafia controls either by the Prefecture or, in cases covered by art.6-bis of Italian Legislative Decree 163/2006, the database established by the Public Contract Oversight Authority (AVCP – Autorità per la Vigilanza sui Contratti Pubblici).

The Role of the Economy: Approaches and Models of Environmental Governance

The economic aspects of environmental issues are increasingly important in our age. This is natural: in fact, the resolution of environmental problems requires the use of substantial (and still growing) economic resources, while a significant change in the characteristics of production and consumption processes and a particular orientation of technological progress are needed to prevent new environmental problems Ignazio Musu (2003) – il Mulino

In the 1970s, due to repeated oil shocks and subsequent periods of economic stagnation and inflation, the scientific world began to question for the first time the dominant model of economic development by opening up the debate on the future of growth. There were many contributions – and criticisms – even from disciplines that were not strictly related to economics, including natural sciences, concerned with the environmental inefficiency of growth models, and the humanities, interested in redefining the concepts of development and well-being by disconnecting them from the utilitarian conception of monetary wealth.

These criticisms arose from the recognition of some of the recognised symptoms of inefficiency, for example the strong link between economic growth and consumption of natural resources, the unequal distribution of wealth, especially in underdeveloped countries, and the identification in many western countries of a trend towards an increase in the gap between the evolution of economic growth rates and improvements in well-being.

Natural sciences highlighted the environmental problem starting from the observation that in the various economic models, whether the capitalist free market system or the planned socialist model, the limited nature of natural resources and, consequently, the need for their conservation were not properly taken into account. Both systems, albeit with very different methods, aimed at generating wealth and well-being through the production and consumption of goods and implicitly considered the environment as an unlimited supplier of raw materials with an unlimited capacity to handle waste.

In the early 1970s the first signs of significant environmental problems began to emerge, such as the increasingly rapid disappearance of animal and plant species, loss of soil fertility, worsening water quality, deforestation and desertification in different parts of the planet. With the UN Stockholm Conference on Human Environment in 1972 the subject of the environment officially became a major international issue. In the same period, the United Nations launched UNEP – United Nations Environment Programme. In those same years, in order to better assess the effects of economic policies, various techniques were identified for calculating the wealth of nations that took into account the environmental costs of economic development (Zamagni and Bruni 2009).

The lively ongoing debate was reflected in the work of the World Commission for Environment and Development (WCED) of 1983, known as the Bruntland Commission, in which the needs of economic development and environmental sustainability were compared, arriving at the definition of the concept of sustainable development as *development that meets the needs of the present without compromising the ability of future generations to meet their needs.*

The implementation of the principles of sustainable development in the construction of economic policy guidelines defined the operational context of two branches of economics, environmental economics and ecological economics.

The former, based on the neoclassical paradigm and inspired by the work of Arthur C. Pigou and the Coase theorem,[2] states that environmental damage is the result of the non-existence of a market for natural resources as they are public goods that exhibit non-rivalry and non-excludability. Starting from this consideration and the definition of the concept of externality, environmental economics proposes various methods to limit the problem: on the one hand, it tries to assign a monetary value to the environment to be introduced into the pricing system through economic policy tools; on the other hand, it tries to attribute property rights to certain types of public goods. As will be discussed below, this approach is at the heart of many environmental policies, including the Emission Trading System (ETS) envisaged by the Kyoto Protocol.

The ecological economy, on the other hand, proposes an integrated knowledge of the links between ecological and economic systems. In this approach, a key role in the development of sustainable models is assumed by various types of constraints (thermodynamics, biophysics, availability of natural resources, pollution absorption, demographics and the planet's carrying capacity), and, to a greater extent, by the limits of current knowledge with regard to the magnitude of these constraints and their influence on the entire human and planetary system. This branch of economic science has made numerous attempts to develop biophysical and social welfare indicators that can make the reading of the state of the environment and society more accurate. These include the Agenda for Sustanable Development and related Sustainable Development Goals and indicators (in continuity with previous Millennium Development Goals), Index of Sustainable Economic Welfare

[2]See: http://www.econlib.org/library/Enc/bios/Coase.html

(ISEW), then transformed into the Genuine Progress Indicator (GPI), the Ecological Footprint (EF) and the eMergia indicators inspired by the work of American eco-worker Howard Thomas Odum.[3] Georgescu-Roegen's bioeconomy is one of the contributions that more courageously sought to create an economic paradigm that could encompass ecological aspects in terms of environmental, social and welfare sustainability.

In any case, the need to know how to combine economic growth, social development and the preservation of the environment in which we live now seems to be unavoidable. In this regard, the existence of indicators that can guide economic policies towards objectives of sustainable development is crucial. In fact the design and implementation of effective policies requires the identification of assessment tools and indicators to guide policy-makers in defining short-, medium- and long-term goals and to measure progress in achieving these goals (Amerighi and Felici 2011).

Over time many scholars and international organisations have sought to achieve statistical tools that can identify the living conditions, development and well-being of societies and individuals better than GDP. Among these must surely be included Amartya Sen's work on the theory of equality and freedoms inspired by the Human Development Index (HDI) and the findings of the Report of the Commission on the Measurement of Economic Performance and Social Progress commissioned in 2008 by the French government to the economists Sen, Fitoussi and Stiglitz. On 8 June 2011 the European Parliament itself adopted a resolution entitled: *Not just GDP – Measuring progress in a changing world.* The recent OECD proposal for a set of indicators to monitor progress towards *green growth*[4] aims to *qualify* GDP by adding other indicators or by orienting it to variables that represent the environmental and social dimension of economic growth.

The *green economy*, invoked as a panacea to economic, climatic and environmental issues, can be the means for creating the necessary preconditions for the progress of society as a whole. At the same time, it is evident that technological, organisational and behavioural innovation represents its driver. In particular, so-called *eco-innovation* will play a key role in the next few decades in favouring a structural change in the economy and society and in affirming sustainable production and consumption models.

Economy, Resource Management and Pollution Control

> *Most people have little regard for the common good. Each thinks more about his own, almost none about common interest and only when concerns about the common good become a burden to the individual. It is always expected that others will act for the common good. Based on these considerations, common interest will be neglected by all.* Aristotle, Politics II

---

[3]Odum's life and work are well illustrated in the Encyclopaedia Britannica, also in the online version: http://www.britannica.com/EBchecked/topic/864021/Howard-Thomas-Odum

[4]OECD, (2011), *Towards Green Growth: Monitoring Progress – OECD Indicators*, May.

In the economic sphere, natural resources are understood as all those physical materials not produced by man that have an economic utility.

The orthodox classification of natural resources distinguishes them first and foremost in *permanent* and *non-permanent.*

Permanence is defined as the characteristic that allows the resource itself to not diminish in quality and intensity neither with the passing of time nor as a result of man's action.

On the contrary, non-permanent resources are those that do not enjoy this characteristic, and these are distinguished as *reproducible* – as it is possible to extract certain quantities without threatening the overall existence – and *not reproducible*, available in fixed amounts in time horizons relevant to human action and therefore resulting in irreversible decreases in stock available for future needs when used.

Examples of permanent natural resources are the sun and tides; non-permanent reproducible: forests, fertility of the soil, biodiversity; non-permanent and non-reproducible: fossil fuels, landscape resources.

The most important resource included from the beginning by the literature among non-permanent and non-reproducible sources is, however, the environment's capacity to handle pollution, understood as its tolerance threshold for the impact of various forms of human activity without irreversibly losing its physical characteristics and resulting economic utility.

The widespread and rooted conception of natural resources as infinite, a source to be drawn from for the satisfaction of economic utility, sparked a vicious cycle that inevitably led to the loss or otherwise minimisation of the awareness of the impact of human activities on the environment, society and every living being.

Sustainable Production and Consumption

Respect and care of the environment in which we live are essential elements for healthy and inclusive growth, not only of our economy but also, above all, of our well-being and that of the generations to come. The effort now being asked of people, as citizens and political decision-makers, as people responsible for the good management of public goods and services, is to change direction quickly and without additional costs to the community and, above all, without further waste that damages our limited natural heritage.

Decisions have to be taken in a hurry because climate change does not grant respite to affected populations, but they must also be taken with clarity, seriousness and profound responsibility because it is no longer a matter of merely making a few adjustments, but rather boldly reversing direction to produce results capable of lasting over time, trying to prevent and not simply manage a deeply rooted evil. Looking at the current Italian economic situation it might seem like an impossible endeavour: but if a crisis is an opportunity, everyone must act to seize it, even taking some risks, always with intelligence and open to debate. There are many examples to choose from: virtuous communities, private companies and associations that each day work to combine their economic well-being with that of the environment are becoming increasingly widespread and should be remembered, imitated and supported.

Consumers' attention to labels on products, choosing products that are truly made in Italy, the ever-increasing need to be informed by businesses about their production methods, including their environmental, ethical and social policies, are clear signals of the change that is taking place.

Health, product quality, the values on which a business is founded must be guaranteed to consumers throughout the entire production cycle, developing the most appropriate forms of communication to meet the need for information of all stakeholders with the objective of establishing a trusted relationship with them and achieving broader consensus.

There are several tools companies can use to communicate with the outside: most of these are initiatives that start from the bottom, in the sense that the companies themselves have codified development models not yet enacted by law but rather developed through direct implementation. Environmental certifications and budgets have been established, just now being recognised by the legislature, due to the virtuous companies' need to stand out in the market, affirming their prestige and their ability to produce in a sustainable and socially ethical way, even with respect to their workers.

Unfortunately, these virtuous attitudes are contrasted by the presence in the market of companies that base their earnings on improper actions, amplified by the phenomenon of globalisation, which has placed goods and services from all over the world on the same level, favouring those with the lowest price notwithstanding a questionable quality and very little respect for the environment and the dignity of people.

The push for delocalisation due to the presence in Italy of one of the highest tax rates in Europe and beyond, as well as the greater efficiency of infrastructure and transport and lower labour costs in other countries, have resulted in a significant loss of economic, financial, intellectual and natural capital, causing the impoverishment of both places and people.

The phenomenon of delocalisation has also caused another serious problem for the marketing of goods produced abroad and offered for sale under the label Made in Italy thanks to a final transformation in Italy but hardly definable as *substantial* as required by European Community customs regulations. In fact, judges of the Court of Cassation have acknowledged in various judgements the aspects of fraud in the behaviour of those who present their products made elsewhere using the colours of the Italian flag, the expressions "Made in Italy" or other marks, for the obvious reason that the consumer is led to believe that it is a product entirely made in Italy.

There are areas of craftsmanship in which our country has achieved unparalleled reputation, despite the many attempts to imitate them: textiles, clothing, food, cars and footwear. These sectors are distinguished not only by excellent product quality but also talent, creativity, passion and great experience rooted in centuries of tradition.

The quality of these products, therefore, is not only the result of the machinery and equipment used, but above all of the knowledge and skills acquired and passed down from generation to generation.

Consequently, while delocalisation can offer an opportunity for businesses in difficulty to improve their sales and increase their production in the short term, in the long run the strategy is likely to result in significant damage to the brand. In fact, we are seeing an inestimable loss of Italian craftsmanship, the continuous closing of artisanal bottegas and local shops, the mass production of low quality goods, the impossibility of companies to attract investment and to be competitive, the inability to offer youth attractive career opportunities. This state of affairs is reflected, inevitably, in a general malaise that is expressed in increasingly widespread degradation of inland areas, and now increasingly also of cities, and, inevitably, in the poverty of the entire society.

It is therefore necessary to rethink the relationship between business and the local area, business and community, business and the environment, so that delocalisation is replaced by the investment of economic activities in the territory where they were born. Indeed, our country is characterised by the presence of small and medium-sized enterprises that have difficulty competing against large European industries, by which they are often swallowed up whole. However, it is the SMEs (small and medium enterprises) that ensure the quality and diversification of products and services, because they preserve traditional methods of production and better meet the needs of consumers since they operate locally and are therefore aware of the needs and expectations of their community.

In this regard, there are many companies that, in order to preserve and possibly improve the relationship of trust with consumers, have invested in activities aimed at enhancing the quality of products and promoting the sustainable nature of their production processes, spontaneously taking on extra responsibility – corporate social responsibility (CSR) – without waiting for legislative constraints.

The implementation of CSR expresses not only the intention of firms to overcome moments of crisis and to withstand the pressure to delocalise, but also the need to be supported in a complex and expensive journey that requires considerable investment. At the same time, CSR is not only a cost, but also an effective competitive tool that the company can use to stand out on the market. In fact, the company that voluntarily demonstrates compliance with certain environmental and social standards obtains several advantages with regard to access to credit, participation in tenders, the best placement of products on the market, destined to be chosen with greater trust by consumers, who are reassured by brands and other distinctive traits that attest to the company's virtuous behaviour.

The implementation of CSR should not, therefore, only be a burden exclusively on businesses, but should become a genuine development model that is used and encouraged by public administrations for the capacity that they have to orient purchases and investments and to attract funding and make businesses competitive.

In this sense the experience of Green Public Procurement (GPP) is a prime example of the ability of public administrations to become promoters of economic development and environmental protection.

Municipalities in particular can play a very important role in combining budgetary policies and respect for the environment through the adoption of minimum environmental criteria in tenders for the supply of goods and services, thus representing a point of reference for the community, businesses and the local area. The ability of governments to direct production and purchases by virtue of the institutional role they play is such as to involve entire communities and influence whole productive sectors. Consider the size of the public sector, the number of people it employs and the quantity of goods and services it needs to support its work. Now consider the difference a public authority could make by deciding to provide canteens of schools, offices and hospitals with only fresh food products from the local area compared to another public institution that accepts, perhaps at lower costs, to enter into contracts for the purchase of preserved, packaged products from other regions and countries.

Green public procurement therefore marks an evolutionary phase in the tender process in terms of sustainability. Under EU pressure, member countries were asked to draw up action plans in which the state government would indicate to the public administrations the activities to be performed for greening their purchases. In our system this was undertaken by the Minister of the Environment, Land and Sea, in consultation with the Ministries of Economy and Economic Development, which adopted the National Action Plan for Green Public Procurement (NAP-GPP) in 2008, updating it in 2013.

In particular, NAP-GPP identifies the sectors requiring greater attention under an environmental profile and delegates to specific decrees the task of identifying the minimum environmental criteria that must be set by contracting entities and respected by the tendering companies at different stages of the call for tenders. The environmental criteria are considered basic because they constitute the minimum elements required for production to be considered sustainable. Added to these are award criteria, which provide additional points when the contract recipient is being decided. These are designed to encourage companies to seek innovative solutions in terms of environmental technologies and to guide public demand toward products or services that produce the least possible impact on the environment throughout the entire product life cycle.

And it is precisely with regard to the life cycle of the products that the purchasing decisions of public authorities must be performed in order to observe the performance of the goods not only in terms of design, production, use and disposal, but also in relation to costs for the community. In fact, this point of view demonstrates how green public procurement can be considered *an instrument for containing public spending in that it assesses not just the production cost of the good but the entire life cycle, as well as offering a cultural model of limiting consumption and dematerialisation.*[5]

Among other things, the involvement of public administration produces a number of positive effects that can be summarised in its ability to act as a role model to

[5]http://www.minambiente.it/pagina/gpp-acquisti-verdi

be imitated and spread, not only in the context of the public sector but also among businesses and consumers. In fact, public procurement plays an important role in the national economy and is therefore able to affect both production and consumption, nudging both towards objectives of sustainability.

References

Amerighi O. & Felici B. (2011, n. 3). Sviluppo Sostenibile e Green Economy: oltre il PIL (pp. 43–48). *EAI Energia, Ambiente e Innovazione*. Roma: ENEA.

Borrelli G. & Sartori S. (1990). Rischi tecnologici e interessi diffusi. *Quaderni ENEA*. Roma: ENEA.

Borrelli G. & Guzzo T. (2011). *Tecnologia, rischio e ambiente*. Acireale: Bonanno Editore.

http://www.britannica.com/EBchecked/topic/864021/Howard-Thomas-Odum

http://www.econlib.org/library/Enc/bios/Coase.html

http://www.legambiente.it/contenuti/dossier/rapporto-ecomafia, considered the primary source on this subject

http://www.minambiente.it/pagina/gpp-acquisti-verdi

Musu I. (2003). *Introduzione all'economia dell'ambiente*. Bologna: il Mulino.

Oecd, (2011), Towards Green Growth: Monitoring Progress – Oecd Indicators, Oecd, Paris.

Zamagni S. & Bruni L. (2009). *Dizionario di economia civile*. Roma: Città Nuova.

Sports and Physical Activities in Europe: How to Measure Active Lifestyles

Antonio Mussino and Riccardo Cosmai

Abstract The paper presents the importance of monitoring participation in sports and physical activities. In fact, the regular practice of physical activity brings physical, psychological and social benefits. The Governments should support the measures taken in this field by the monitoring, control work, preparation of appropriate tools and platforms, evaluation and research. We analyse the results from Special Eurobarometer survey (2014) and discuss their limits, suggesting new strategies to improve their use to individualize patterns and rankings of the 28 EU countries in sports participation. For this purpose, we did not analyse issued results, but reprocess the individual record file in a different way, using COMPASS strategy to help us. We applied a multivariate statistical model (logistic regression) to study which are the determinants of sport participation in the European Union.

Introduction

According to the voluntary targets established in the "Global action plan for the prevention and control of non-communicable diseases WHO 2016–2025 (2015)," the Regional Office for Europe of the WHO (World Health Organization) has developed a strategy to promote active lifestyles (through the practice of sports and physical activities) to improve citizens' health and welfare.

Governments should encourage these activities by ensuring adequate and accessible infrastructures, sport facilities and public spaces. They should also ensure equal opportunities for all citizens, regardless of gender, age, education, ethnicity, income, disability and so on.

In fact, the regular practice of physical activity starting in childhood or adolescence brings physical and psychological benefits, both immediately and in the medium to long term, and can predict an active lifestyle in adulthood.

A. Mussino (✉) · R. Cosmai
Department of Statistical Sciences, Sapienza University of Rome, Rome, Italy
e-mail: antonio.mussino@uniroma1.it

A. Bianco et al. (eds.), *Italian Studies on Quality of Life*, Social Indicators Research Series 77, https://doi.org/10.1007/978-3-030-06022-0_25

The WHO's goal is to achieve a 10% reduction in sedentary lifestyles by 2025, which would allow the achievement of three objectives: a 25% relative reduction in premature mortality due to cardiovascular diseases, cancers, diabetes and chronic respiratory diseases; a 25% relative reduction in the prevalence of hypertension; and an end to the rise of diabetes and obesity.

In this context, the 5th priority area in the European strategy (WHO 2015) refers to the need to "support the measures taken by the monitoring, control work, preparation of appropriate tools and platforms, evaluation and research". To meet this goal, it is necessary to have reliable and timely information to evaluate national and local policies, as well as to translate them into synthetic indicators to compare the various situations and to study changes due to public interventions in this field.

In this framework, the European Commission commissioned a survey on Sports and Physical Activity (Special Eurobarometer 412, 2014). Given this data, and considering the important role that sports play in society, the aim of this work is to answer the following research questions:

- Which tools are available to categorise citizens' participation in sports and physical activities in a broad sense?
- How can the Eurobarometer surveys be used to study sport participation in Europe?
- Which are the best strategies to process and analyse data on sport participation in various countries and at various times?
- What are the determinants of sport participation in the enlarged European Union (28 state members)?

The organization of this paper is as follows: after the Introduction, in section "Theoretical background", we propose a short historical overview of past studies and the strategies used in them; in section "The data from the Eurobarometer surveys and their limits", we present the data and outline a new strategy for processing and analysing those data. Section "Reprocessing data according to the COMPASS model" is devoted to the results, section "Multivariate Analysis"presents the application of a multivariate statistical technique, and section "Conclusions" provides a concluding summary.

Theoretical Background

At the end of the 1970s, in many European countries, we find the first research studies on sport demand, which refers to the population's behaviour in sport participation. The subjects that the researchers analysed included the participants (and the ways they participated), their social patterns, motivations for participation and for nonparticipation, and rankings of sport activities. This approach was necessary to evaluate the characteristics of sport supply, to optimize resources and to rationalize sport policy choices.

Sport models changed significantly in those years. The modern sport model, which is based on organization, selection, competition, membership, measures, rankings and so on, was losing popularity in favour of the postmodern sport model, which is characterized by sport-for-all activities, in which millions of citizens participate with varied individual models, in the hope of finding new relationships between bodies and the environment.

The possibility of measuring the complexity of these activities represented a new challenge for statisticians. Before that point, only organised, competitive sport activities were measured (and these were very easy to measure).

In those years, the Council of Europe was a driving force for many researchers, who tried to monitor changes in sport participation and to measure the levels and characteristics of that participation. These researchers, including Castejon Paz and colleagues (1973), Rodgers (1977), and Claeys (1982), proposed studies on sport policies and transnational surveys on participation and the motivation to participate in sports.

Starting from this point, many countries organised surveys to monitor their citizens' participation in sports, but each country had its own methodology. Only in 1996 did a common project try to coordinate the various methodologies: the Anglo-Italian project COMPASS (Co-ordinated Monitoring of Participation in Sports; Gratton et al. 1999; Mussino 1999, 2004).

> The main goal of the project was to examine existing systems for the collection and analysis of sport-participation data in European countries. COMPASS aimed at promoting the harmonisation of these statistics by persuading countries to adopt some aspects of a common methodology in the collection of survey data. Thus, greater comparability of data from different countries would become possible (Mussino 2014).

A crucial point is that the statistical boards in charge of collecting data on sport participation do so through national surveys, which use questionnaires to register information on a range of specified sporting activities over a specified period.

This was not the only strategy for collecting data to meet this goal. In fact, there are some supranational surveys (including Eurobarometer) performed concurrently. In national surveys, the questionnaires, sampling strategies, age limits, and years of the surveys, among other characteristics, are different. In a supranational survey, such differences were eliminated, as the survey takes place at the same time and uses the same questionnaire and the same methodology.

A cost-benefit analysis of the two strategies therefore points to the supranational approach as superior. The national approach, however, has the advantage of being more respectful of cultural differences, as it takes into account the sporting traditions in each country. In the supranational case, these traditions level out concepts, definitions and questions. This case also suffers from problems deriving from the translation of the questionnaire into many languages.

The supranational approach is also expensive, and the number of units sampled in each country is small. Therefore, we cannot disaggregate the individual-country analyses with respect to structural variables such as age, education level, gender or region of residence.

The COMPASS project ended in 2005. Therefore, as we wait for a new version of project COMPASS (Gratton et al. 2011), we must be satisfied with other supranational surveys; the Special Eurobarometer 412 is the most recent one that is useful for our goals. In the analysis of this survey's results, we can still use the COMPASS strategy to mitigate some of the survey's faults.

The Data from the Eurobarometer Surveys and Their Limits

To answer the research questions, we reprocessed the original Eurobarometer survey's data, applying the COMPASS general model strategy and suggesting various indexes that could be valid indicators of national trends in sport participation. Afterwards, we applied a multivariate analysis strategy to the data (record file) to individualize the various patterns in the determinants of sport participation amongst European citizens, as measured according to the COMPASS strategy.

The Special Eurobarometer 412 was carried out by TNS Opinion & Social Network on behalf of the Directorate-General for Education and Culture's Sport Unit. The survey was conducted in the 28 member states of the European Union between 23 November and 2 December 2013. The sample comprised 27,919 European citizens from various social and demographic groups; the participants were interviewed face-to-face at their homes in their mother tongues.

First, we have to point out some limits of this survey (Mussino 2014).

The two key questions in English are "How often do you exercise or play sport?" (Q1) and "How often do you engage in a physical activity outside sport such as cycling or walking from one place to another, dancing, gardening . . . ?" (Q2).

In French, the situation is rather different: "Tous le combien faites-vous du sport ou de l'exercice physique?" (Q1) and "Et tous le combien exercez-vous une activité physique qui ne soit pas du sport, comme faire du vélo, marcher d'un endroit à un autre, faire du jardinage . . . ?" (Q2). It is true that the second question still leaves out any kind of sport activities, but the interviewed persons could have interpreted their participation in any physical activity as applying to the first question!

Moreover, determining what is a sport activity and what is a physical activity is a subjective choice that depends on a country's sport culture, not only on individual opinion.

A third problem is that the respondents' classification with respect to participation is coded as follows: "5 or more times a week" (regularly), "3–4 times a week" (with some regularity), "1–2 times a week" (with some regularity), "1–3 times a month" (seldom), "less than once a month" (seldom), "never" (never), and "do not know" (missing). Thus, "3–4 times a week" is not considered regular participation, as it is in the last WHO statement (WHO 2007); moreover, in the official results, the second and third items are presented together (i.e., "1–4 times a week").

It is possible to overcome these problems only by using individual records to reprocess the data. In fact, if we want to measure the levels of involvement in active lifestyles against the levels of sedentary lifestyles, we jointly analyse Q1 and Q2 in the crosstab in Table 1.

Table 1 Contingency table: Q1 ("How often do you exercise or play sports?") × Q2 ("How often do you engage in a physical activity?"), in total %

		Q2: How often do you engage in a physical activity outside . . . ?							
		5+ times a week	3–4 times a week	1–2 times a week	1–3 times a month	Less than once a month	Never	Don't know	Total
Q1: How often do you exercise or play sport?	5+ times a week	3.7^{a}	1.2^{a}	1.2^{a}	0.4^{a}	0.7^{a}	1.0^{a}	–	8.2
	3–4 times a week	2.1^{a}	4.3^{a}	3.0^{a}	0.9^{a}	1.2^{a}	1.0^{a}	–	12.5
	1–2 times a week	2.8^{b}	2.8^{b}	8.4^{c}	2.0^{c}	2.2^{c}	1.9^{c}	–	20.1
	1–3 times a month	0.6^{b}	0.6^{b}	1.5^{c}	1.8^{d}	0.6^{d}	0.4^{d}	–	5.5
	Less than once a month	1.2^{b}	1.3^{b}	1.9^{c}	1.6^{d}	4.5^{e}	1.0^{e}	–	11.5
	Never	4.3^{b}	2.7^{b}	4.1^{c}	2.2^{d}	3.9^{e}	24.9^{f}	–	42.1
	Don't know	–	–	–	–	–	–	0.1^{g}	0.1
	Total	14.7	12.9	20.1	8.9	13.1	30.2	0.1	100

Reprocessing Data According to the COMPASS Model

Using the WHO's statements, we constructed a COMPASS-like model from the Eurobarometer data,[1] starting with the results presented in Table 1. The people who participated 3 or more times a week in an activity were placed in COMPASS groups 1 and 2 (more than 150 times a year), according to the new classification proposed in Table 2. The difference between these two groups is related to the kind of activity that the people participate in. We gave the same importance to sports and other physical activities.

This first group, A1, corresponds to the first two rows (labelled[(a)]) in Table 1. People, who exercise or play sports less frequently but who engage in a physical activity 3 or more times a week [(b)] are placed in the second group, A2.

The third group, B, matches COMPASS groups 3 and 4; it corresponds to those people who participate in sports and/or physical activities 1–2 times a week[(c)].

We can easily match the rest of the cells with the other COMPASS groups: group C[(d)] corresponds to COMPASS group 5; group D[(e)] corresponds to COMPASS group 6; and group E[(f)] (24,9) corresponds to COMPASS group 7.

As for the missing values ("don't know"), we considered this option only for people who did not reply to both Q1 and Q2[(g)]; in other cases, we substituted "never" for "no reply". Therefore, the rate of non-response was minimal (0.1), and this included only those who did not answer both Q1 and Q2.

Table 2 COMPASS model recoding, in %

	Percentages	Valid percentages 2013	Old COMPASS levels	Valid percentages 2009	
A1[(a)] Regular sport activity	20.7	20.7	1	21.2	
A2[(b)] Regular physical activity	16.3	16.3	2	27.8	(*)
B[(c)] Almost regular activity	22.0	22.0	3–4	21.4	(*)
C[(d)] Irregular activity	6.6	6.6	5	7.2	(*)
D[(e)] Occasional activity	9.4	9.4	6	9.4	(*)
E[(f)] No activity	24.9	25.0	7	13.0	
Total	99.9	100.0		100.0	
Missing	0.1				
Total	100.0				

(*) In this reprocessing of the 2009 survey data (Mussino 2014), the categories were assembled in a different way, giving greater priority to the frequency of sport activities than to the frequency of physical ones

[1]According to the results for the three components (quality, quantity and organization), the COMPASS levels of participation are: (1) regular sport, (2) regular recreation, (3) almost-regular sport, (4) almost-regular recreation, (5) irregular, (6) occasional, and (7) nonparticipation.

The results proposed in Table 2 may lead to new COMPASS levels. Within this framework, we can better define European citizens' levels of participation without an a priori definition of both sports and physical activities.

The first item to note is that 25% of the EU population is completely inactive (i.e., has a sedentary lifestyle). This outcome, of course, is a subset of both the 42.1% non-sportive population (from the responses to Q1), and the 30.2% inactive population (from the responses to Q2), as proposed in the official Eurobarometer report.

With respect to the similar survey performed in 2009 (Mussino 2014), we notice that the percentage of inactive people ("no activity") has almost doubled, from 13% to 25% (+12%). This increase depends only marginally on the decrease in "regular sport activity" (−0.5%), which in turn depends mainly on decreases in the intermediate categories. We cannot compute the differences relative to the 2009 survey, as the classifications were different.

The causes of these differences are certainly numerous and complex. Our opinion is that the economic crisis makes available to European citizens fewer resources to engage in leisure time: those who are persuasive, persistent, and committed to their sport activity do not distract economic resources from this. Those who are less involved, or only practise physical activities, do not consider it important to engage the residual economic resources.

Comparing the results of such classification in the 28 countries is rather interesting, as we can study trends from a sport-oriented point of view or from an active-lifestyle point of view (Table 3).

The results may in fact be read according to different rankings: that of the regular participation predominantly with sport features (A1), of the regular participation (A1 + A2), of the active lifestyle (A1 + A2 + B), of the sedentary lifestyle (D + E), of the failure to practice (E), and so on.

The readers may prefer to build their own rankings: here we report, for each of the proposed ones, the nations in the top three positions (the "podium") and those in the last three positions (the potential "drop out" from sportive Europe).

As for the regular sport participation (A1), on the podium are Sweden, Finland and Denmark; at the bottom are Romania, Malta and Bulgaria (last).

As for the complete regular participation (A1 + A2), the Netherlands, Sweden and Denmark are in the first positions; at the bottom are Bulgaria, Portugal and Italy (last).

As for those who are active (A1 + A2 + B), the first positions are the same, that is the Sweden, Netherlands and Denmark, whereas the last ones are Italy, Bulgaria and Portugal (last).

As for the sedentary percentages (D + E), the ranking reverses: therefore, on the podium are Sweden, Denmark and the Netherlands; the last countries are Bulgaria, Italy and Portugal. The same goes for the non-practice (E), which is negligible mainly for Sweden, Denmark and the Netherlands; in the last positions, there are Bulgaria, Malta and Portugal.

Table 3 Contingency table: Country × COMPASS recode, in row%

		COMPASS recode						
		A1	A2	B	C	D	E	Total
Country	Austria	17.6	12.0	29.5	11.8	15.3	13.8	100
	Belgium	22.6	18.7	25.5	6.2	11.5	15.4	100
	Bulgaria	5.7	18.3	13.1	6.7	7.0	49.2	100
	Croatia	20.0	17.1	20.6	7.0	22.2	13.1	100
	Cyprus	22.1	6.1	17.2	4.9	5.0	44.6	100
	Czech Republic	12.3	15.4	28.2	9.3	17.7	17.0	100
	Denmark	35.8	26.6	24.8	6.1	3.4	3.4	100
	Estonia	18.3	21.6	25.7	7.9	10.5	16.0	100
	Finland	37.3	22.8	25.0	3.6	6.0	5.4	100
	France	19.1	20.4	25.1	7.5	5.9	22.1	100
	Germany	21.6	22.5	27.8	6.5	9.8	11.7	100
	Great Britain	25.9	14.4	24.3	9.3	8.5	17.5	100
	Greece	17.6	9.2	19.9	5.5	8.4	39.4	100
	Hungary	26.1	16.6	15.6	5.2	12.0	24.5	100
	Ireland	32.3	11.4	21.2	5.6	9.3	20.2	100
	Italy	12.3	8.0	19.3	3.8	10.2	46.4	100
	Latvia	15.7	29.1	19.5	10.4	12.9	12.2	100
	Lithuania	23.3	16.7	18.2	7.6	11.9	22.3	100
	Luxembourg	28.2	16.8	30.1	7.7	6.6	10.7	100
	Malta	11.2	14.9	15.6	4.1	4.0	50.2	100
	Netherlands	27.6	43.1	18.2	4.3	2.6	4.3	100
	Poland	13.2	11.4	18.2	9.7	13.4	34.0	100
	Portugal	15.7	5.7	14.2	3.8	7.3	53.4	100
	Romania	12.0	19.0	15.9	8.3	12.4	32.5	100
	Slovakia	13.3	21.3	26.6	8.6	13.3	16.8	100
	Slovenia	28.7	16.9	24.4	5.5	14.8	9.7	100
	Spain	30.9	7.2	17.1	2.4	7.4	35.0	100
	Sweden	37.7	27.4	24.1	6.1	2.7	1.9	100
Total		20.7	16.3	22.0	6.6	9.4	25.0	100

Multivariate Analysis

For the last research question, we decided to apply a well-known multivariate analysis method (logistic regression model) to study the determinants of sporting participation.

Logistic regression (Agresti 2010; Harrell 2001) is a special case of a generalized linear model, in which the dependent variable is dichotomous (that is, it can take only two categories, which are usually coded as 0 and 1) and is assumed to have a Bernoulli distribution. We measured the effects that some independent variables (determinants) had on the probability of changing status from 0 to 1.

We believe that this is the best method for processing data and displaying results. The first reason is the nature of the variables (categorical ones in our case); the second reason is that the output is easily readable for sport policymakers.

Therefore, we considered three models, through which we analysed the relationships between a set of independent categorical variables and various dependent variables. In the first model, we studied the probability of passing from a category of "irregular, occasional or no participation" to one of "regular or almost regular participation," in either sports or physical activities. In the second model, the categories were "almost regular, irregular, occasional and no participation" and "regular participation according to the classification of the WHO"[2]. In the last model, we analysed the dichotomy between physical activities and sport activities amongst regular participants.

The independent variables in the models are the following: *Sex* (2 categories), *Age* (6 categories), *Welfare typology* in the country of residence (5 categories[3]), *Occupation* (3 categories), *Life satisfaction* (3 categories), and *Years of study* (4 categories). For each variable, we defined a reference category: "male" (*Sex*); "15–24" years (*Age*); "liberal" *(Welfare typology)*; "not employed" *(Occupation)*; "not satisfied" *(Life satisfaction)*; and "still studying" *(Years of study)*.

In addition, we computed a synthesis variable concerning the individuals' perceptions of the participation opportunities available in their areas. We created this variable by adding a positive or negative score,[4] depending on whether their areas had "opportunities for sport participation" and "opportunities at a local sport club," as well as whether the "local authorities do not do enough to improve sport participation".[5] The added variable *Condition* has 3 categories: "unfavourable" (reference category, with individual scores between -6 and -2, inclusive), "indifferent" (between -1 and $+1$), and "favourable" (between $+2$ and $+6$).

The results for all models, in terms of the significance on certain tests, are shown in Table 4.

Therefore, it is interesting to analyse the effects of the single variables; except for *Occupation* in the third model, they are all significant (see Table 5).

[2]At least three times per week.

[3]Porro (2013) proposed a *welfare* typology for the European Union's state members using this classification: "corporative" (Austria, Belgium, France, Germany, Luxembourg, and the Netherlands); "social democratic" (Denmark, Finland, and Sweden); "ex-communist" (Bulgaria, Croatia, Czech Republic, Estonia, Hungary, Latvia, Lithuania, Poland, Romania, Slovakia, and Slovenia); "family" (Cyprus, Greece, Italy, Malta, Portugal, and Spain); and "liberal" (Great Britain and Ireland).

[4]For these three questions, the possible answers (with their relative scores) were: "totally disagree" (-2); "tend to disagree" (-1); "tend to agree" ($+1$); "totally agree" ($+2$); and "don't know" (0; also includes missing answers).

[5]The ranking in the third question is reversed, as people with favourable conditions should tend to reply negatively to this question.

Table 4 Results for the likelihood ratio, score and wald test

	Model 1		Model 2		Model 3	
Test	Chi-square	*p-value*	Chi-square	*p-value*	Chi-square	*p-value*
Likelihood ratio	3932.81	<.0001	2097.34	<.0001	961.71	<.0001
Score	3649.68	<.0001	2045.93	<.0001	918.16	<.0001
Wald test	3174.72	<.0001	1895.55	<.0001	846.11	<.0001

Table 5 Type 3 analysis of effects

	Model 1		Model 2		Model 3	
	Wald		Wald		Wald	
Effect	Chi-Square	*p-value*	Chi-Square	*p-value*	Chi-Square	*p-value*
Sex	76.26	<.0001	78.95	<.0001	28.14	<.0001
Age	136.24	<.0001	46.63	<.0001	107.43	<.0001
Welfare	811.61	<.0001	478.89	<.0001	287.88	<.0001
Occupation	19.26	<.0001	29.04	<.0001	1.78	0.4109
Life satisfaction	448.79	<.0001	302.54	<.0001	59.29	<.0001
Years of study	289.37	<.0001	76.96	<.0001	66.50	<.0001
Condition	197.26	<.0001	146.90	<.0001	66.96	<.0001

For the estimated coefficients, the results are shown in Table 6. An asterisk code in the Sign column mean that this category influences the probability of changing from 0 to 1 (e.g., from sedentary to active, from not regular to regular; or from regular activity to regular sport), with $p < 0.05$ or better.[6] Remember that each variable has a reference category that is not in the output.

However, the simplest way to communicate the results of these elaborations is by analysing the odds ratios, as in Table 7. Remember that the relationships proposed are valid only if the corresponding coefficient is significant.

The odds ratios indicate whether a category has lower, equal or higher probability, with respect to the category of reference, to have a score of 1 for the dependent variable. For instance, for the variable *Sex*, the category of reference is "male," which has an odds ratio if 1; "female," on the other hand, has an odds ratio of 0.793 (Model 1): this means that, for every 1000 men who participate in a "regular or almost regular way" (either actively or as a sport), there are only 793 women. That is, men participate much more than women do; this relationship is significant according to the p value in Table 6.

If an odds ratio is greater than 1, that category has a higher probability to participate. For instance, those who declared that they live in "favourable conditions" have an odds ratio of 1.267 (Model 1), which means that 1267 people in "favourable conditions" participate in a regular or almost regular way for every 1000 people who participate while living in "unfavourable conditions" (the category of reference).

[6] $***p < 0.001$; $**p < 0.01$; $*p < 0.05$. If the coefficient is not significant, the cell is empty.

Table 6 Analysis of maximum-likelihood estimates

Parameter	Category	Model 1			Model 2			Model 3		
		Estimate	S.E.	Sign	Estimate	S.E.	Sign	Estimate	S.E.	Sign
Intercept		0.938	.086	***	−0.342	.078	***	0.962	.128	***
Sex	Female	−0.232	.026	***	−0.230	.026	***	−0.217	.041	***
Age	25–34 years	−0.207	.067	**	−0.253	.063	***	−0.251	.099	*
Age	35–44 years	−0.341	.067	***	−0.314	.064	***	−0.623	.101	***
Age	45–54 years	−0.398	.067	***	−0.264	.063	***	−0.781	.099	***
Age	55–64 years	−0.399	.067	***	−0.217	.064	***	−0.778	.100	***
Age	65+ years	−0.687	.069	***	−0.403	.066	***	−0.676	.104	***
Welfare	Corporative	0.390	.052	***	0.241	.051	***	−0.813	.083	***
Welfare	Ex-communist	0.006	.049		0.088	.049		−0.636	.081	***
Welfare	Family	−0.484	.054	***	−0.368	.055	***	0.265	.097	**
Welfare	Social democratic	1.165	.069	***	0.784	.059	***	−0.321	.089	***
Occupation	Employed	−0.015	.035		−0.162	.035	***	0.056	.055	
Occupation	Self-employed	0.220	.057	***	0.036	.055		−0.032	.084	
Life satisfaction	Fairly satisfied	0.454	.033	***	0.304	.035	***	0.407	.061	***
Life satisfaction	Very satisfied	0.920	.044	***	0.722	.042	***	0.529	.070	***
Years of study	Up to 15	−1.022	.089	***	−0.406	.079	***	−0.661	.126	***
Years of study	16–19	−0.826	.084	***	−0.304	.073	***	−0.562	.115	***
Years of study	20+	−0.470	.087	***	−0.107	.075		−0.279	.118	*
Conditions	Indifferent	−0.456	.057	***	−0.488	.063	***	0.044	.113	
Conditions	Favourable conditions	0.237	.032	***	0.186	.033	***	0.427	.055	***

Table 7 Odds-ratio estimates

		Model 1	Model 2	Model 3
Variable	Effect	Estimate	Estimate	Estimate
Sex	Female *vs.* Male	0.793	0.795	0.805
Age	25–34 years *vs.* 15–24 years	0.813	0.776	0.778
Age	35–44 years *vs.* 15–24 years	0.711	0.730	0.536
Age	45–54 years *vs.* 15–24 years	0.672	0.768	0.458
Age	55–64 years *vs.* 15–24 years	0.671	0.805	0.459
Age	65+ years *vs.* 15–24 years	0.503	0.669	0.508
Welfare	Corporative *vs.* Liberal	1.477	1.272	0.444
Welfare	Ex-communist *vs.* Liberal	1.006	1.092	0.529
Welfare	Family *vs.* Liberal	0.616	0.692	1.304
Welfare	Social democratic *vs.* Liberal	3.205	2.190	0.726
Occupation	Employed *vs.* Not employed	0.986	0.851	1.057
Occupation	Self-employed *vs.* Not employed	1.246	1.036	0.969
Life satisfaction	Fairly satisfied *vs.* Not satisfied	1.575	1.355	1.503
Life satisfaction	Very satisfied *vs.* Not satisfied	2.509	2.059	1.697
Years of study	Up to 15 *vs.* Still studying	0.360	0.666	0.517
Years of study	16–19 *vs.* Still studying	0.438	0.738	0.570
Years of study	20+ *vs.* Still studying	0.625	0.898	0.757
Conditions	Indifferent *vs.* Unfavourable conditions	0.634	0.614	1.045
Conditions	Favourable conditions *vs.* Unfavourable conditions	1.267	1.205	1.532

The analysis of the odds ratios was, therefore, very simple, and we noticed a confirmation of the traditional determinants of participation. Because of Rodgers, we knew that, in Europe, men and younger people participate in sports at higher rates than women and older people do.

However, in our results, we found interesting differences amongst the three models and in the effects of the other variables, with the exception of *Occupation* in Model 3.

As for the *Welfare* variable, in the first two models, we found that the highest levels of participation were in the "social democratic" countries of Northern Europe, whilst the lowest levels were in the "family"-based Mediterranean countries. In the third model, the situation was reversed: We considered only people who participated in a regular way (according to the WHO's definition), and we found a higher odds ratio in Mediterranean ("family") countries ((1.304), than in "liberal" (1.000), "social democratic" (0.726), "ex-communist" (0.529) or other countries. In other words, proportionally, more people participate in sports than in other physical activities in the "family" countries.

The results for *Occupation* and *Years of study* are dependent on *Age*, as the youngest people were mainly in the "not employed" and "still studying" categories, respectively. These results underestimate the predictive role that education plays in participation. We reprocessed the data, eliminating those who were under 35 years, and the results confirmed that there is concordance between the number of years of study (a proxy for educational level) and the probability of being active, including the probabilities of being regularly active and of being active in sports specifically.

It is interesting to observe that there is a concordance between the levels of *Life satisfaction* and the odds ratios. This means that the probability of being more regularly active is higher for those who are satisfied with their lives; however, there is no such concordance between regular sport activities and regular physical activities (see the third model).

The local *Conditions* (facilities, organizations and sport policies) do not affect the odds ratios for the first two models, but do affect those of the third model, as people need facilities, organizations and sport policies so that they can practice sports.

There are varying patterns based on level of activity; these would have been impossible to find using the traditional output of the Eurobarometer surveys.

Conclusions

We wanted to measure the levels in which EU citizens are involved in active lifestyles. However, we only had information from the Eurobarometer surveys, and neither the data-processing nor the results-submission methods used for these surveys were valid for our aims.

Therefore, we did not analyse the issued results directly; instead, we reprocessed the individual records by analysing both the sport activities and the physical ones. During this process, the COMPASS strategy helped us. The main result of this step was a ranking of the 28 countries with regard to certain indicators of active lifestyle, sport participation and sedentary lifestyle.

Moreover, we propose three models for studying patterns of participation in relation to a set of both traditional and new determinants: demographic, social, economic, territorial and so on.

The study's results provide useful tools for ranking and clustering European countries and for understanding the main relationships between the analysed variables.

In sport policy, there is a strong need to identify indicators for national levels of sport participation. Given the opportunity to process the Eurobarometer survey data, we are able to monitor the evolution of European citizens' active lifestyles and to compare the results for many countries.

We stress the usefulness of the results obtained in this study: the European Union and the governments of the state members should utilize these results to ensure equal opportunities for participation in sports and physical activities for all citizens, regardless of gender, age, education, ethnicity, income, disability and so on.

References

Agresti, A. (2010). *Analysis of Ordinal Categorical Data*, Second Edition. Wiley Series in Probability and Statistics.

Castejon, Paz B., de Dios Garcia Martinez, J., Carbalada, R. (1973). *Rationalising Sports Policies. Outline of a Methodology*. Strasbourg: Council of Europe.

Claeys, U. (1982). *Rationalising Sports Policies. Sport in European Society: a Transnational Survey into Participation and Motivation*. Strasbourg: Council of Europe.

European Commission (2014). *Sport and physical activity. Special Eurobarometer 412*. Brussels: European Commission DG Education and Culture.

Gratton, C., et al. (1999). *COMPASS 1999. A project seeking the co-ordinated monitoring of participation in sports in Europe*. London: UK Sport.

Gratton, C., Rowe, N., Veal, A. J. (2011). *International Comparisons of Sports Participation in European Countries. An Update of the COMPASS Project*. European Journal of Sport & Society 8 (1–2), 99–116.

Harrell, F. E. (2001). *Regression Modelling Strategies*. Springer.

Mussino, A. (1999). *Conceptual and Operational Problems in Measuring Participation in Sports*. Bulletin of the International Statistical Institute, 52nd ISI Session LVIII (2), 345–346. Helsinki: ISI.

Mussino, A. (2004). *L'armonizzazione delle statistiche sulla partecipazione sportiva: una sfida europea*. Rivista Italiana di Economia, Demografia e Statistica LVIII (1–2) (2004),. 149–176.

Mussino, A. (2014). *Levels and Typologies of Participation in Sports in Europe: Methodological and Operational Challenges*. Journal of Sports Science, vol. 2, pp. 32–46, ISSN: 2332-7839.

Porro, N. (2013). *Europa, sistemi sportivi e integrazione comunitaria*. In Pioletti, A.M. & Porro, N. (Eds.) *Lo sport degli europei. Cittadinanza, attività, motivazioni* (pp. 17–71). Milano: Franco Angeli.

Rodgers, B. (1977). *Rationalising Sports Policies. Sport in its Social Context: International Comparisons*. Strasbourg: Council of Europe.

World Health Organisation (2007). *HEPA Europe*. Copenhagen: WHO Regional Office for Europe.

World Health Organisation (2015). *Physical activity strategy for the WHO European Region 2016–2025*. Copenhagen.

The Emergence of the Middle Class and Improving Quality of Life in the Global South

Adele Bianco

Abstract Thanks to globalization a remarkable growth rate has been achieved since 1990 in some regions of the Global South and an overall Middle Class (MC) is rising. The paper aims to address the question if the per capita income and the level of consumption could be considered the key indicators to describe the rise of the MC and the improvement of the quality of life in the Global South. In so doing, the paper stresses the role played by cultural variables.

The paper is structured as follows. The first section is devoted to the theoretical background. The second focuses on the Kahras' definition of the global MC. In the third section, we make an empirical test. I selected from the World Bank database two set of indicators referring to typical dimensions of a MC society. Then I separately processed these data with a two-step principal component analysis. I extracted two factorial indexes supposed to indicate the modernity of the labour market and the social status of women.

Evidence shows that the condition for the rise of the MC are a modern economic system and a social context where gender gaps are reduced and where women are respected and empowered. In sum, the rise of the MC is a multidimensional phenomenon, where cultural variables play a crucial role.

Introduction

The paper aims to address theoretical and methodological questions. Could *per capita* income and the level of consumption be considered the key indicators to describe the rise of the Middle Class (MC) and the improvement of the quality of life (QoL) in the Global South (GS)?

Thanks to globalization a remarkable growth rate has been achieved since 1990 in some regions of the GS (Gilpin 2001). The increasing average income and the

A. Bianco (✉)
Department of Psychological, Health and Territorial Sciences, University G. D'Annunzio Chieti-Pescara, Chieti, Italy
e-mail: adele.bianco@unich.it

A. Bianco et al. (eds.), *Italian Studies on Quality of Life*, Social Indicators Research Series 77, https://doi.org/10.1007/978-3-030-06022-0_26

reduction of inequality improved the standard of living and the QoL of a consistent proportion of the world population which used to live in extreme poverty. The domestic markets and consumption in goods and services have been improved in the GS. An overall MC is rising and it could be considered a source of economic growth and a driver of social change.

In this paper I am going to stress the role played by cultural variables in the emergence of the occupational and social groups called MC.

This paper is structured as follows. The first section is devoted to the theoretical background. The second paragraph focuses on the Kahras' definition of the global MC. In the third section, we make an empirical test. I selected from the World Bank (WB) database two set of indicators referring to typical dimensions of a MC society. Then I separately processed these data with a two-step principal component analysis. I extracted two indexes, supposed to indicate the modernity of the labour market and the social status of women. The correlations between the two indexes and some economic and social indicators are higher than those between the economic indicators and the *per capita* income. This regards especially the social status of women index that seems to be a more valid indicator of MC than the *per capita* income. It is more closely related to the life expectancy of women and men, i.e. two relevant indicators of the QoL. In sum, the rise of the MC is a multidimensional phenomenon, where cultural variables play a crucial role.

Theoretical Background

This section is devoted to the theoretical background concerning the two central issues of this paper: the QoL topic and the concept of "social class".

A definition of the QoL in the emerging economies is a complex issue both theoretical and methodological (Land et al. 2012; Camfield et al. 2009). From a theoretical point of view, we can say that QoL is the new definition of "development", because many variables and indicators are an enlargement of this concept focused on the economic dimension as well as on the empowerment and well-being of people (Nohlen and Nuscheler 1992, 55–75; Menzel 2016, 13–18). From a methodological point of view, many researchers use qualitative methods such as participatory research to evaluate subjective QoL in developing countries (Camfield 2012). Quantitative methods make it possible to compare different data sources, to analyze developmental trends and to construct social progress indexes. We adopt the UNDP QoL definition based on the Human Development Index (HDI). It is composed of three different dimensions: «a) life expectancy, b) educational achievement, and c) command over the resources needed for decent living» (UNDP 2013, 1).

For the sociological tradition, social classes are a particular type of power distribution within (modern) society (Weber 1922, chp. 4; Parkin 1979). In modern society social mobility is possible and often encouraged, unlike a society based on status groups. Since the late nineteenth century the Western social development model has witnessed the reduction of (economic, social, political) gaps between the social classes. Thanks to the regulation of the labor market, and the enlargement of social and civil rights (Marshall 1950, 46ff; Esping Andersen 1990) the abovementioned gaps have been reduced, though not disappeared. Several social groups previously excluded — i.e. women — have been admitted to the rights of citizens and benefitted from them. In this framework, social and occupational groups labeled MC could emerge and develop within contemporary society. In the historical Western experience, the MC designates a set of social classes that enjoys:

(a) a relatively high standard of living;
(b) an upper-intermediate education level leading to quality jobs. In terms of content, employment is mainly in the service sector and the working conditions involve clerical and freelance activities;
(c) the ownership of a certain number of durable goods;
(d) the opportunity and the attitude to access consumer services such as culture and tourism (Gimenez 1991, 143–5).

In a classic book, following Max Weber, David Lockwood (1958) pointed out that the definition of a class should make a distinction between at least three dimensions: the market situation, working conditions and status.

Unlike the historical Western experience, the MC in the GS was often unable to bring in modern dynamism and social transformations but used to act more as an élite (Goetze 1976, 176–195). Despite this record, the recent rise of MC in the EC (emerging countries) marks a bettering of living conditions, coming out of poverty and raising the level of consumption. The consumption propensity of today's MC is considered the way to promote development UNDP (2013).

It is difficult to describe what exactly is a MC in the developing countries. Firstly because of its puzzling diversity (Lange and Meier 2009). Secondly, in comparison with the bureaucratic élites (Elsenhans 1981) or the *strategische Gruppen* in South East Asia (Evers 1988), today's MC in EC seems to benefit from globalization (Scrase and Scrase 2009; Cheng 2010; Lin 2011; Yuan et al. 2011; Donner 2012). Economic reforms have been an opportunity for professionals and entrepreneurs. Many MC members accepted the reform process of modernization, in contrast to the experience in South America (Germani 1971, 1975). There are different ways to define and evaluate this kind of consensus (e.g. Dayton-Johnson, 2015 Ch. 1, referring to Latin America; Rocca 2017 and Yuk-Ha Tsang's 2014 to China; Nissanov 2017, Ch. 1, particularly pp. 7ff. to Russia).

Several authors, particularly economists, have drafted a profile of the MC, distinguishing between a relative and an absolute definition (Easterly 2001; Kharas and Gertz 2010, 34ff; Ferreira et al. 2013, 29–37). The absolute definition is based on income distribution. Starting from the poverty line of the developing countries (2US$ daily), Banerjee and Duflo (2007a, b) consider as belonging to the MC those who earn between 2US$ and 10US$ per person daily (2005 Purchasing Power Parity – PPP). According to Birdsall's appraisal (2010) the starting line for the MC is US$10 income a day, excluding the richest people in the top 5% of the income distribution.

The relative definition considers spending on consumption and purchasing power, and makes possible cross-country comparisons. It considers as members of the MC in the EC those who can spend up to 20 US$ daily. This implies many differences within the MC in terms of household's income levels and quality of consumption. Below this limit there are poor people, i.e. those who have an availability of daily spending of less than 2US$.

Ravaillon considers as belonging to the MC those in the EC who can spend daily between 2US$ and 13 US$ (2005 PPP). He adds that «the lower bound is the median poverty line of developing countries while the upper bound is based on the US poverty line» (2009, 17). Sumner (2012) sets the line between 4US$ and 10 US$. That means that there are *vulnerable* people, out of poverty but not fully part of the MC.

The Global MC and Its Limits

An often cited definition of the MC is proposed by Kharas. He considers the *global* MC as a culturally diversified and geographically vast social group. Despite of its internal differences, the *global* MC is homogenous in terms of income, lifestyle, quality and quantity of consumption (2010, 11–13). Its basket consumption reflects a typical urban standard of living and covers a set of semi-durable goods with a strong technological content (Fernandes 2006; Jaffrelot and van der Veer 2008; Chua 2009). According to Kharas' appraisal those who belong to the global MC are people with a purchasing power from 10 to 100 US$ a day (2010, 8–9, 2017, 3).

Concerning the evolution of the global MC, the population expanded from 26 to 58% between 1990 and 2010 (Chun 2010, 8). According to Kharas' calculation «there were about 3.2 billion people in the MC at the end of 2016» (2017, 2). Moreover, he forecasts that «around 2020, the MC will become a majority of the global population for the first time ever» (Id., 11).

Table 1 estimates the progression of the global MC up to 2030 by geographical area. It is going to increase in number but the share of the population belonging to it will be different by region. Stagnant or lightly decreasing in the advanced countries — as an outcome of the demographic decline and aging population (Kharas 2017, 2, 10, 16) and of the diminishing relevance of the West in the world economy (PWC 2015, 3) — and stable in Central, Southern America and in Africa, the global MC will rise in Asia. Nearly two thirds of it will be concentrated in this continent.

Concerning consumption and spending capacity, the projections estimate that by 2030 more than 80% of the world's MC will be based in the GS accounting for 70% of total consumption expenditure, despite great disparities among them. As can be seen from Table 2, more than half of the spending capacity of the global MC will be concentrated in Asia by 2025.

Melber (2016) is critical of Kharas and other institutions like the African Development Bank which consider income and purchasing power as the base

Table 1 Middle class in different world regions. Absolute values (millions) and share 2015 (actual) – 2030 (estimates)

	2015	%	2020	%	2025	%	2030	%
North America	335	11	344	9	350	8	354	7
Europe	724	24	736	20	738	16	733	14
Central and South America	285	9	303	8	321	7	335	6
Pacific Asia	1,380	46	2,023	54	2,784	60	3,492	65
Sub-Saharan Africa	114	4	132	4	166	4	212	4
Middle East and North Africa	192	6	228	6	258	6	285	5
World	3,030	100	3,766	100	4,617	100	5,412	100

Source: Kharas (2017, 14)

Table 2 Spending by the global middle class (PPP constant of 2011) Billion US$ and shares 2015 (actual) – 2030 (estimates)

	2015	%	2020	%	2025	%	2030	%
North America	6,174	18	6,381	15	6,558	13	6,681	10
Europe	10,920	31	11,613	27	12,159	23	12,573	20
Central and South America	2,931	8	3,137	8	3,397	8	3,630	6
Pacific Asia	12,332	36	18,174	43	26,519	51	36,631	57
Sub-Saharan Africa	915	3	1,042	2	1,295	2	1,661	3
Middle East and North Africa	1,541	4	1,933	5	2,306	4	2,679	4
World	34,814	100	42,279	100	52,234	100	63,854	100

Source: Kharas (2017, 15)

dimension of the MC (AfDB 2011). According to Melber, the Kharas' range of daily income or expenditure is too «generous». Less optimistically, he observes that such definition includes social groups which in the advanced countries have been affected in recent decades by precarization and fallen into poverty.

An Empirical Test

These MC features are one-dimensional from a sociological point of view. In fact they focus on households' and individuals' available income, ignoring other dimensions of social classes. It is therefore appropriate to consider some indicators stressing two other dimensions, the labour market and the social status of people, with particular attention to the situation of women.

The hypotheses of this paper are the following. First, I propose that a robust MC could be a driver of economic growth above all in a modern economic system, with a developed service sector and (relatively) equal opportunities for men and women. Indeed, a robust MC could develop when the labor market has modern features. Secondly, MC development could be fulfilled if the women are empowered, i.e. when their social status is enhanced and their needs are satisfied. Thirdly, a modern labour market and the empowerment of women could be associated with a better and general QoL. Fourthly, education plays a role in facilitating or hindering the two abovementioned processes (OECD 2014, 30). This facilitates a lowering of the birth rate and childhood mortality rates. More educated women, with fewer children, could care better for them. Equal opportunities on the labor market allow a significant proportion of skilled women to be employed. This could facilitate the economic growth and the development of a robust MC. This trend has recently been confirmed by the European Central Bank (2017) stressing that «the increase in the labour force during the economic recovery [in Europe] has been driven by the participation of women [and] [. . .] has been dominated by the highly skilled» (ibid, 46–48).

My purpose is to evaluate in which countries a MC is actually arising. I realized two principal component analysis, analyzing a set of indicators selected from the WB database (http://data.worldbank.org/indicator) referring to the year 2014 and to all the world's countries (n = 217).[1] These variables could be associated to the MC

[1]For the first PCA the selected variables, regarding the economy and labour market situation were in a first step:

1. Access to electricity (% of total population)
2. Electricity power consumption KWh *per capita*
3. Employment in services, female (% of female employment)
4. Employment in services, male (% of male employment)
5. Energy use (kg oil per capita)
6. GDP per capita (constant 2010 US$)
7. Government expenditure on education, total (% of GDP)
8. Labor force, female (% of total labor force)
9. Literacy rate, adult total (% of people ages 15 and above)
10. Mobile cellular subscriptions (per 100 people)
11. Rural population (% of total population)
12. Share of women in wage employment in the nonagricultural sector (% of total nonagricultural employment)
13. Technicians in R&D (per million people)
14. Unemployment Total (% of total labor force) (modeled ILO estimate)
15. Unemployment, female (% of female labor force) (modeled ILO estimate)
16. Urban population (% of total population)
17. Vulnerable employment, female (% of female employment)
18. Vulnerable employment, male (% of male employment)
19. Wage and salaried workers female (%of female employment)
20. Wage and salaried workers, total (% of total employment).

The second PCA considered variables concerning the status and the social role of women. Here is the list of the variables used in the first phase of the analysis:

1. School enrollment, primary and secondary (gross), gender parity index
2. Maternal mortality ratio (modeled estimate, per 100,000 live births)
3. Fertility rate (birth per woman)
4. Life expectancy at birth, female (years)
5. Life expectancy at birth, male (years)
6. Mortality rate, neonatal (per 1000 live births)
7. Adolescent fertility rate (births per 1000 women ages 15–19).

profile and to typical aspects of its lifestyle. Since the WB offers only aggregated data nation based — the data have to do with countries not with social actors — these variables could be interpreted as a proxy of social class. Unfortunately some important indicators (e.g. Gini index) could not be considered because many countries have missing data, also regarding other relevant variables. That could distort the results of the analysis presented in this paper.

With a two-step principal component analysis (Marradi and Di Franco 2013) two factors were separately extracted. The first one concerns *Labour Market Modernization* (LMM) and consequently the state of the economic system. The second is associated to the social status of women. The five components of the first factor are indicators of the LMM level. The variables are:

1. wage and salaried female workers (.224);
2. wage and salaried workers (.222);
3. women employed in services (2013 data) (.210);
4. male workers employed in services (.197);
5. vulnerable employment female (−.219).

The first four variables of this factor are negatively correlated with the vulnerability of female employment (ILO 2017).[2]

The second factor concerns women's status in the society, i.e. the consideration and reputation, and their living conditions. Its four components are the following:

1. fertility rate per woman (.279);
2. maternal death (.276);
3. neonatal mortality rate (.273);
4. adolescent fertility (.265)[3]

The results highlight an index that could be called *Women's Subordination* (WS). It is associated with high maternal and neonatal death rates, and a high fertility rate both among adult and adolescent women.

My hypothesis was corroborated by the data presented by Table 3. It shows the correlations between the two factorial indexes — the GDP per capita and some relevant indicators of economic and social development (literacy rate; percentage of population living in urban settlement; percentage of population having access to electricity; percentage of population with mobile cellular subscription) — and two indicators of QoL: male and female life expectancies.

[2]The score of the KMO test is 0.78; the results obtained by the Barlett test are the following: Chi square 723.83; DL 10, sign.000). The number of cases is 80. The range of variation of the MML index, a standardized variable, is −3.0 and 1.25.

[3]The score of the KMO test is 0.853 and the results obtained by the Barlett test are quite good (Chi square 626.26; DL 6, sign.000). The number of the cases is 184. The range of variation of the WS index, a standardized variable, is −1.12 and 2.75.

Table 3 Correlation coefficients between two factorial indexes (LMM and WS), some social and economic development indicators (literacy rate, access to electricity, mobile cellular subscription), indicators of the QoL (male and female life expectancies) and GDP per capita in emerging and advanced countries, World Bank data 2014

		Labour Market Modernization (LMM)	Women Subordination (WS)	Literacy rate adult >15 years	% Urban population	Access to electricity % of population	Mobile cellular phone per 100 people	Life expectancy female	Life expectancy male	GDP per capita
Labour Market Modernization (LMM)	Pearson Correlation	1	−699**	.449**	.674	.473**	.396**	.663**	.634**	.671**
	N	80	77	55	79	80	79	80	80	80
Women Subordination	Pearson Correlation	−.699**	1	−.827**	−561**	−843**	−554**	−914**	−874**	−.529**
	N	77	184	149	183	184	183	184	184	178
Literacy rate adult >15 years	Pearson Correlation	.449**	−.827**	1	.500**	.742**	.444**	729**	.657**	.406**
	N	55	149	156	155	156	155	154	154	148
% Urban population	Pearson Correlation	.674**	−561**	.500**	1	.564**	.481**	.607**	.608**	.576**
	N	79	183	155	214	211	204	196	196	192
Access to electricity % of population	Pearson Correlation	.473**	−843**	.742**	.564**	1	.560**	.815**	.780**	.410**
	N	80	184	156	211	214	203	198	198	192

Mobile cellular phone per 100 people	Pearson correlation	.396**	−554**	.444**	.481**	.560**	1	.505**	.497**	.440**
	N	79	183	155	204	203	205	193	193	185
Life expectancy female	Pearson correlation	.663**	−914**	.729**	.607**	.815**	.505**	1	.971**	.597**
	N	80	184	154	196	198	193	199	199	183
Life expectancy male	Pearson correlation	.634**	−874**	.657**	.608**	.780**	.497**	.971**	1	.652**
	N	80	184	154	196	198	193	199	199	183
GDP per capita	Pearson correlation	.671**	−529	.406**	.576**	.410**	.440**	.597**	.652**	1
	N	80	178	148	192	192	185	183	183	193

**Correlations are significant at 0.01 (two tiers)

More specifically:

(a) Pearson's correlation coefficient between the two indexes is strongly negative (−0.7) and significant at. 000 (two tiers).
(b) The correlation coefficients between the two factors and the abovementioned indicators of economic and social development (literacy, urban population etc.) are in general higher than those between GDP per capita and the same indicators. This is clearly evident for the WS index.
(c) The correlation coefficients between the two factorial indexes and the indicators of QoL (life expectancies) are also higher than those between GDP and the same indicators.[4]

In other words, it seems that the social and economic development of a country and its QoL, and hence the rise of social and occupational groups generally labelled MC, are more validly indicated by the LMM and WS indexes, rather than the GDP per capita. In other words, a cultural variable such as the social status of women seems to be crucial as a driver of social and economic development of a country.

There is also a strong association between the two factors and the groups of countries taken into consideration. The association is particularly strong when considering the index of the condition of women (Table n. 4).

The data on Table 4 (and other data not presented here) confirm my hypothesis.

- The *advanced countries* are the place where the labour market (mean of WS index: –.96) has more modern features. In the advanced countries a high degree of QoL is confirmed also by male and female life expectancies. Literacy covers virtually the whole adult population; everybody has access to electricity; nearly 80% of population live in urban settlement, and the per capita GDP is the highest in the world.
- In *Asia*, there is a remarkable difference of the WS index between *China* (−0.88) and *India* (1.06). China seems to be more women-friendly than India[5] and this diverging situation could have an impact on the economic development chances of both countries.
- In the *Russian Federation* despite widespread literacy among the adult population, the general access to electricity and a WS index above the general mean (−48), the mean of LMM index is quite low (–.65).
- In the *Middle East* and in *Northern Africa* the per capita GDP is higher than in other groups of EC but the fertility and the maternal and neonatal death rates are high, the level of women's education low, the mean of LMM is above the general

[4]As mentioned above, there are, unfortunately, many missing cases, probably due to a deficit in the statistical data collection. Reliable data can be attributed only to 80 countries in relation to the LMM factor. Those concerning the WS were calculated on the data of 184 countries.

[5]The number of rapes reported each year in Delhi has more than tripled over the last 5 years, registering an increase of 277% from 572 in 2011 to 2155 in 2016, according to data released recently by the Delhi Police, http://www.delhipolice.nic.in/PDF/CRIME%20IN_%20DELHI.pdf

Table 4 Analysis of univariate variance

Groups of countries		LMM	WS
Advanced countries	Mean	.75	−.96
	N	35	35
	Std. Dev.	.29	.11
Emerging ex URSS	Mean	−.65	−.48
	N	6	12
	Std. Dev.	.99	.31
Emerging Asia	Mean	−1.09	−.13
	N	8	24
	Std. Dev.	.94	.45
China	Mean	Missing	−.88
India	Mean	Missing	.106
Emerging Europe	Mean	−.15	−.85
	N	11	11
	Std. Dev.	.68	.13
Emerging Latin America	Mean	−.27	−.20
	N	12	29
	Std. Dev.	.61	.32
Middle East and North Africa	Mean	−.61	.05
	N	4	27
	Std. Dev.	1.31	.95
Subsaharan Africa	Mean	−1.55	1.30
	N	4	44
	Std. Dev.	1.58	.84
Total	General mean	0.0	0.0
	N	80	184
	Std. Dev.	1.00	1.00

Groups of countries with different degrees of economic development (advanced vs. emerging) of different geographical areas. (World Bank classification) Standardized variables, 2014
Association measures
Eta = 0.744 (LMM * groups of countries); 0.810 (WS * groups of countries)
Eta squared = 0.554; 0.655

mean (WS index .05). In fact, even if the GDP per capita in Saudi Arabia is high, only recently was the driving ban for women removed.

- In *Sub-Saharan Africa* the LMM index (−1.55) as well as women's social status (1.30) are clearly under the average level general means.

Concluding Remarks

The starting point was the emergence of the MC in the GS as a dimension of better living conditions. I assumed that income and consumption level could not be the key indicators of the emergence of the MC.

In the WB database I selected two different set of indicators referred (i) to labour market and economic development and (ii) to the women status in society. I processed the data with two principal component analysis and extracted two factors. I called the first LMM. Its five components regard the expansion of the service sector and female employment. The LMM factor is negatively correlated to the second factorial index composed of four variables and called WS. A high WS is a driver for a strong informal sector where women are mostly vulnerable workers, affected by inequality in working condition and persisting gender gap (Nohlen and Sturm 1982, 92–116; Klemp 1992; ILO 2017; Martin 2010; Nuscheler 2016, 303–306).

Conversely, women's empowerment is correlated to two relevant dimensions of QoL, such as female and male life expectancies (Table 3). More empowered and proactive women could get access to several social spheres and in so doing they contribute to building the well-being of the society. In sum, a MC could arise in a modern economic system if and when the gender gaps are reduced, i.e. when challenging gender barriers and segregation are removed. The gender issue has been discussed for years by the literature (Boserup 1970; Moser 1995). It is today a consolidated assumption of the scientific literature and a topic in the agendas of institutions devoted to development (World Bank 2013), aiming at supporting women and girls for the collective wellbeing (UNFA 2016, ch. 4; ILO 2018).

In conclusion, the results show that not only the income and consumption level but cultural variables, such as the status of women, are crucial in promoting socio-economic conditions favorable to the emergence of a MC and in bettering the overall QoL. These results suggest once more to policy makers that supporting women and reducing gender gaps are the best way to promote social development, stimulate the internal consumption level, and support the domestic market.

References

African Development Bank (AfDB) (2011). *The Middle of the Pyramid: Dynamics of the Middle Class in Africa*. http://www.afdb.org/fileadmin/uploads/afdb/Documents/Publications/The%20Middle%20of%20the%20Pyramid_The%20Middle%20of%20the%20Pyramid.pdf

Banerjee, A. V. & Duflo, E. (2007a). The Economic Lives of the Poor. *Journal of Economic Perspectives*. DOI: https://doi.org/10.1257/jep.21.1.141.

Banerjee, A. V. & Duflo, E. (2007b). *What is middle class about the middle classes around the world?*https://economics.mit.edu/files/2081

Birdsall, N. (2010). *The (Indispensable) Middle Class in Developing Countries; or, the Rich and the Rest, Not the Poor and the Rest, in* Ravi, K., Spence, M. (eds.), *Equity in a Globalizing World* Washington: World Bank. http://siteresources.worldbank.org/EXTPREMNET/Resources/489960-1338997241035/Growth_Commission_Equity_Growth_Globalizing_World.pdf

Boserup, E. (1970). *Woman's role in economic development.* London: George Allen & Unwin.

Camfield, L. (2012). *Quality of Life in Developing countries.* In Land, K.C., Michalos, A. C., Sirgy, M. J. (Eds.), 399–432.

Camfield, L., Crivello, G. &, Woodhead, M. (2009). Wellbeing Research in Developing Countries: Reviewing the Role of Qualitative Methods. *Social Indicators Research.* doi:https://doi.org/10.1007/s11205-008-9310-z.

Cheng, L., 2010, *Introduction: The Rise of the Middle Class in the Middle Kingdom.* in Id. (Ed.). *China's Emerging Middle Class. Beyond Economic Transformation*, Brookings Institution Press, Washington. D.C. : 3–31.

Chua, B.C. (2009). *From Small Objects to Cars: Consumption Expansion in East Asia*, in Lange, Meier (Eds.), 101–115.

Chun, N. (2010). *Middle Class Size in the Past. Present. and Future: A Description of Trends in Asia.* Asian Development Bank, Economics Working Paper Series 217.

Dayton-Johnson, J. (2015). *Latin America's emerging middle classes: economic perspectives.* London: Palgrave Macmillan.

Donner, H. (Ed.) (2012). *Being Middle-class in India. A Way of Life.* London: Routledge.

Easterly, W. (2001). The Middle Class Consensus and Economic Development. *Journal of Economic Growth*, 6(4), 317–35.

Elsenhans, H. (1981). *Abhängiger Kapitalismus oder bürokratische Entwicklungsgesellschaft.* Frankfurt am Main: Campus Verlag.

Esping-Andersen G. (1990). *The three worlds of welfare capitalism.* Woodstock: Princeton University Press.

European Central Bank (2017). *Economic Bulletin.* Issue 6. https://www.ecb.europa.eu/pub/pdf/ecbu/eb201706.en.pdf?dab5b01c961114783aba4ddf7e7cc5722

Evers H.D. (1988). *Strategische Gruppen. Vergleichende Studien zu Staat. Bürokratie und Klassenbildung in der Dritten Welt.* Berlin: Reimer.

Fernandes, L. (2006). *India's New Middle Class. Democratic Politics in an Era of Economic Reform.* Minneapolis. London: University of Minnesota Press.

Ferreira, F.H.G. et al. (2013). *Economic Mobility and the Rise of the Latin American Middle Class.* Washington, D.C.: The World Bank.

Germani, G. (1971). *Sociologia della modernizzazione.* Bari: Laterza.

Germani, G. (1975). *Autoritarismo. fascismo e classi sociali.* Bologna: Il Mulino.

Gilpin, R. (2001). *Global Political Economy: Understanding the International Economic Order.* Woodstock: Princeton University Press.

Gimenez, M. E. (1991). Middle Class. In Darity, W.A. Jr. (ed). *International Encyclopedia of the Social Sciences.* (143ff.) New York: MacMillan.

Goetze, D. (1976, 2002^2). *Entwicklungssoziologie.* München: Goldmann.

ILO (2017). *World Employment and Social Outlook: Trends for women 2017.* – Global snapshot. Geneva: ILO

ILO (2018).*World Employment and Social Outlook: Trends for Women 2018* – Global snapshot. Geneva: ILO.

Jaffrelot, C. & van der Veer P. (2008). *Patterns of Middle Class Consumption in India and China.* London: SAGE.

Kharas, H. (2010). *The Emerging Middle Class in Developing Countries.* http://www.oecd.org/dev/44457738.pdf.

Kharas, H. (2017). *The Unprecedented Expansion of the Global Middle Class. An Update.* Global Economy & Development Working Paper 100. https://www.brookings.edu/research/the-unprecedented-expansion-of-the-global-middle-class-2/
Kharas, H. & Gertz, G. (2010). *The New Global Middle Class: A Crossover from West to East.* In Cheng, L. L. C. (Ed.). *China's Emerging Middle Class. Beyond Economic Transformation* (pp. 32–51). Washington, D.C: Brookings Institution Press.
Klemp, L. (1992). Frauen im Entwicklungs- und Verelendungsprozeß. In Nohlen, D. & Nuscheler, F. (Eds.). *Handbuch der Dritten Welt.* vol. 1. *Grundprobleme – Theorien – Strategien* (pp. 287–303). Bonn: J.H.W. Dietz Nachf.
Land, K., Michalos, A. & Sirgy M. (Eds.) (2012). *Handbook of Social Indicators and Quality of Life Research.* Dordrecht: Springer.
Lange, H. & Meier, L. (2009). Who are the New Middle Classes and why are they Given so Much Public Attention? In Id. (Eds.). *The New Middle Classes: Globalizing Lifestyles. Consumerism and Environmental Concern* (pp. 1–26). New York, Heidelberg: Springer.
Lin, G. C. S. (2011). *Developing China, Land, Politics and Social Conditions.* London, New York: Routledge.
Lockwood, D. (1958). *The Blackcoated Worker.* Clarendon Press: Oxford University Press.
Marradi, A. & Di Franco, G., 2013, Factor analysis and principal component analysis, Milano, Angeli.
Marshall, T.H. (1950). *Citizenship and Social Class.* Cambridge: Cambridge University Press.
Martin, J. P. (2010). *Inequality in Emerging Economies: What Role for Labour Market and Social Policies*? OECD Employment. Labour and Social Affairs. http://www.oecd.org/
Melber, H. (ed.) (2016). *The Rise of Africa's Middle Class: Myths. Realities and Critical Engagements.* London: Zed Books.
Menzel, U. (2016). Was ist Entiwcklungstheorie? In Stockmann, R., Menzel, U., Nuscheler, F. (Eds.) *Entwicklungspolitik* (pp. 13–46). Oldenburg: De Gruyter.
Moser, C.O.N. (1995). *Gender planning and development. Theory, practice and training.* London: Routledge.
Nissanov, Z. (2017). *Economic Growth and the Middle Class in an Economy in Transition. The Case of Russia.* New York: Springer.
Nohlen, D. & Nuscheler, F. (1992). Was heiβt Entwicklung? In Id. (Eds.), *Handbuch der Dritten Welt. I. Grundprobleme-Theorien-Strategien* (pp. 55–75). Bonn: Verlag J.H.W. Dietz Nachf
Nohlen, D. & Sturm, R. (1982). Über das Konzept der strukturellen Heterogeneität. In Nohlen, D. & Nuscheler F. (Eds.), *Handbuch der Dritten Welt.* vol. 1. *Unterentwicklung und Entwicklung: Theorien - Strategien – Indikatoren* (pp. 92–116). Hamburg: Hoffmann und Campe.
Nuscheler, F. (2016). Das Armutproblem als entwicklungspolitisches Schlüsselproblem. In Stockmann R., Menzel U., Nuscheler, F. (Eds.) *Entwicklungspolitik* (pp. 295–318). Oldenburg: De Gruyter.
OECD (2014). *Education at a Glance 2014: OECD Indicators.* https://doi.org/10.1787/eag-2014-en
Parkin, F. (1979). *Marxism and Class Theory.* London: Tavistock.
PWC (2015). *The World in 2050 Will the shift in global economic power continue*?. https://www.pwc.com/gx/en/issues/the-economy/assets/world-in-2050-february-2015.pdf
Ravaillon, M. (2009). *The Developing World's Bulging (but Vulnerable) "Middle Class".* Policy Research Working Paper 4816, The WB, https://openknowledge.worldbank.org/bitstream/handle/10986/4013/WPS4816.pdf
Rocca, J.L. (2017). *The Making of the Chinese Middle Class.* London: Palgrave Macmillan.
Scrase, G. R. & Scrase, T. J. (2009). *Globalisation and the Middle Classes in India. The Social and Cultural Impact of Neoliberal Reforms.* London: Routledge.
Sumner, A. (2012). *Global poverty reduction*, EADI Working paper. https://www.eadi.org/typo3/fileadmin/Documents/Publications/EADI_Policy_Paper/EADI_policy_paper_december_2012.pdf
UNDP (2013). *Human Development Report 2013. The Rise of the South.* http://hdr.undp.org
UNFA (2016). *The State of World Population.* http://www.unfpa.org/swop

Weber, M. (1922). *Wirtschaft und Gesellschaft*. In *Max Weber-Gesamtausgabe* (1984ff.). Tübingen: J.C.B. Mohr (Paul Siebeck).

World Bank (2013). *World Bank Gender Overview*. www.worldbank.org

Yuan, Z., Wan, G. & Khor, N. (2011). *The Rise of the Middle Class in the People's Republic of China*. Asian Development Bank. http://www.adb.org/publications/rise-middle-class-peoples-republic-china

Yuk-Ha Tsang, E. (2014). *The New Middle Class In China. Consumption. Politics and the Market Economy*. London: Palgrave Macmillan.

If you have any concerns about our products, you can contact us on
ProductSafety@springernature.com

Springer Nature Customer Service Center GmbH
Europaplatz 3, 69115 Heidelberg, Germany

Hamburg, Germany

MIX
Papier aus verantwortungsvollen Quellen
Paper from responsible sources
FSC® C105338

If you have any concerns about our products,
you can contact us on
ProductSafety@springernature.com

In case Publisher is established outside the EU,
the EU authorized representative is:
Springer Nature Customer Service Center GmbH
Europaplatz 3, 69115 Heidelberg, Germany

Printed by Libri Plureos GmbH
in Hamburg, Germany